# Endoscopic Ultrasonography

This book is due for return on or before the last date shown below.

# Endoscopic Ultrasonography

*Edited by*

**Frank G. Gress, MD, FACP, FACG**

Associate Professor of Medicine
School of Medicine
State University of New York at Stony Brook
Chief of Endoscopy
Division of Gastroenterology and Hepatology
Winthrop University Hospital
Long Island, New York

**Ishan Bhattacharya, MD**

Chairman, Division of Gastroenterology
South Bend Clinic & SurgiCenter
South Bend, Indiana

*b*

**Blackwell
Science**

©2001 by Blackwell Science, Inc.

Editorial Offices:
Commerce Place, 350 Main Street, Malden, Massachusetts 02148, USA
Osney Mead, Oxford OX2 0EL, England
25 John Street, London WC1N 2BL, England
23 Ainslie Place, Edinburgh EH3 6AJ, Scotland
54 University Street, Carlton, Victoria 3053, Australia

Other Editorial Offices:
Blackwell Wissenschafts-Verlag GmbH, Kurfürstendamm 57, 10707 Berlin, Germany
Blackwell Science KK, MG Kodenmacho Building, 7–10 Kodenmacho Nihombashi, Chuo-ku, Tokyo 104, Japan

Distributors:
*USA*
    Blackwell Science, Inc.
    Commerce Place
    350 Main Street
    Malden, Massachusetts 02148
    (Telephone orders: 800-215-1000 or 781-388-8250; fax orders: 781-388-8270)
*Canada*
    Login Brothers Book Company
    324 Saulteaux Crescent
    Winnipeg, Manitoba R3J 3T2
    (Telephone orders: 204-837-2987)
*Australia*
    Blackwell Science Pty, Ltd.
    54 University Street
    Carlton, Victoria 3053
    (Telephone orders: 03-9347-0300; fax orders: 03-9349-3016)
*Outside North America and Australia*
    Blackwell Science, Ltd.
    c/o Marston Book Services, Ltd.
    P.O. Box 269
    Abingdon
    Oxon OX14 4YN
    England
    (Telephone orders: 44-01235-465500; fax orders: 44-01235-465555)

Acquisitions: Chris Davis
Development: Julia Casson
Production: Louis C. Bruno, Jr.
Manufacturing: Lisa Flanagan
Marketing Manager: Anne Stone
Cover design by Linda Willis
Typeset by Pre-Press Company, Inc.
Printed and bound by Sheridan Books/Ann Arbor

Printed in the United States of America
00 01 02 03 5 4 3 2 1

**Library of Congress Cataloging-in-Publication Data**

Endoscopic ultrasonography / edited by Frank G. Gress, Ishan Bhattacharya.
  p. ; cm.
  ISBN 0-86542-565-5
  1. Endoscopic ultrasonography. 2. Gastrointestinal system—Diseases—Diagnosis. 3. Gastrointestinal system—Ultrasonic imaging. I. Gress, Frank G. II. Bhattacharya, Ishan.
  [DNLM: 1. Endosonography. WN 208 E567 2001]
  RC804.E59 E62 2001
  616.3'307543—dc21                        00-056421

# Contents

# Foreword

Transcutaneous ultrasonography is a widely applied technique for the evaluation of gastrointestinal, gynecological, cardiac, urological, and peripheral vascular diseases. Endoscopic ultrasound of the gastrointestinal tract initially struggled to gain a foothold as a diagnostic tool. Instruments were of large diameter, had rigid tips, and durability and resolution were suboptimal. Diagnostic sonographic information correlated but did not equate with final histologic diagnoses. The technique was not readily available in most institutions. Managing physicians had little experience with it; therefore, confidence in the techniques and diagnoses generated was relatively low.

Fortunately, times have changed. Patients in the new millennium will benefit from a new era of endoscopic ultrasound. Many of the aforementioned limitations have been addressed and improved or resolved. Technical improvements include endoscopes with linear and circumferential arrays, decreased instrument diameter, and Doppler capabilities. Biopsy capability and other limited therapeutics have been added. Currently there are approximately 250 endoscopic ultrasound units in the United States. Although many of these units do not have well-trained staff, this number is improving as the number of training centers with ultrasound expertise is increasing.

Dr. Gress has brought together a group of authors with experience in many areas of endoscopic ultrasonography to create this textbook. The authorship is divided between U.S. and international experts. Authors include members of the old guard endoscopists and the younger generation. The text begins with the basics of ultrasound principals and moves on to equipment and room setup. The main body of the text discusses endoscopic ultrasound applications for specific pathologic conditions or organ systems. There is a nice balance between technique and interpretation of images. The very important area of tissue sampling is presented well. There are discussions of what the future of endoscopic ultrasound applications may hold, including treatment of achalasia, gastroesophageal reflux disease (GERD), tumor ablation, and suture placement. Miniprobes have yet to gain extensive application and need further refinement.

The editor and authors are to be congratulated for their excellent work in producing this text. It is a must for those training in endoscopic ultrasound today.

Glen A. Lehman, MD
Professor of Medicine and Radiology
Indiana University Medical Center
Indianapolis, IN

# Preface

The pace of development of medical innovation applied to the management of human diseases in the 20th century can be only described as astonishing. In that context, the advances in diagnostic and interventional endoscopic technology in the area of gastrointestinal disease over the past decade have been equally amazing. The development of the first fiberoptic endoscopic instrument, followed by videoendoscopy and the universal availability of these instruments, has allowed the gastroenterologist and gastrointestinal endoscopist the ability to evaluate thoroughly and treat a multitude of gastrointestinal disorders. Interventional endoscopic techniques now permit minimally invasive therapies to be applied with decreased morbidity, improved outcomes, and in many cases, greatly improved quality of life for patients.

Endoscopic ultrasound (EUS) was first conceptualized more than 20 years ago during the early years of endoscopy and was developed in an attempt to improve ultrasound imaging of the pancreas. The first EUS prototype was designed and manufactured in the early 1980s. Endoscopic ultrasound evolved into first, an accepted and valuable endoscopic adjunct and subsequently, a therapeutic modality for the management of many gastrointestinal disorders. Unfortunately, as with most new technologies, a lack of skilled experienced endosonographers has limited the availability of this important tool.

*Endoscopic Ultrasonography* is our effort to bridge this gap in the EUS training process and to provide interested gastrointestinal endoscopists with an authoritative, yet practical approach to the role of EUS in the management of specific digestive disorders. The primary purposes of this text are to first, allow a complete and thorough understanding of the current state of endoscopic ultrasonography and second, help guide the reader in learning both basic and advanced endoscopic ultrasound techniques. Both diagnostic and therapeutic applications of endoscopic ultrasonography are thoroughly reviewed. We have emphasized a practical "how to" approach to learning endoscopic ultrasound and have made great efforts to present each chapter in extensive detail. Each chapter individually discusses a specific aspect of EUS as it relates to a particular gastrointestinal disorder or organ system. The experts who have graciously contributed to the book have identified current references in their chapters and more importantly, have purposefully included their own particular styles, practices, and opinions as to how EUS should be performed. This individualized approach provides a diverse introduction to the role of EUS in gastroenterology today without obscuring key concepts in both the theory and performance of this procedure.

The target audience for this text includes all gastroenterologists and trainees wishing to know more about endoscopic ultrasound and its role in managing digestive disorders. More importantly, for those interested in learning or training in endoscopic ultrasound, the text provides a technical "how to" approach to learning this advanced endosocopic procedure. In fact, this text would be appropriate not only for gastroenterologists but also gastrointestinal surgeons, surgical residents, medical housestaff, and oncologists who deal with gastrointestinal malignancies. We have chosen the contributors primarily for their expertise and experience with endoscopic ultrasound. They are all experts in gastroenterologic endosonography and have proven track records as scientists, clinicians, and educators. Their collective experience in applying endoscopic ultrasonography in the management of gastrointestinal diseases is unsurpassed. In fact, many of the contributors are "second-generation" endosonographers, having been trained by the early pioneers of EUS. A tremendous amount of effort on the part of each individual author has led to the final product, this book. They are the true masters of gastrointestinal endoscopy. We are deeply grateful to them for their outstanding collaboration.

# Acknowledgments

We would like to take this opportunity to acknowledge our mentors, all of whom have inspired us throughout our training and careers as gastroenterologists. We are indebted to our endoscopic training directors: Maurice Cerulli, Robert Hawes, Glen Lehman, and John P. Cello, all of whom nurtured in us patience, persistence, and the importance of the scientific method in the area of endoscopy. Their leadership and inspiration have driven us to become advanced endoscopists. We also would like to express our sincere appreciation to our secretaries Nancy Ruiz-Torchon and Donna Ellzey for their unending efforts as the liaisons among the many people involved in the process. Their meticulous attention to detail made our task less stressful and more tolerable. In addition, we extend our gratitude to the staff at Blackwell Science including Lou Bruno, Senior Production Editor, Amy Novit, Book Production Editor, and Julia Casson, Editorial Assistant. Most particularly, we thank Christopher Davis, the Executive Editor of Medicine at Blackwell for his direction and patience during the development of this text. All of them were instrumental in coordinating the development of this work from its inception to the final product. Finally, we wish to thank our wives Debra Gress and Jacqueline J. R. Wisner for their unending support, understanding, and sacrifice during the many hours we have spent completing this text. We dedicate this book to our wives and to our children, Travis, Erin, Morgan, Katherine, and Allison for their love, kindness, and patience that sustain us every day.

Frank G. Gress, MD
Ishan Bhattacharya, MD

# Contributors

**John Affronti MS, MD**
Associate Professor of Medicine
Emory University School of Medicine
Director of Endoscopy
Emory University Hospital
Atlanta, Georgia

**Sandeep Bhargava, MD**
Fellow in Gastroenterology
Columbia-Presbyterian Medical Center
The New York Presbyterian Hospital
Columbia University, College of Physicians
    and Surgeons
New York, New York

**Ishan Bhattacharya, MD**
Chairman, Division of Gastroenterology
South Bend Clinic & SurgiCenter
South Bend, Indiana

**Manoop S. Bhutani, MD, FACG, FACP**
Director, Center for Endoscopic Ultrasound
Director, Center for Experimental Endoscopy
Associate Professor of Medicine
University of Florida
Gainesville, Florida

**Kenneth F. Binmoeller, MD**
Associate Professor of Medicine and Surgery
Director, Gastrointestinal Endoscopy
University of California, San Diego,
San Diego, California

**Richard A. Erickson, MD, FACP, FACG**
Associate Professor of Medicine
Texas A&M Health Science Center College of Medicine
College Station, Texas
Director, Division of Gastroenterology
Scott and White Clinic and Hospital
Temple, Texas

**Douglas O. Faigel, MD**
Assistant Professor of Medicine
Oregon Health Sciences University School
    of Medicine
Portland, Oregon
Director of Gastrointestinal Endoscopy
Portland VA Medical Center
Portland, Oregon

**Paul Fockens, MD, PhD**
Associate Professor of Medicine
Director of Endoscopy
Department of Gastroenterology
Academic Medical Center
University of Amsterdam
Amsterdam
The Netherlands

**Klaus Gottlieb, MD, MBA, FACP, FACG**
Spokane Digestive Disease Center
Spokane, Washington
Clinical Associate Professor
University of Washington School of Medicine
Seattle, Washington

**Frank G. Gress, MD, FACP, FACG**
Associate Professor of Medicine
School of Medicine
State University of New York at Stony Brook
Chief of Endoscopy
Division of Gastroenterology and Hepatology
Winthrop University Hospital
Long Island, New York

**Michael B. Kimmey, MD**
Professor of Medicine
University of Washington
Director of Gastrointestinal Endoscopy
University of Washington Medical Center
Seattle, Washington

**Michael L. Kochman, MD, FACP**
Associate Professor of Medicine
University of Pennsylvania School of Medicine
Director, Gastrointestinal Oncology
Division of Gastroenterology
Hospital of the University of Pennsylvania
Philadelphia, Pennsylvania

**Charles J. Lightdale, MD**
Columbia University, College of Physicians
    and Surgeons
Columbia-Presbyterian Medical Center
The New York Presbyterian Hospital
New York, New York

**Michael Bau Mortensen, MD, PhD**
Senior Registrar
Department of Surgical Gastroenterology
Odense University Hospital
Odense, Denmark

**Ian D. Norton, MBBS, PhD**
Assistant Professor of Medicine
Division of Gastroenterology and Hepatology
Mayo Clinic and Foundation
Rochester, Minnesota

**Bonnie J. Pollack, MD**
Assistant Professor of Medicine
State University of New York at Stony Brook School
    of Medicine
Division of Gastroenterology and Hepatology
University Hospital
Stony Brook, New York

**Thomas J. Savides, MD**
Associate Professor of Clinical Medicine
Division of Gastroenterology
University of California at San Diego School
    of Medicine
San Diego, California

**Harry Snady, MD, PhD**
Pancreatobiliary Treatment Group
Division of Gastroenterology and Hepatology
North Shore University Hospital
Manhasset, New York

**Peter D. Stevens, MD**
Director, Gastrointestinal Endoscopy
Assistant Professor of Clinical Medicine
Columbia University, College of Physicians
    and Surgeons
Director, Endoscopy Unit
Columbia-Presbyterian Medical Center
The New York Presbyterian Hospital
New York, New York

**Brian R. Stotland, MD**
Assistant Professor of Medicine
Department of Gastroenterology
Boston University School of Medicine
Director of Endoscopic Ultrasound
Boston University Medical Center Hospital
Boston, Massachusetts

**Peter Vilmann, MD, DSc**
Head of Endoscopy, Associate Professor of Surgery
Department of Surgical Gastroenterology
Gentofte University Hospital
Hellerup, Denmark

**Maurits J. Wiersema, MD**
Associate Professor of Medicine
Director, Endoscopic Ultrasound
Division of Gastroenterology and Hepatology
Mayo Clinic and Foundation
Rochester, Minnesota

**Notice:** The indications and dosages of all drugs in this book have been recommended in the medical literature and conform to the practices of the general community. The medications described and treatment prescriptions suggested do not necessarily have specific approval by the Food and Drug Administration for use in the diseases and dosages for which they are recommended. The package insert for each drug should be consulted for use and dosage as approved by the FDA. Because standards for usage change, it is advisable to keep abreast of revised recommendations, particularly those concerning new drugs.

# History of Endoscopic Ultrasonography

**Ishan Bhattacharya**

The arrival of the new millennium marks the twentieth anniversary of endoscopic ultrasonography (EUS). The marriage of ultrasonography and endoscopy began in March, 1980 when Eugene DiMagno and colleagues published the first report of a gastroscope equipped with an ultrasonic probe (1). This prototype instrument had an 80-mm-long rigid tip, precluding use in humans. In the canine model, however, high-resolution images of the great vessels, portions of the esophagus and stomach, the spleen, hepatic and portal veins, and the liver were obtained with far greater clarity than was possible with conventional transcutaneous ultrasonography. Later that year, Strohm and colleagues reported their experience with "ultrasonic tomography" of the abdomen in 18 patients with known biliary, pancreatic, and hepatic disorders or postoperative anatomic changes (2). In half of their patients, the aorta and vena cava were identified, two of the landmarks now considered essential for an accurate EUS exam. The pancreas was also seen in 50% of the patients studied and patients with known pancreatic malignancy had their lesions visualized. The ability to identify the distal common bile duct, often obscured by bowel gas during transcutaneous ultrasound exams, was a perhaps unexpected benefit.

Why was endoscopic ultrasound developed? As described by Terada, one of the chief engineers of the EUS revolution, this technology emerged in the early 1980s not as a "need based" medical device like fiberoptic scopes but as a "seed based" project—an innovative engineering design looking for a purpose (3). The practical limitations of transcutaneous ultrasound—lack of penetration and interference by bony structures, intra-abdominal gas, and adipose tissue—were well understood 20 years ago. At the same time, fiberoptic technology, although amazing for its time, still did not permit evaluation of extraluminal pathology except by infer-

ence. Researchers hoped that EUS would combine the best of both technologies and "reveal a new potential demand among medical doctors" (3). Two endoscope manufacturers took the lead with Olympus Corporation in Japan and ACMI in the United States being the early competitors.

Progress during the 1980s was slow. Initial applications of this new technique were dedicated to defining the normal anatomical appearance of various digestive organs and structures. This was a challenging problem because in the United States, ultrasonography is not a part of training programs in gastroenterology. As a consequence, few endoscopists are expert in the interpretation of ultrasonographic images obtained in conventional transabdominal studies. To make matters more difficult, even experienced ultrasonographers had never seen images of gastrointestinal anatomy from such a unique intraluminal perspective. Interpretation of these high-resolution, close proximity images of the gastrointestinal tract also required correlation with the mural histology of the gastrointestinal tract—the mucosa, submucosa, muscularis propria, and adventitia or serosa. Consensus on such basic questions was not reached until 1989 (4). Standard viewing angles or positions had to be established so that reproducible imaging was possible in serial exams of the same patient as well as to identify the range of normal variation of anatomy, especially of vascular structures (see Chapters 5, 8, 10, 11). During these early years, formal training in EUS was not available and the learning curve was (and is) very steep (see Chapter 15). The medical convention of "see one, do one, teach one" does not apply.

At the same time, advances in EUS engineering were slow to develop. Even in the late 1980s most EUS instruments were by definition, prototypes. Fragile, bulky, and expensive to buy and maintain, they were

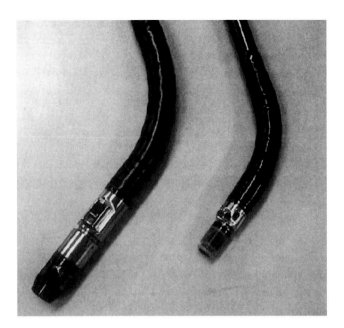

**Figure 1-1.** Comparison of the first EUS prototype and current Olympus GF-UMP230 scope. (From Terada M, Tsukaya T, Saito Y. Technical advances and future developments in endoscopic ultrasonography. Endoscopy 1998;30 [suppl 1]: A4, with permission.)

cumbersome for operators and less than comfortable for patients. Prone to failure, a prominent gastroenterologist as late as 1988 stated that it would "be prudent to regard EUS as investigative until its merits as well as limitations are more precisely defined" (5). The cheerful optimism of Tytgat that "this novel imaging technology will become standard in major hospitals in the not too distant future" seemed entirely misplaced (6).

By the early 1990s however, two factors had combined to produce an explosion of interest in the field. Technological progress was a key determinant. A new EUS instrument was developed that utilized linear array technology. Advances in miniaturization allowed ultrasound transducers to be more easily accommodated on endoscopes, and fiberoptic equipment was replaced by the videoendoscope, in which a charge coupled device (CCD) chip transmits images electronically to a video processor (see figures in Chapter 3). The scopes became much thinner and more flexible, allowing easier manipulation with less patient trauma (Figure 1-1). By this time, both sector scanning and linear array EUS scopes had optimized the balance between transducer size and frequency, allowing exceptionally high resolution images to be obtained with relative ease. The durability of EUS scopes increased as well.

At the same time, an impressive body of data had been collected on the EUS appearance of both normal anatomy and gastrointestinal pathology. By 1994, published data from EUS examinations on more than three

thousand patients clearly showed that EUS was the most accurate imaging modality for staging gastrointestinal malignancies of the esophagus, stomach, duodenum, rectum, ampulla of Vater, extrahepatic bile ducts and the pancreas (6).

This new "gold standard," however, had an Achilles heel. The radial scanning echoendoscope was the most commonly used instrument for performing EUS worldwide. It provides a 360-degree image of superb resolution perpendicular to the long axis of the instrument. Early experimentation with prototype biopsy needles, however, revealed that when passing a needle through the biopsy channel of the radial scanning scope, the image of the needle appeared only as an echogenic dot and the depth of insertion of the needle into the tissue being sampled could not be accurately determined. Attempts to use this technique for fine needle aspiration (FNA) tissue sampling produced inconsistent results and a high complication rate.

The development of linear array EUS scopes that scan parallel to the axis of the instrument and can visualize the full length of an FNA needle and track it during the biopsy procedure brought on the era of interventional EUS. The first large series was reported in 1995 by Giovannini (7). In a recent update of his results on 522 patients with a variety of gastrointestinal neoplasms (8), the positive and negative predictive values of FNA were 99.7% and 62.8%, respectively. The same investigators have reported that EUS-guided FNA made more invasive diagnostic tests superfluous in almost 40% of cases. Such optimistic assessments must be balanced with a more critical review of patient selection and sources of systematic bias in reporting results. Nevertheless, an accuracy rate of 85% overall for EUS-guided tissue sampling in patients with gastrointestinal tumors is probably a realistic figure and exceeds that reported even with modern magnetic resonance imaging and helical computed tomography (CT)-guided tissue FNA or biopsy.

In the past two years, there have been several dozen reports on a wide variety of therapeutic applications of EUS FNA. These have included such diverse approaches as EUS-guided celiac plexus neurolysis for patients with intractable pain from pancreatic cancer or chronic pancreatitis, injection of botulinum toxin into the lower esophageal sphincter in achalasia, and local immunotherapy for pancreatic carcinoma. Minimally invasive therapy using radio frequency waves and microwaves for ablation of tumor tissue is under development, though no trials in human beings have been reported yet. The ability of EUS to precisely define the depth of superficial mucosal esophageal tumors has indirectly allowed the recently developed method of endoscopic mucosal resection for esophageal cancer to become a viable clinical option, sparing the patient an esophagectomy.

The first "progeny" of the union of endoscopy and ultrasound is the catheter miniprobe. This, "through the scope probe," can be passed through the biopsy port of a conventional videoendoscope; a dedicated echoendoscope is not required, and, in theory, any gastrointestinal endoscopist could use it. Because of its small size and narrow diameter, the probe operates at a high frequency and, as a consequence, has a depth of penetration of, at best, 2 cm; however, it has exceptionally high resolution, substantially better than conventional EUS instruments. The miniprobe is ideally suited for the examination of small superficial cancers and fluid-filled tubular structures such as the biliary and pancreatic ductal systems. It has also been used to examine esophageal varices and stenotic malignant lesions. At present, the utility of the miniprobe remains limited and the price is high. The initial assumption that the miniprobe would allow widespread patient access to EUS (i.e., outside referral centers) has been diminished by the realization that accurate miniprobe EUS-image interpretation by endoscopists with little prior training in ultrasound remains a formidable obstacle.

Furthermore, advances in computing technology and raw processing power should allow three-dimensional reconstruction of EUS images within the near future, although the clinical usefulness of such images is unknown. From a therapeutic perspective, we have already seen several innovative applications for EUS as a result of the linear scope and FNA biopsy technique. In the future, as EUS evolves from a diagnostic modality to an interventional/therapeutic tool, we should see the continued transition of this technology toward therapeutics and treatment guided techniques. For example, high-intensity-focused ultrasound for ablation of abnormal tissue has been successful in early animal experiments. Nevertheless, the utility of gastrointestinal EUS in the new millennium will ultimately require proof of a favorable influence on clinical outcomes (9). The information base for EUS must also grow: one of the world's most accurate medical imaging technologies is still a secret to the general medical community and to the general public. Much work remains to "get the word out" about EUS and teach and train future endoscopists to competently perform this technically challenging procedure.

## References

1. DiMagno EP, Baxton JL, Regan PT, et al. Ultrasonic endoscope. Lancet 1980;1:629–631.
2. Strohm WD, Phillip J, Classen M, et al. Ultrasonic tomography by means of an ultrasonic fiberendoscope. Endoscopy 1980;12:241–244.
3. Terada M, Tsukaya T, Saito Y. Technical advances and future developments in endoscopic ultrasonography. Endoscopy 1998;30(suppl 1):A3–A7.
4. Kimmey MB, Martin RW, Haggit RC, et al. Histologic correlates of gastrointestinal ultrasound images. Gastroenterology 1989;96:433–441.
5. Sivak MV. Is there an ultrasonographic endoscope in your future? Gastrointest Endosc 1988;34:64–65.
6. Tytgat GNJ. Transintestinal ultrasonography—present and future. Endoscopy 1987;19:241–242.
7. Giovannini M, Seitz JF, Monges G, et al. Fine-needle aspiration cytology guided by endoscopic ultrasonography: results in 141 patients. Endoscopy 1995;27:171–177.
8. Giovannini M, Monges G, Bernardini D, et al. Diagnostic and therapeutic value of the endoscopic ultrasound (EUS) guided biopsy. Results in 522 patients. Gastroenterology 1998;114: A16. Abstract.
9. Nickl N. Endosonography at a crossroads: the outcomes obligation. Gastrointest Endosc 1999;50:875–878.

# 2

# Basic Principles and Fundamentals of Endoscopic Ultrasound Imaging

## Michael B. Kimmey

An understanding of the fundamental mechanisms of ultrasound (US) is useful to both the beginning and experienced endosonographer. It is not necessary to be a physicist or an electrical engineer to appreciate some basic principles of US imaging. These principles can guide the endosonographer in both obtaining the best representation of a tissue structure with endoscopic ultrasound (EUS) and in interpreting the images. Knowing these fundamental concepts also aids in the recognition and avoidance of artifacts.

In this chapter the principles of ultrasound imaging will be reviewed. An emphasis will be placed on their practical application to endosonography rather than on the derivation of formulas and equations, which will soon be forgotten.

## How Ultrasound Images Are Made

Sound is a physical force that is transmitted as a wave through a fluid or solid medium (1,2). Unlike electromagnetic waves (e.g., radio, light, and x-ray), sound waves cannot be transmitted through a vacuum. The energy must be transmitted via its impact on the molecules of the transmitting medium.

The periodicity or frequency of sound waves per unit of time varies widely and is measured in the number of cycles of the wave that are formed in one second, termed a *hertz* (Hz). Each wave cycle has both a positive and a negative component. Sound higher in frequency than can be heard by the human ear is called ultrasound (Figure 2-1). The frequencies of waves commonly used in medical imaging are between 3.5 and 20 million Hz, usually abbreviated as 3.5 to 20 megahertz (MHz). Even higher-frequency waves can be used in microscopy to define tissue ultrastructure.

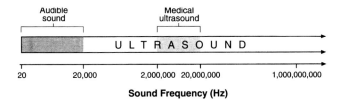

**Figure 2-1.** The frequencies of audible sound and ultrasound.

The high-frequency sound waves used in imaging have some interesting properties that affect how they are used. Unlike lower-frequency audible sound waves that travel well through air, high-frequency sound is more readily absorbed by air and is strongly reflected at the boundary between tissue and air. This is why gas-filled lungs and bowel limit the use of transcutaneous US in imaging of mediastinal and retroperitoneal structures.

### How US Waves Are Made

Sound waves are made by applying pressure to a medium. When this pressure is applied with controlled fluctuations, sound waves are created. A radio speaker vibrates at variable speeds or frequencies to create sound waves in air, which we hear as sound. Higher-frequency ultrasound waves are made by crystals that vibrate to produce a wave within a body fluid or tissue. These crystals are made from a special ceramic material because it can be made to vibrate at a high frequency when a high-frequency alternating polarity charge is applied to it. This property is termed *piezoelectric* and is also responsible for the crystal's ability to detect sound waves returning from the tissue and convert them back into an electrical signal.

4

Ultrasound transducers are composed of either one large crystal or, more commonly, multiple crystals aligned in an array. These transducers change an electrical signal to a sound wave and also receive the reflected sound wave back from the tissue. Ultrasound transducers typically emit a series of waves or a pulse, and then stop transmitting while they wait to detect the returning echo.

### What Happens When US Waves Encounter Tissue

Ultrasound waves propagate through tissue at a speed that is determined by the physical properties of the tissue (3,4). The speed of transmission is largely determined by the stiffness of the tissue: the stiffer the tissue, the faster the speed. For soft tissue, the variation in speed is only approximately 10 percent, ranging from 1460 meters per second in fat to 1630 meters per second in muscle (5–7).

Ultrasound waves are reflected back to the transducer when the sound wave encounters a tissue that is more difficult to pass through. For example, water easily transmits US, but air and bone do not. A sound wave that travels through a water-filled structure like the gallbladder is likely to reach the opposite gallbladder wall unless it encounters a gallstone that reflects the acoustic wave back to the transducer. Other solid tissues reflect sound waves to a variable extent depending on the tissue properties. Fat and collagen are more reflective to US than are muscle and lean solid organs. Sound waves are also reflected when they encounter a boundary or interface between two tissues with different acoustical properties (see following section).

### How Images Are Made from Reflected US Waves

Sound waves that are reflected by tissue components back to the transducer are detected by the same piezoelectric crystals that created them. These crystals then translate the waves back into electrical signals for processing into an image.

The transducer detects the returning echo as a function of the time that passed from when the sound pulse was emitted. The duration of time for an echo to return is a function of the speed of sound in the tissue and the distance from the transducer of the part of the tissue from which the sound wave is being returned. Because the speed of sound in lean tissue varies only by approximately 10 percent, the time between transmission of and return of an echo is a good marker for the distance the sound wave has traveled. Thus, for medical imaging, distance or location of a reflector within a tissue can be approximated by the delay observed in the return of an ultrasound pulse.

The returning waves or echoes can be displayed in a number of ways or *modes*. The simplest display plots the intensity or amplitude of echoes according to the time at which they are detected. This is termed *A-mode* and is infrequently used for medical imaging. If the amplitude of the returning signals is displayed as the brightness of a dot on the image, a *B-mode* image is created. If the transducer is moved across the tissue or if the transducer contains numerous crystals, a two-dimensional image is created out of the dots, which reflect echo amplitude; one dimension is the location or depth of the reflector causing the echo and the other dimension represents the span of tissue being imaged (Figure 2-2).

The precise time when a returning echo is detected is also a function of the orientation of the target tissue and the transducer. A more accurate representation of tissue structure is obtained when the ultrasound wave propagates in a direction that is perpendicular to the target. The reflected wave is then perpendicular to the transducer as well. If the US wave encounters the target from another angle or tangentially, then the returning wave is detected later and thus is displayed at a distance on the image that overestimates its actual position (see following section on artifacts).

## How Transducer Properties Affect the Image
### US Frequency and Axial Resolution

When high US frequencies are used, more waves can be transmitted per unit of time and the duration of the pulse of US energy can be proportionately reduced. This allows the US transducer to receive returning echoes more often. The result is a better ability to discriminate between two points in the target tissue that are within the direction of the US beam. This distance between distinguishable points in the direction of the US beam is termed *axial* or *range resolution* (Figure 2-3). In general, the higher the US frequency, the better the axial resolution. Most endoscopic US systems have axial resolutions that are approximately 0.2 mm. However, tissue penetration is also reduced with higher US frequencies (Table 2-1).

**Table 2-1.** Effect of US Frequency on Axial Resolution and Tissue Penetration

| US Frequency (MHz) | Axial Resolution (mm) | Tissue Penetration (cm) |
|---|---|---|
| 5 | 0.8 | 8 |
| 10 | 0.4 | 4 |
| 20 | 0.2 | 2 |

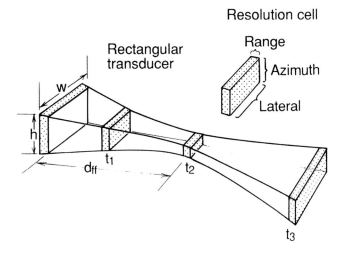

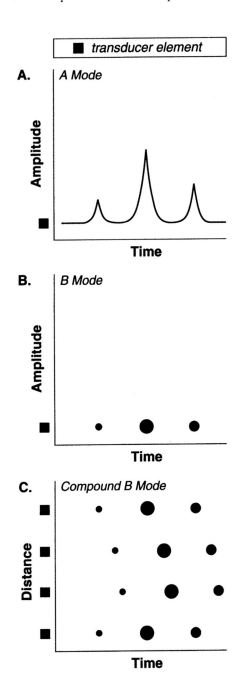

**Figure 2-2.** The basic types of ultrasound images. **A.** An A-mode image plots the amplitude of a returning echo versus the time when it returns relative to the transmitted ultrasound wave. Because the velocity of sound through soft tissue is relatively constant, the time of a returning echo can be converted into the distance or depth into the tissue from which the echo originated. **B.** A B-mode image displays the amplitude of an echo as the brightness of a dot. **C.** When multiple transducers are used or when a single transducer is moved over an area, the multiple single-line B-mode images can be converted into a rectilinear or compound scan.

## Transducer Size and Lateral Resolution

The lateral resolution makes it possible to distinguish between two points in the lateral dimension (see Fig-

**Figure 2-3.** The resolution in three dimensions (resolution cell) for a pulse of ultrasound energy as it propagates from a rectangular-shaped transducer of defined width ($w$) and height ($h$). The duration of the pulse, defining the axial or range resolution, stays the same as the wave propagates and is illustrated at three times: $t_1$, $t_2$, and $t_3$. Changes in the beam pattern produce changes in the lateral and azimuthal resolutions at the three time points, however. The near–far field transition point ($d_{ff}$) is the point with the smallest resolution cell (in this case, illustrated at time $t_2$) and offers the best overall resolution. (Reproduced from Kimmey MB, Martin RW. Fundamentals of endosonography. Gastrointest Endosc Clin North Am 1992;2:560, with permission from WB Saunders.)

ure 2-3). The magnitude of this resolution is dependent on the diameter of the transducer. In general, larger transducers have poorer lateral resolution. The lateral resolution is not constant but varies according to the distance of the target reflector from the transducer. The location of the best lateral resolution is often referred to as the *focal zone* of the transducer, and is the point at which the beam is focused and the lateral resolution is optimized. With most US endoscopes, this distance is between 2 and 3 centimeters from the transducer.

The frequency of an US transducer also affects the lateral resolution. Small-diameter transducers used on catheter probes are especially vulnerable to this effect. With other variables being equal, higher-frequency small-diameter transducers have a narrower focal zone over a broader distance from the transducer than do lower frequency transducers of the same diameter (Figure 2-4). This is the primary reason why catheter probes are made with higher-frequency (12 to 20 MHz) transducers.

## Attenuation and Tissue Penetration

*Attenuation* refers to the loss of strength of the US beam over time or distance traveled. The degree of attenuation is dependent on the properties of both the US transducer and the tissue, but the most important

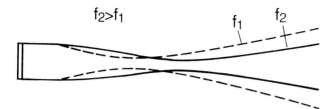

$f_2 > f_1$     $f_1$   $f_2$

**Figure 2-4.** The effects of ultrasound frequency ($f$) on the beam pattern of a transducer. For the same size transducer, a beam (solid lines) with a higher ultrasound frequency ($f_2$) produces a near–far field transition point that is further from the transducer and also causes a narrower beam width in the far field. A beam (dashed lines) with a lower frequency ($f_1$) is illustrated for comparison. (Reproduced from Kimmey MB, Martin RW. Fundamentals of endosonography. Gastrointest Endosc Clin North Am 1992;2:561, with permission from WB Saunders.)

factor is the US frequency. Higher US frequencies are maximally attenuated and hence do not penetrate as far into the tissue. Higher frequencies are also attenuated to a greater degree by specific tissue components, such as fat. For example, a lipoma within the GI wall can attenuate a 12 or 20 MHz US beam so effectively that no US energy reaches the deep aspect of the lesion (Figure 2-5). The entire lipoma therefore may not be represented on the US image. In these situations, a lower-frequency US transducer might be preferable.

Since all tissue attenuates US to some degree, returning echoes from deeper tissue structures will have

lower amplitude than those from more superficial structures. This is due to attenuation of both the transmitting US wave and the returning echo. Medical US imaging systems compensate for this effect by amplifying the echoes that return later to the transducer (Figure 2-6). Amplification of these echoes from deeper tissue structures is called *time gain compensation* (TGC). TGC can be controlled by the sonographer by changing settings on the US processor. The goal is to make similar tissue have the same US appearance irrespective of location within the tissue.

Knowledge of attenuation can also be useful in image interpretation. Most bodily fluids (blood, urine, and bile) attenuate an US beam very little. Thus, when imaging a fluid-filled structure, more US energy is transmitted to the tissue deep to the structure in comparison to the tissue deep to the adjacent solid tissue. There are then more returning echoes from the tissue deep to the fluid-containing structure, making this tissue brighter on the image. This *through-transmission enhancement* can be used to help distinguish between

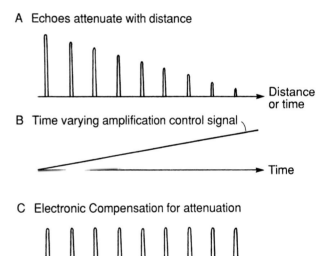

A  Echoes attenuate with distance

Distance or time

B  Time varying amplification control signal

Time

C  Electronic Compensation for attenuation

Distance

**Figure 2-6.** The concept of time varying gain (TVG) compensation is illustrated. The vertical axis represents the amplitude of the received echoes (*A* and *C*) and the control signal (*B*). **A.** Ultrasound echoes with the same amplitude at the reflection site are received by the transducer as lower amplitude signals according to how far the reflector is from the transducer because of attenuation of both the transmitted and the reflected ultrasound waves. **B.** The received echo can be electronically amplified according to when it is received, as shown by the linear increase in the control signal. **C.** When amplification of the control signal exactly compensates for tissue attenuation, echoes from similar reflectors have the same amplitude at all distances from the transducer. (Reproduced from Kimmey MB, Martin RW. Fundamentals of endosonography. Gastrointest Endosc Clin North Am 1992;2:563, with permission from WB Saunders.)

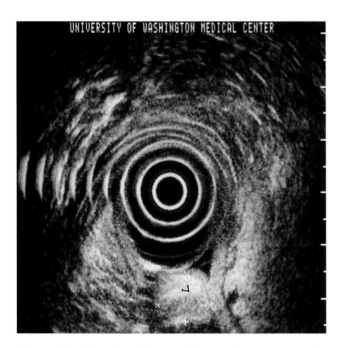

UNIVERSITY OF WASHINGTON MEDICAL CENTER

**Figure 2-5.** A duodenal lipoma (*L*) strongly attenuates the 12.5 MHz ultrasound beam producing an acoustic shadow (*arrows*) in the tissue deep to the lipoma.

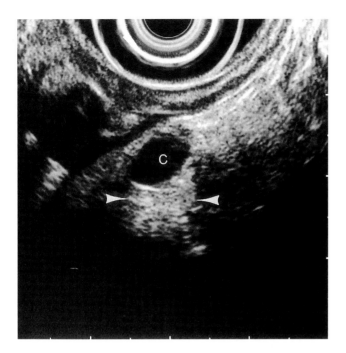

**Figure 2-7.** Fluid within this small pancreatic cyst (*C*) does not reflect much of the US beam, leading to more echoes being seen in the tissue deep to the cyst (between arrows). This is the *through-transmission artifact.*

fluid-filled and solid structures. For example, images of a cyst will show brighter echoes in the area of tissue deep to the cyst (Figure 2-7).

# How Tissue Properties Affect Images: The GI Wall

The composite image of a tissue depends on properties of the tissue as well as the US transducer and system used. US imaging of the GI tract wall is a good example of how these various factors interact.

## Frequency Dependence

Early reports of imaging of the GI wall with transcutaneous US transducers described a three-layered structure. These layers represented luminal contents (echo rich), the wall itself (echo poor), and the surrounding tissues (echo rich). The axial resolution of these low-frequency (3 to 5 MHz) systems was too poor to detect the different components of the wall itself. With the development of endoscopic US systems with higher frequency (7.5 to 12 MHz) and better resolution transducers, the GI wall was usually imaged as a five-layered structure, due to the different US properties of the mucosa, submucosa, and muscularis propria (8). Most recently, 20 MHz catheter-based EUS systems routinely image the GI wall as a seven- or nine-layered

structure due to better resolution, which allows the muscularis mucosae and the intermuscular connective tissue of the muscularis propria to be distinguished (9, 10).

Higher US frequencies also produce brighter echoes from specular reflectors (see following section). This also contributes to the improved resolution seen with higher-frequency US systems.

## Specular and Nonspecular Reflectors

There are two types of tissue reflectors that are sources of echoes on US images. These are termed *nonspecular* and *specular reflectors*. Echoes from nonspecular reflectors are produced by tissue components that scatter the US wave. Echoes from specular reflectors are produced when the US wave encounters two adjacent tissues with different acoustical properties. The US image is a composite of echoes from both types of reflectors. For example, the US image of a mixture of oil and water is homogeneous and echo rich. Echoes are reflected from nonspecular reflectors caused by the small oil droplets mixed in the water. After separation of the oil and water, however, only a thin echoic line is seen from the specular reflector at the interface between the oil and the water.

### Nonspecular Reflectors (Scatterers)

Fat and collagen are the most reflective tissue components of the GI wall. These tissue components are responsible for the bright layer seen in the center of the GI wall on EUS images. The submucosa is a dense network of collagen fibrils that provide structural support and allow for sliding of the overlying mucosa during motility. There is sometimes fat present in the submucosa as well. The other bright layer on EUS images of the bowel wall is from tissue just deep to the muscularis propria. In most areas of the body, this is from fat in the subserosa. In the esophagus, which is not covered by serosa, the bright layer is due to fat in the mediastinum. In the rectum, fat and collagen in the pelvis creates the bright layer.

### Specular Reflectors (Interface Echoes)

Early interpretations of US images of the GI wall associated the echo-poor second layer with the muscularis mucosae. However, careful measurements later demonstrated that this US layer was much too thick to be the muscularis mucosae (8). Further measurements also suggested that the central echoic layer was too thick to be the submucosa and the deep echo-poor, or fourth, layer was too thin to represent the muscularis propria. These observations were reconciled by considering the contribution to the image of specular reflectors produced at the interface between tissue layers of the bowel wall (8).

The thickness of an interface echo is determined by the pulse length or axial resolution of the US transducer. The beginning of an interface echo corresponds with the location of the interface so that the thickness of the interface echo itself will colocate with the most superficial aspect of the deeper tissue layer. Thus, an interface echo will add thickness to a more superficial echo-rich layer like the submucosa but subtract from the apparent thickness of a deeper echo-poor layer like the muscularis propria. When layer measurements are corrected for the presence of interface echoes, an accurate interpretation of the images is possible (Figure 2-8).

These principles can also be applied to the interpretation of seven- or nine-layered images of the GI wall that are obtained with higher US frequencies. Better axial resolution and thinner interface echoes allow the muscularis mucosae to be visualized as a thin echo-poor layer superficial to the submucosa. The interface echo between the lamina propria and the muscularis mucosae divides the mucosa into four layers: an interface echo at the mucosal surface, the lamina propria, an interface echo between the lamina propria and muscularis mucosae, and the remainder of the muscularis mucosae that was not obscured by the interface echo (9,10). The additional three layers in a nine-layered GI wall are due to the division of the muscularis propria

into inner circular and outer longitudinal components by a line of nonspecular echoes from a thin layer of connective tissue (Figure 2-9).

## Detection of Tissue Movement: Doppler Imaging

When an US wave encounters a moving object the US frequency is shifted. This frequency change is termed the *Doppler shift*, and the use of this principle in detecting tissue movement is called *Doppler imaging*. Movement of red blood cells within blood vessels is the most common application of Doppler imaging. The direction of the frequency shift can also be used to determine the direction of the movement (i.e., toward or away from the transducer).

A few special principles of Doppler physics need to be recalled to optimize use of this technique. First, the Doppler frequency shift is maximal when the US wave encounters the moving objects at a tangential rather than a perpendicular angle. This is contrary to

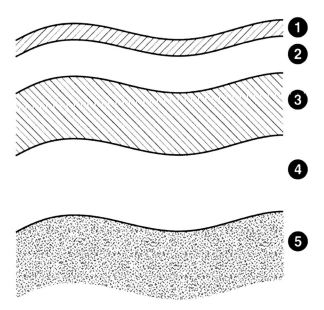

**Figure 2-8.** The five layers of the normal gastrointestinal wall as imaged with most endoscopic ultrasound equipment. From the mucosal surface at the top, layer 1 is produced by the interface between luminal fluid and the mucosal surface. Layer 2 is from the remainder of the mucosa. Layer 3 is from the submucosa and its interface with the muscularis propria. Layer 4 is the remainder of the muscularis propria. Layer 5 is from subserosal fat and connective tissue.

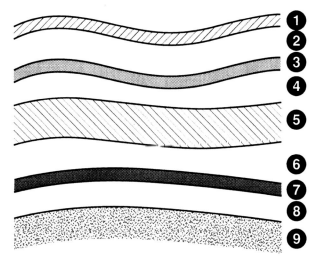

**Figure 2-9.** High-frequency ultrasound transducers may image the gastrointestinal wall as a nine-layered structure. From the mucosal surface at the top, layer 1 is produced by the interface between luminal fluid and the mucosal surface. Layer 2 is from the remainder of the lamina propria. Layer 3 is from the interface of the lamina propria and the muscularis mucosae. The remainder of the muscularis mucosae is visualized as a hypoechoic fourth layer only if the muscularis mucosae is thicker than the pulse length or axial resolution of the US transducer used. Layer 5 is from the submucosa and its interface with the muscularis propria. Layer 6 is the remainder of the inner circular component of the muscularis propria. The intermuscular connective tissue produces a thin echoic layer 7. The outer longitudinal component of the muscularis propria is responsible for layer 8. Layer 9 is from subserosal fat and connective tissue.

the principle of US imaging that tissue structure is reproduced most faithfully by an US wave that is perpendicular to the tissue. It is therefore often necessary to move the transducer in real time to simultaneously obtain optimal imaging and Doppler information.

There are two basic types of Doppler instruments: pulsed Doppler and continuous wave Doppler. Pulsed Doppler equipment sends an US wave intermittently so the detection of the returning Doppler shifted wave is not limited by further transmitting waves. This leads to a more reliable detection of the depth of the moving object. For example, pulsed wave Doppler probes have been shown to reliably detect the location of blood vessels in the gastrointestinal wall (11).

Doppler information can be displayed in a number of ways. The Doppler shift of moving blood is approximately 15,000 Hz. Because this is within the range of human hearing, the signal can be amplified into an audible signal. The Doppler signal can also be superimposed on a B-mode scan so that the location of the moving objects can be determined by looking at the B-mode image. This is called *duplex scanning* and is commonly used in endoscopic ultrasound. The presence of a Doppler signal is good evidence that a cystic anechoic structure on B-mode imaging is a blood vessel. The direction of the Doppler shift can also be codified with color in a technique called *color Doppler*. Red is commonly used to represent flow toward the transducer and blue to represent flow away from the transducer.

## Imaging Artifacts

There are a number of artifacts that should be recognized when performing endoscopic ultrasound imaging. *Artifacts* are echoes seen on an image that do not reliably reproduce the actual tissue structure. Failure to recognize artifacts can lead to image misinterpretation and errors in patient management. This section will highlight some common artifacts and discuss how to recognize, or if possible, avoid them.

### Reverberation Artifacts

Strong echoes are produced when an US wave encounters solid nontissue objects. The most common example of this is reverberation of the US beam from the casing of the transducer. This produces a characteristic series of echoes at equal intervals radiating out from the transducer—the *ring artifact* (Figure 2-10). It is seen more commonly with the radial scanning echoendoscope than the curvilinear array instrument, and in some situations can interfere with the near-field image. Reducing overall and near-field gain helps to minimize this artifact. Moving the transducer away from the area

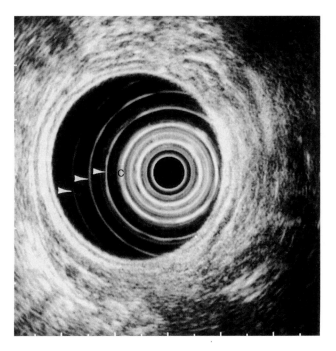

**Figure 2-10.** The plastic casing (*C*) around the US transducer produces a strong reverberation of the US beam between the transducer and the casing. This results in a series of circular rings (*arrows*) of equal spacing and diminishing amplitude around the transducer.

of interest by filling the balloon or bowel lumen with water may also help move the artifact away from the area of interest.

Another problem created by reverberation is the *mirror image artifact* (12). In this situation, ultrasound waves bounce off of an interface between water and air (Figure 2-11). This is typically seen when imaging within a partially water-filled organ such as the stomach or rectum. The ultrasound waves bounce back and forth between the transducer and the air–water interface, creating a mirror image of the transducer on the opposite side of the air–water interface (Figure 2-12). This effect is similar to observing both a mountain and its inverted reflection in a lake. The artifact is easily recognized and can be avoided by removing air and adding more water into the lumen.

### Tangential Scanning

As previously discussed, distances and therefore tissue thickness are most accurate when the US wave is perpendicular to the area of interest. When the US wave is tangential, tissue layers appear artificially thickened (Figure 2-13). This artifact can result in tumor "overstaging," especially in the esophagus and gastroesophageal junction, and particularly when the radial scanning US endoscope is used (Figure 2-14). To avoid the problem, the endoscope should be carefully maneuvered so that the US wave is perpendicular to the tissue. The normal

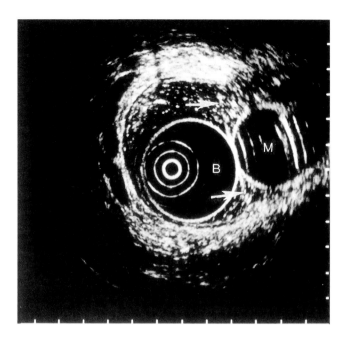

**Figure 2-11.** A mirror image (*M*) of the US transducer and water-filled balloon (*B*) is produced by reverberation between the transducer and the interface (*arrow*) between water and air within the gastric lumen.

wall layers should appear symmetric and of uniform thickness. When imaging abnormal tissue, care must be taken that the findings are reproducible and not altered by small deflections of the endoscope tip.

### Attenuation Artifacts

Other artifacts are caused by attenuation of the US wave, but attenuation artifacts facilitate image interpretation in some cases. For example, lack of transmission of US through a gallstone or pancreatic duct stone is a key feature of cholelithiasis, choledocholithiasis, and pancreaticolithiasis. Soft tissue can also attenuate the US waves, making it difficult to image deep into the tissue, especially when high-frequency transducers such as those on catheter probes are used. This can limit the ability to image the deep aspects of tissue masses.

Another common artifact is due to attenuation by air bubbles. Bubbles develop in several unwanted locations, including the oil surrounding the transducer within the transducer housing, the water in the balloon on the outside of the transducer housing, in water placed into the gastrointestinal lumen, and air within the lumen itself. The transducer casing should be

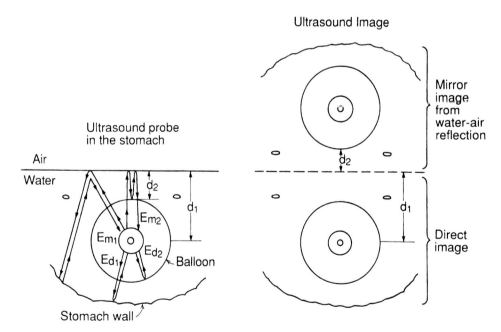

**Figure 2-12.** How reverberation of echoes from a water–air interface produces a mirror image artifact. The water–air interface reflects so strongly that ultrasound energy is redirected back to the transducer like a mirror redirects light. In the illustration at the left, the echoes $E_{m1}$ and $E_{m2}$ result from a double reflection, one from the water–air interface and one from a reflection from the stomach wall or balloon (or transducer case), respectively. The ultrasound processor records the position of the echo according to the time it receives the signal; the double reflection path takes longer and therefore causes the echo to appear further away from the transducer as if it were a reflection in a mirror (diagram at left). The echoes received by the transducer directly (for example, $E_{d1}$ and $E_{d2}$) are displayed on the image in the expected location. The distance from the transducer to the water–air interface ($d_1$) and the distance from the balloon or transducer case to the interface ($d_2$) also are illustrated. (Reproduced from Kimmey MB, Martin RW. Fundamentals of endosonography. Gastrointest Endosc Clin North Am 1992;2:570, with permission from WB Saunders.)

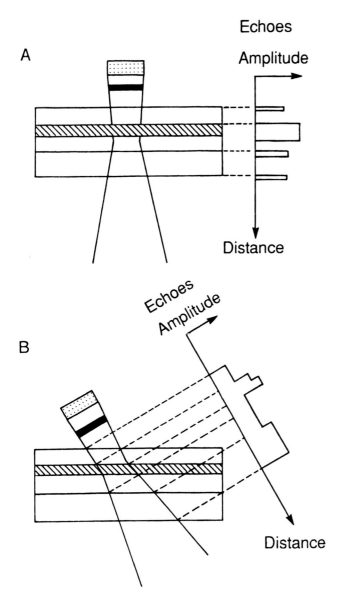

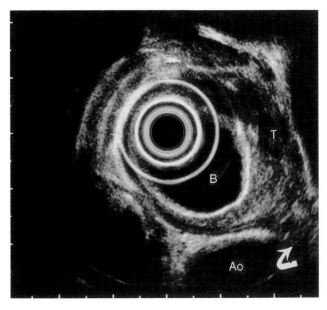

**Figure 2-14.** This EUS image of an esophageal cancer (*T*) appears to show invasion of the descending aorta (*Ao*) at the arrow. This is an artifact caused by nonperpendicular or tangential scanning. A clue to this is the eccentrically-located water-filled balloon (*B*). The transducer and balloon should be positioned in the center of the esophagus with the transducer in the center of the balloon to avoid this artifact and avoid tumor over-staging.

**Figure 2-13.** Why artifactual layer thickness increases with tangential scanning. **A.** The amplitude and spatial duration of the echoes from the interfaces and specular reflectors in the normal gastrointestinal wall are shown in the case when the ultrasound beam is at right angles to the wall. The diagonally-hatched region represents a tissue type with nonspecular echoes (for example, the submucosa); the remaining echoes are produced by interfaces between tissue layers (specular echoes). The duration of the interface echoes is the same as the duration of the ultrasound pulse or the range resolution of the system (illustrated as a black rectangle in the beam). The echoes (displayed at the right) are spatially separated and distinguishable from each other. **B.** When the ultrasound beam is not perpendicular to the wall, both the lateral and range resolution affect the duration of the echoes from each layer. In the extreme situation illustrated here, echoes from each layer overlap and cannot be distinguished individually. (Reproduced from Kimmey MB, Martin RW. Fundamentals of endosonography. Gastrointest Endosc Clin North Am 1992;2:572, with permission from WB Saunders.)

inspected for air bubbles prior to each procedure; removing these bubbles requires a minor repair by the manufacturer. Air bubbles in the balloon can be avoided by using degassed water and by repetitive filling and suctioning of the balloon prior to use. Air in water placed into the lumen can be avoided by using degassed water and by having the patient drink a simethicone "cocktail" before the procedure (13).

## Side Lobe Artifacts

These artifacts are characterized as nonshadowing echoes within an otherwise anechoic or fluid-filled structure (14). They can be confused with biliary sludge in the gallbladder or a mass within a pancreatic cyst (Figure 2-15). Side lobe artifacts are caused by low-amplitude components of the transmitted US beam that are not perpendicular to the target. If these echoes are reflected by solid tissue outside the fluid-containing target, they may be displayed by the US processor as having come from the fluid-filled structure. When imaging solid tissue, low-amplitude side lobe echoes are obscured by the echoes from the solid tissue and do not pose a problem in image interpretation. However, when an anechoic structure is being imaged, these echoes become visible and can artifactually suggest the presence of a solid component. They are

**Table 2-2.** Using US Principles to Optimize Image Quality

| Principle | Practice |
| --- | --- |
| US frequency affects penetration depth | Use lower US frequency for distant targets |
| US frequency affects axial resolution | Use highest US frequency that provides adequate penetration |
| Lateral resolution varies with distance from the transducer | Position transducer so target is in the optimal focal zone |
| Attenuation is greater with higher US frequencies | Use lower frequency for fatty and fibrous structures |
| The same tissue type should appear the same throughout the US image | Adjust the time gain compensation on the US processor |
| Air transmits high-frequency US poorly | Eliminate air bubbles in the water-filled balloon and in the lumen |
| Images are more reliable if the US beam is perpendicular to the tissue | Recognize and avoid tangential scanning artifacts |
| Doppler shift is greatest with a tangential US beam | Adjust the transducer position to optimize Doppler signal |

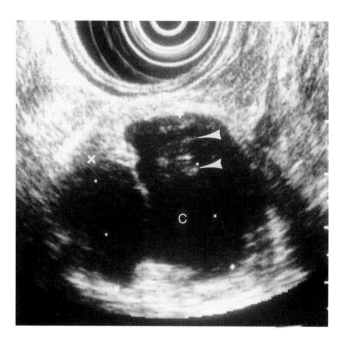

**Figure 2-15.** This pancreatic cyst (*C*) appears to have echoes within it (*arrows*) suggesting a solid component. These echoes are caused by side lobe artifacts and are recognized because they are not consistently imaged when the transducer is maneuvered into another imaging plane.

easily recognized because they disappear with transducer movement and are eliminated by scanning from other angles.

## *Doppler Artifacts*

Artifacts associated with Doppler imaging can lead to signals being detected when no flow is present and, conversely, a lack of signal when flow is present. Flow can be artifactually seen when the Doppler gain is set too high. Under those conditions, bowel wall and transmitted cardiac and respiratory motion can be amplified and give the appearance of flow. However, this false signal is usually easy to recognize because the Doppler signal is diffuse and not localized to a specific structure.

False negative Doppler signals can occur if the US beam is perpendicular to the target. Doppler shift is best detected with an US beam that is less than 60 degrees incident to the target. Doppler can also miss low levels of venous flow if the US processor's wall filter is improperly set. This filter is meant to reduce noise from vessel wall motion but can sometimes indiscriminately delete clinically important low-frequency echoes.

## Using US Principles to Obtain Better Images

The principles of US that have been discussed can be used to facilitate better endosonographic scanning and produce images that more accurately reproduce tissue structure. The importance of a standardized preprocedure checklist and consistent procedure technique cannot be overemphasized. The basic steps in achieving an optimal examination, based on the principles discussed in this chapter, are summarized in Table 2-2.

### References

1. Curry TS, Dowdey JE, Murry RC Jr. Ultrasound. In: Christensen's introduction to the physics of diagnostic radiology 4th Ed. Philadelphia: Lea & Febiger, 1990.
2. Powis RL, Powis WJ. A thinker's guide to ultrasonic imaging. Baltimore: Urban & Schwarzenberg, 1984.
3. Kimmey MB, Silverstein FE, Martin RW. Ultrasound interaction with the intestinal wall: esophagus, stomach, and colon. In: Kawai K, ed. Endoscopic ultrasonography in gastroenterology. Tokyo: Igaku-Shoin, 1988: 35–43.
4. Kimmey MB, Martin RW. Fundamentals of endosonography. Gastrointest Endosc Clinics of North Am 1992;2:557–573.
5. Fields S, Dunn F. Correlation of echographic visualizability of tissue with biological composition and physiological state. J Acoust Soc Am 1973;54: 809–812.

6. Goss SA, Johnston RL, Dunn F. Comprehensive compilation of empirical ultrasonic properties of mammalian tissues. J Acoust Soc Am 1978;64:423–457.

7. Goss SA, Johnston RL, Dunn F. Compilation of empirical ultrasonic properties of mammalian tissues II. J Acoust Soc Am 1980;68:93–108.

8. Kimmey MB, Martin RW, Haggitt RC, et al. Histological correlates of gastrointestinal endoscopic ultrasound images. Gastroenterology 1989;96:433–441.

9. Wiersema MJ, Wiersema LM. High resolution 25-megahertz ultrasonography of the gastrointestinal wall: histologic correlates. Gastrointest Endosc 1993;39: 499–504.

10. Ødegaard S, Kimmey M. Localization of the muscularis mucosae in gastric tissue specimens using high frequency ultrasound. Eur J Ultrasound 1994;1:39–50.

11. Matre K, Ødegaard S, Hausken T. Endoscopic ultrasound Doppler probes for velocity measurements in vessels in the upper gastrointestinal tract using a multifrequency pulsed Doppler meter. Endoscopy 1990; 22:268–270.

12. Grech P. Mirror-image artifact with endoscopic ultrasonography and reappraisal of the fluid-air interface. Gastrointest Endosc 1993;39:700–703.

13. Yiengpruksawan A, Lightdale CJ, Gerdes H, Botet JF. Mucolytic-antifoam solution for reduction of artifacts during endoscopic ultrasonography: a randomized controlled trial. Gastrointest Endosc 1991;37: 543–546.

14. Laing FC, Kurtz AB. The importance of ultrasonic side-lobe artifacts. Radiology 1982;145:763–776.

# 3

# Endoscopic Ultrasound Instrumentation, Procedure Room Setup, and Assistant Personnel

## John Affronti

The echoendoscopes used by endosonographers are among the most versatile and sophisticated imaging devices ever made and have literally added a new dimension to endoscopy. These ultrasound devices produce high-resolution images of the gastrointestinal wall as well as surrounding structures. The echoendoscope also allows collection of real-time color and pulse Doppler data, and permits fine-needle aspiration of extraluminal lesions that are simply not detectable by any other imaging modality. Furthermore, the latest instrument prototypes allow a forward endoscopic view and have the ability to take intraluminal biopsies.

State of the art technology is a prerequisite for the manufacture of these precise instruments and the engineering accomplishments involved in order to achieve the above are amazing. For example, the EUS transducer is less than 5 mm long, and some are as small as a pinhead. In order to generate ultrasound images, some of these transducers rotate radially at a precise and constant speed despite being located on the end of a flexible tube—the standard endoscope—that is being manipulated and maneuvered around acute angles. Other echoendoscopes utilize an electronic curved linear transducer that is fixed to the tip of the scope without any moving parts. In order to create a medium that permits the uniform transmission of ultrasound waves, these endoscopes are designed to allow extremely fine adjustments in transducer position while instilling water into the lumen to displace air as well as aspirating unwanted gas or liquid. All this, in addition to transmitting light (without heat) through the same endoscope shaft so it can be reflected, detected, and displayed on a video screen and guide the endoscopist safely through the human gastrointestinal tract.

EUS instrumentation is constantly being upgraded and improved. Real-time three-dimensional ultrasonog-raphy and computer assisted 3-D ultrasound image reconstruction are on the horizon. Accessories for performing fine-needle aspiration or injection are being constantly upgraded and "therapeutic" EUS equipment is already available as protoypes (1). This chapter's description of the EUS instruments available today is meant to provide a practical foundation for assessing new developments in this field.

## Physics of Endoscopic Ultrasonography

It is useful to briefly review some basic properties of ultrasound in order to appreciate the function and limitations of EUS equipment. For a more detailed review the reader is referred to Chapter 2 on the principles of ultrasonography. Several comprehensive ultrasound textbooks are also available (2,3,4)

Sound energy is substantially different from other forms of energy used to create medical images. Unlike x-rays and other types of electromagnetic radiation that can travel through a vacuum, ultrasonic waves require a medium for propagation. An ultrasound transducer converts electrical energy into a mechanical disturbance within a medium in a constant repetitive (vibratory) manner. Waves of molecular compression and a rebound expansion of the medium are produced. These waves then travel through the medium (Figure 3-1). The transmitted waves can then be reflected back toward the transducer by the mechanisms outlined in the following paragraphs. The same transducer that created the disturbance can convert these waves into electrical energy. This process is called the piezoelectric effect. The electrical impulse created by this process can be amplified and utilized to produce ultrasound images. In most imaging applications, an electrical impulse lasting just a few microseconds is applied

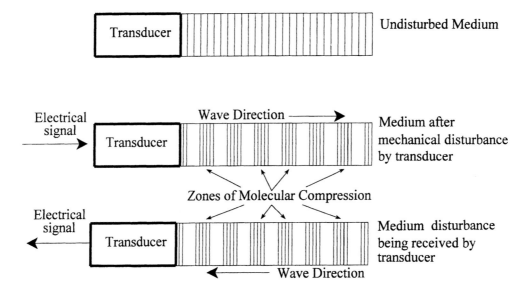

**Figure 3-1.** Ultrasound transducer function. An ultrasound transducer generates ultrasound waves and detects the waves that are reflected back to it.

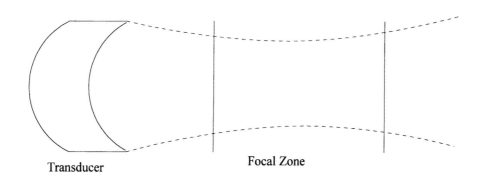

**Figure 3-2.** Ultrasound beam. The ultrasound beam or wave path can be focused to produce optimal image resolution in the focal zone.

to the transducer in order to create a burst of ultrasound energy. The same transducer then remains quiescent for a few milliseconds while it "listens" for echoes to return from reflected areas. This cycle of alternating transmission and reception occurs many times each second.

Transducers are usually made of thin crystals that can be slightly curved into a concave shape to help direct the beam. This produces a directed beam of ultrasound waves that can be focused or concentrated at a certain length from the transducer (Figure 3-2). It is within this area of wave concentration (the focal zone) that the spatial resolution of the structure being imaged is optimal. A transducer with a larger diameter can generate a larger ultrasound beam, which has a larger focal zone. The spatial resolution in both the lateral and axial dimensions of the ultrasound beam improves as the frequency of the beam increases. However, as the ultrasound beam frequency is increased the beam is at-

tenuated more rapidly by surrounding soft tissue. Moreover, at higher frequencies the depth of ultrasound wave penetration through soft tissue is significantly reduced.

EUS devices are engineered to capitalize on these physical principles. The echoendoscopes and probes allow for the placement of the transducer relatively close to the area of interest so the ultrasound waves have to travel only a short distance prior to being reflected. Therefore, higher ultrasound frequencies can be employed to generate high-resolution images. Many EUS instruments use frequencies of 7.5 to 12 MHz. For echoendoscopes, 4 cm is the usual depth of ultrasound penetration. In contrast, EUS probes commonly utilize frequencies of 12 or 20 MHz. As a consequence, echoprobes have focal zones that are closer to the transducer, and the depth of ultrasound wave penetration is often significantly less for probes as compared with the standard echoendoscope.

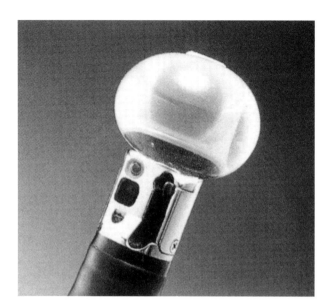

**Figure 3-3.** An EUS balloon assembly. A balloon surrounding the transducer can be inflated with water to improve ultrasound transmission. Courtesy Olympus America, Inc.

The ease with which an ultrasound wave passes through a medium or substance is determined by the acoustic impedance of that substance. As an ultrasound wave passes through the soft tissues surrounding the lumen of the gastrointestinal tract, the different impedances of the various structures are encountered. At the interface of differing impedances some of the ultrasonic energy is reflected back toward the transducer and some is transmitted past the interface. The transducer converts the reflected ultrasonic energy into an electrical signal that can be used for generating images.

For a target lesion to be imaged optimally, it is best if the medium between the target lesion and ultrasound transducer is as homogenous and as free from impedance interfaces as possible. For practical reasons, degassed or deaerated water has often been used as a coupling medium to conduct ultrasound waves between the transducer and the target tissue or structure. Therefore, device manufacturers have developed relatively elaborate methods for instilling and aspirating water into the gastrointestinal lumen. Also, water-filled balloon systems have been engineered to surround the transducer with water while the scope is being positioned close to the area of interest. These modifications have been very helpful in enhancing the quality of EUS images (Figure 3-3).

Most EUS instruments utilize a real-time imaging technique that is similar to a B-mode (brightness modulation) display format. In this display arrangement, a real-time image is constructed from a series of small dots or pixels on a monitor screen. Each dot represents a single reflected ultrasound pulse. The brightness of each

pixel varies approximately with the amount of reflected ultrasound energy. The location of the pixel represents the position of the reflecting interface. Consequently, on the display, intensely reflecting areas appear white (hyperechoic) and areas of low reflection are dark (hypoechoic). Substances of intermediate reflectivity are displayed as various shades of gray.

Different EUS transducer designs are available to allow for the emitted ultrasound beam to scan through the patient's anatomy at various angles. Using the standard approach, the region of interest is scanned by a relatively thin ultrasound beam and the reflections of the beam are used to create an image in the manner already described. If the transducer is mechanically rotated, however, a sweeping circular ultrasound image can be generated. Using this method, radial scan images (full circle views) or sections of the circle in the form of pie-shaped sector scan images can be rendered. A variation of this design employs a rotatable acoustic mirror to alter the direction of the ultrasound beam generated from a stationary transducer (a *mechanical sector* scanner). An alternative design arranges multiple small transducers in an array on a curved surface to form the *linear array* scanner. With the linear array technique, multiple transducers are sequentially activated via time delay circuits in such a manner that an ultrasound beam sweeps through the target area in a wedge-shaped geometric plane. Actually, the region being imaged is being exposed to a series of narrow, nearly parallel ultrasound beams in rapid succession. Therefore, the displayed image is similar to those generated by mechanical rotating scanners.

Ultrasound waves reflected from objects moving toward the ultrasound source are reflected back at a higher frequency, and those reflected from objects moving away return at a lower frequency. This is the well-known Doppler effect. This shift in ultrasound frequency between the transmitted and received waves can be used to determine the direction and velocity of movement at a specified location in the ultrasound beam. Some EUS devices are able to provide Doppler measurements of moving fluids. The design of the linear array EUS device is ideal to provide this information, because multiple transducers remain stationary. Also, the linear array setup permits simultaneous display of real-time ultrasound imaging and Doppler information, which can be used to help identify blood vessels and differentiate vascular from cystic structures during the EUS procedure.

A basic familiarity with the physics of ultrasound is essential if an endosonographer is to make informed decisions on current and future equipment purchases and at the same time maintain realistic expectations regarding the information that EUS can provide. This knowledge will not only help one assess the EUS equipment that is currently available but also will allow for

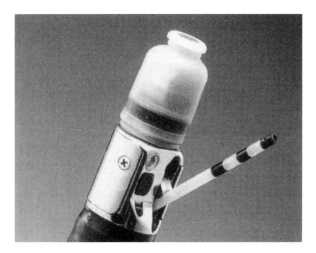

**Figure 3-4.** An EUS radial scanning transducer assembly. The transducer (*black disk*) is seen in the oil-filled plastic capsule. Courtesy Olympus America, Inc.

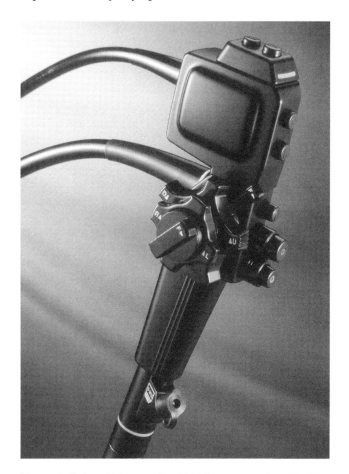

**Figure 3-5.** A radial scanning EUS instrument handle. The square portion of the handle contains the motor that drives the rotating transducer cable. Courtesy Olympus America, Inc.

the critical analysis of future modifications and new EUS accessories, which are continually enhancing this imaging modality.

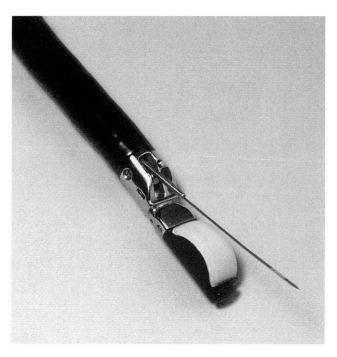

**Figure 3-6.** A linear array transducer. This configuration provides a scan plane parallel to the shaft of the endoscope. Courtesy Pentax Instruments, Inc.

## Endoscopic Instruments

Over the last several years, much progress has been made in the development of endoscopes that possess built-in ultrasound transducers (i.e., echoendoscopes). Three basic EUS designs are currently sold: scopes with mechanically rotating transducers, linear array devices, and most recently, mechanical sector scanners. Each design has particular strengths and weaknesses for endosonography.

The primary constraint on all EUS instruments is the limitations imposed on the size and shape of the transducer that can be introduced safely and comfortably into the gastrointestinal system. One manufacturer (Olympus America, Inc., Melville, NY) has addressed this problem by encasing a small transducer in a tapered, oil-filled plastic capsule mounted on the tip of the endoscope shaft (Figure 3-4). The transducer rests on a revolving cylinder so that the plane of the scan is perpendicular to the shaft of the scope. A cable extends from a motor in the endoscope handle through the shaft of the instrument to the tip and drives the transducer rotation (Figure 3-5). This radial scanning configuration is the only EUS design that produces a 360-degree ultrasound image display. Many endosonographers prefer this instrument because a large portion of the anatomy can be viewed while the instrument is stationary. Also, the images obtained are oriented

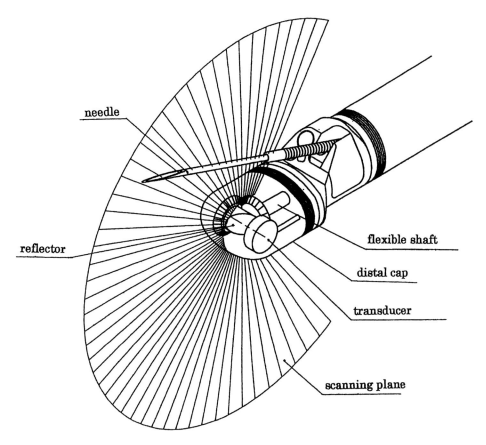

**Figure 3-7.** An EUS transducer with rotating reflector. This alternative configuration provides a scan plane parallel to the shaft of the endoscope. Courtesy Olympus America, Inc.

spatially in the same way as images obtained by computed tomography. These instruments can also be manufactured with two different transducers on opposite sides of the rotating cylinder, each operating at a particular frequency. The operator then has the option to utilize the beam frequency optimally suited for the target lesion in terms of depth of penetration, focal zone, and image resolution. At present, only 7.5 MHz and 12 MHz frequencies are available on these switchable frequency instruments.

The most important disadvantage of a perpendicular scanning plane is the inability to "track" or guide needle biopsy devices when they are extended out from the working channel of the instrument. In order to optimally monitor and guide these working channel tools, the ultrasound plane must be parallel to the shaft of the instrument. Also, it is important for the ultrasound beam to be relatively wide. A wide ultrasound beam permits continued scanning of these tools even when there are slight deviations in their trajectory. This "wiggle factor" occurs because the tools are slightly deviated by various forces as they are maneuvered through soft tissue to the target area.

The EUS instruments with a linear array transducer configuration provide ultrasound scanning parallel to the shaft of the scope. These instruments were initially used to refine methods of EUS-guided FNA (Figure 3-6). Subsequently, instruments with mechanically rotatable acoustic mirrors were produced, which scanned parallel to the shaft (Figure 3-7). Although one group has reported fine-needle aspiration (FNA) with radial scanning equipment (5), most still prefer using linear array technology, which not only facilitates invasive procedures but also has Doppler capability.

Some practical issues regarding these endoscopic instruments deserve emphasis. First, the size constraints on the transducers mentioned have forced most of these devices to be manufactured as side viewing instruments. Although the optics of the side viewing esophagus and gastric EUS instruments are similar to that of standard duodenoscopes, the endoscopic view provided by EUS devices is directed more toward the tip of the scope—a "forward oblique" orientation. Manipulating these instruments is not difficult for an endoscopist experienced in biliary and pancreatic endoscopy, because the side viewing duodenoscope used

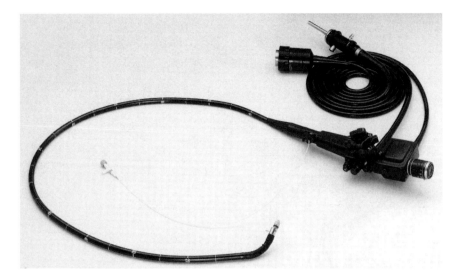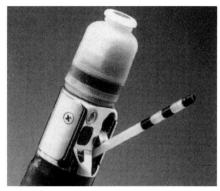

**Figure 3-8.** An ultrasonic duodenoscope (left). A side viewing objective lens and elevator are designed to facilitate biliary and pancreatic duct cannulation. At right is a closeup of the catheter tip. Courtesy Olympus America, Inc.

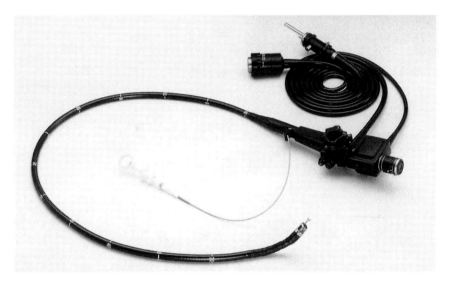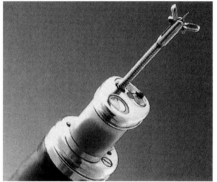

**Figure 3-9.** An ultrasonic colonoscope (left). The objective lens on the tip (right) of this assembly provides a forward endoscopic view. Courtesy Olympus America, Inc.

for ERCP is very similar to the EUS instrument. Nevertheless, the "forward oblique" perspective can be disorienting. In fact, most endosonographers still perform standard endoscopy to inspect the esophagus, stomach, and duodenum prior to an EUS exam. Duodenoscopes that allow for biliary and pancreatic duct cannulation as well as EUS imaging are available (Figure 3-8).

For colonoscopic exams, a forward viewing design is essential for safely reaching the cecum. However, the colonoscopic EUS instruments currently available have compromised the conventional full radial display in order to place the forward viewing optic components in the tip of the endoscope (Figure 3-9). This has resulted in a 300-degree display for colonoscopic EUS instruments as opposed to a full 360-degree display.

The tip of EUS instruments is generally less flexible due to the ultrasound transducer components, which must coexist in the same proximal location as the standard optical components of the endoscope. These space restrictions initially prevented adequate electrical shielding for the video CCD chip used in state of the art endoscopes. Interference from the operation of the ultrasound transducer disrupted the CCD chip function and resulted in an unacceptable endoscopic image. Therefore, earlier EUS instruments employed fiber-optic methods for displaying endoscopic views. With continued advances in material science, however, proper shielding is now possible without enlarging the diameter of the endoscope. EUS instruments are now available with a CCD chip, which pro-

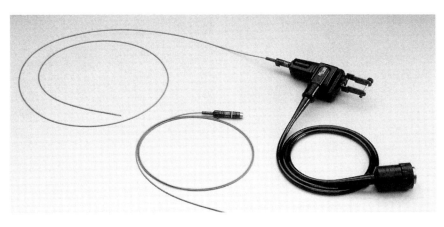 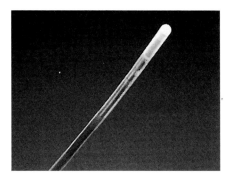

**Figure 3-10.** An ultrasonic probe (left). The transducer rotates inside this catheter. At right is a closeup of the catheter tip. Courtesy Olympus America, Inc.

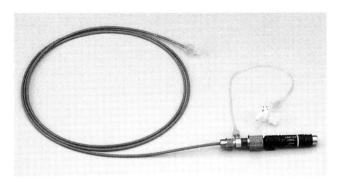

**Figure 3-11.** An ultrasonic probe with a balloon sheath. This assembly provides improved coupling for ultrasound transmission. Courtesy Olympus America, Inc.

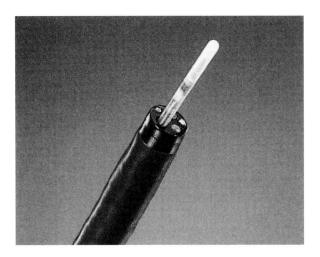

**Figure 3-12.** An ultrasound probe and endoscope. The ultrasound probe can be passed though the working channel of an endoscope. Courtesy Olympus America, Inc.

vides a larger, more detailed endoscopic view than their fiber-optic counterparts.

The maintenance of EUS instruments also deserves consideration. The radial scanning echoendoscopes are motor driven, have many moving parts, and require frequent repair. The transducer itself is surrounded by a light oil and encased in a polyurethane housing so periodic oil changes and processor calibration are a necessity. The linear array ultrasound transducers have no moving parts and, in theory, require less maintenance. In addition, both types of instruments are submitted to the torquing and twisting forces used during endoscopy and eventually require a complete overhaul.

## Probes

Recently, a catheter-based ultrasound technology has been developed. Although the technology is similar to dedicated echoendoscopes, these tiny probes can be passed through a standard endoscope for ultrasound imaging of normal and abnormal structures. A commonly-used design for EUS probes involves a sheathed cable with a small-diameter transducer placed at the tip of the cable (Figure 3-10). The cable is turned within the sheath in order to rotate the transducer. Because the transducer is small, the depth of ultrasound penetration is limited. The focal zone is relatively close to the transducer, typically within 1 to 2 cm. Some probes have inflatable water-filled balloons that facilitate acoustic coupling in the manner previously described (Figure 3-11). Probes that do not have balloons can be placed into the water-filled gut lumen and over the target area. Probes are now available with an external diameter small enough to permit the passage of the entire assembly through the working channel of standard endoscopes (Figure 3-12). Other larger-diameter probes have been

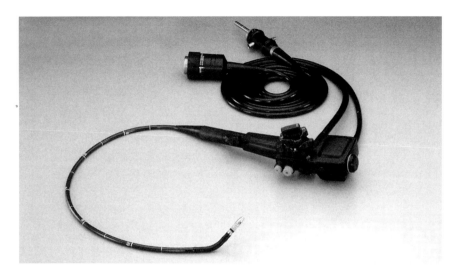
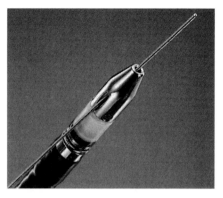

**Figure 3-13.** A blind ultrasonic probe and wire. This probe accepts a guide wire to facilitate passage through stenotic areas. At right is a closeup of the catheter tip. Courtesy Olympus America, Inc.

designed that can be passed blindly into the GI tract or advanced over a guide wire (Figure 3-13).

The thin diameter of the latest probes permits their use within narrow lumenal structures such as the biliary system or pancreatic duct, areas that can be studied with high-frequency, high-resolution ultrasonography (6). In fact, several investigators have also found EUS probes to be superior to conventional endoscopy when studying the common bile duct and the pancreas, as well as esophageal varices and achalasia because there is less displacement and distortion of the structures being studied (7).

EUS probes offer a convenient, relatively inexpensive means of evaluating soft tissue areas that are relatively close to the mucosal surface. Most probes available in the United States are compatible with several different standard ultrasound processors that are already used in most radiology departments. Although there is substantial cost savings by using miniprobes, their life span is limited. The probes are thin and easily damaged. This is especially true for probes that are passed through the working channel of a duodenoscope and maneuvered with the instrument's elevator. These issues need to be considered when determining the long-term cost of EUS probe use.

## Processors and Consoles

Currently, the ultrasound processors and consoles manufactured for EUS use differ significantly between manufacturers. Historically, manufacturers have developed EUS systems independently from each other and do not share transducer configurations. Also, each type of transducer used (radial or linear scanning) requires its own particular customized processor. Linear array transducers also generate Doppler data, which must be displayed separately from the ultrasound and endoscopic images. As a consequence, consoles must be designed to meet the different functional capabilities of the transducer configuration preferred for a particular examination. Even if the same manufacturer offers both linear array and rotating transducer devices, the consoles have to be device-specific. Some endosonographers have purchased two entire systems: a linear array/Doppler system for its ability to monitor tools extended from the working channel, and a rotating transducer system to provide enhanced anatomic images similar to what is seen in CT imaging. One manufacturer now produces an EUS instrument that reorients the ultrasound scan plane of a rotating transducer so that it is parallel to the shaft of the scope (Figure 3-14). Nevertheless, the limited versatility—and the necessary added cost—of current EUS equipment remains a significant financial handicap, preventing more widespread use of this technology.

The consoles for all available EUS systems provide "user-friendly" tools to adjust the ultrasound image (Figure 3-15). The amplification or attenuation of ultrasound signals reflected from various distances can be altered as needed to improve the image contrast displayed on the monitor. Various labeling functions enable the operator to mark points of interest in a relatively detailed manner, and a body locator is available to mark the position of the scope during imaging. Image freezing provides the ability to more closely inspect and label ultrasound findings. It also allows for an accurate measurement of structures using methods specific to each console. The image can be enlarged as well as rotated and inverted on some systems. Most systems now produce images in formats

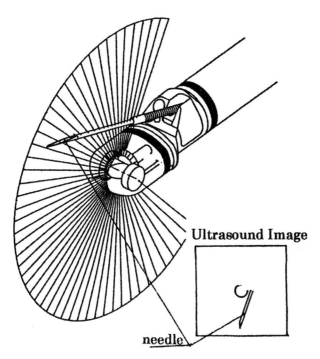

**Figure 3-14.** An EUS instrument and needle. This instrument can monitor the puncture path of a needle and is compatible with a console for radial scanners. Courtesy Olympus America, Inc.

that can be utilized by other accessory devices such as moving image recorders and still image printers. This ability is becoming more important as image manipulation and image transfer over the Internet become more popular.

## Auxiliary Equipment

Water irrigation devices are essential for EUS because relatively large volumes of water need to be instilled into the GI tract during an exam for optimal ultrasound conduction. Simple homemade devices involving enema bags attached to catheters, which are then connected to the endoscope's working channel, have been in use for years. Foot-controlled water pumps with large fluid reservoirs are also available (Figure 3-16).

As linear array technology has advanced, equipment for fine-needle aspiration has been developed that will function reliably in this rather unique environment. Straight needles that are long enough to access target areas well beyond the gastrointestinal tract wall but small enough to traverse the curves of an endoscope's working channel have been refined (Figure 3.17). One of the major advances that made this equipment possible was the improvement of the metal sheath that protects the working channel from puncture damage. Many costly repairs were required for these expensive instruments before the need for a

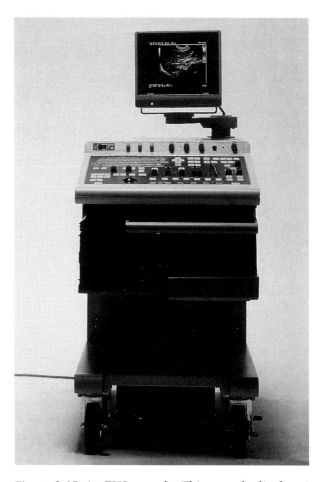

**Figure 3-15.** An EUS console. This console displays images from a linear array transducer with Doppler capability. Courtesy of Pentax, Inc.

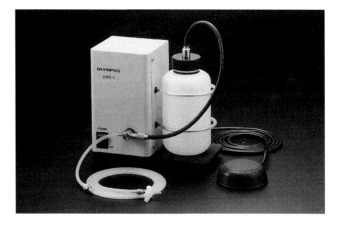

**Figure 3-16.** A water supply unit. A foot pedal activates a motorized pump that transports water from the reservoir to the endoscope channel. Courtesy Olympus America, Inc.

properly-positioned metal sheath was appreciated. These needles may also be used for therapeutic injections (8). More information about tissue aspiration devices is provided in Chapter 12.

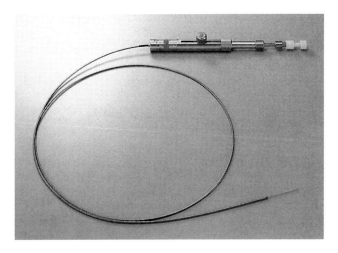 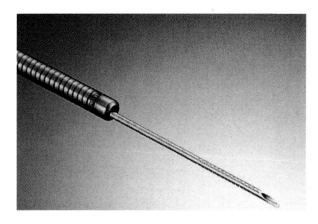

**Figure 3-17.** Aspiration needle with metal sheath (left). The sheath and needle can be passed through the working channel to a target lesion under ultrasound guidance. At right is a closeup of the catheter tip. Courtesy Olympus America, Inc.

Image management is a particularly important component of a successful EUS study. In addition to displaying real-time ultrasound images simultaneously with live endoscopic views, recording these images in various formats is important for the purpose of documenting each EUS exam. Color and monochrome printers are available that produce paper copies of selected images. The video signal produced by these processors can also be converted into standard ultrasound hard copies on celluloid. Many find this to be a convenient storage medium because the images can be stored in the patient's radiology folder and kept in the radiology department's file room.

Image conversion to a digital form is also becoming more popular. A standard format for radiological imaging is DICOM (Digital Imaging Communication in Medicine). Images stored in this format, as well as other digital formats, can be reproduced and manipulated without image quality degradation and can also be transmitted easily to remote printers or display monitors over various internal networks or the Internet. The digital files can be electronically enhanced as desired using computer software to produce a variety of images for patient reports, publications, and presentations. Videotape recorders still remain the standard tool for capturing real-time images. Digital recordings of moving EUS images are possible, but large files are generated. As methods of image file compression become more efficient and reliable, long-term storage of these digitally recorded moving EUS images will become less expensive and more widely used and use of analog devices such as VCRs for this purpose will gradually disappear.

## Procedure Room Setup

The importance of a thoughtfully arranged EUS system and exam room should not be underestimated. Time-consuming preprocedure preparations, cramped working conditions, and complicated equipment connections that limit functionality can raise the frustration factor for each EUS exam to the point that those who are participating perceive it as a negative experience. Moreover, time constraints and "windows of opportunity" can be narrow; often, a quick, efficient study by an experienced endosonographer can have enormous impact on patient outcome. A well-organized layout for a procedure area is a necessary prerequisite for maintaining high levels of quality and efficiency in an EUS practice.

Even though there is additional equipment necessary for EUS, the standard recommendation for endoscopy room setup (9) remains the most sensible for the endoscopist and assistants. Slight modifications are appropriate in order to provide easy access to the keyboard/ultrasound processor and an ultrasound image display, in addition to the endoscopic image (Figure 3-18). Having the keyboard for the ultrasound processor console comfortably within reach of the endoscopist's dominant hand while the endoscopist holds the EUS instrument in the other hand is particularly helpful. Also useful is the ability to project both the ultrasound and the endoscopic image simultaneously and adjacent to each other. This can be achieved by a split-screen image on one monitor, or simply by placing two monitors side by side in the direct line of sight for the endoscopist.

Taking advantage of ceiling space can remedy many practical problems that are encountered when setting up a room for EUS exams. Suspending a weight-balanced monitor cradle from the ceiling allows for more free space in the endoscopy area and facilitates patient access by endoscopy assistants. Hanging oxygen and suction tubing as well as monitor wiring from the ceiling eliminates dangerous trip lines on the floor. Many blood pressure monitors and oximeters are small

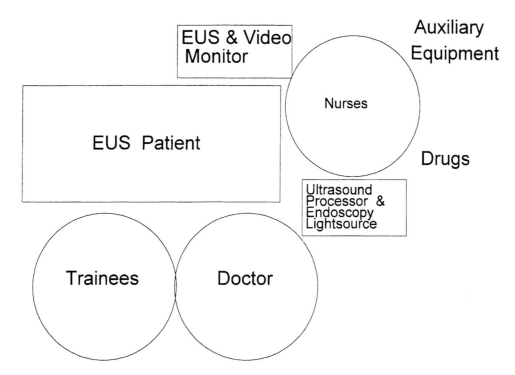

**Figure 3-18.** EUS room setup. Modifications to the standard endoscopy setup allows for efficient EUS exams.

enough that they can be placed or clamped on the gurney near the patient's face. This provides the endoscopy nurse and endoscopist with the ability to quickly assess the patient's face for signs of discomfort or inadequate sedation as well as monitor blood pressure, pulse, oxygen saturation, and so on in the same field of view. Placing these devices so that they are behind the patient and below the line of sight to the ultrasound/video monitors is ideal. This also eliminates the need for wires and tubing being strung from the stretcher to the wall where they can potentially cause injuries to personnel or cause equipment damage. The use of an easily adjustable endoscopy stretcher (or motorized table), which facilitates patient positioning, is also important. The endosonographer may want to change the patient's position several times during an exam in order to optimize the water conduction of ultrasound and improve the EUS image.

The volume and type of EUS exams done in an endoscopy unit determines whether or not a room will be dedicated exclusively for endosonography. If a multipurpose endoscopy room is used and EUS equipment must be moved into place prior to each exam, it is imperative that the process of setting up for an EUS exam be made as simple as possible. Having one mobile EUS cart on which all the needed equipment is permanently wired in the desired manner is very helpful. Rigging the equipment so that only one power cord needs to be plugged into the wall outlet is ideal. In

short, minimizing the number of cables that need to be connected and disconnected when preparing the room is critical. A complicated setup process can be intimidating to some assistants, cause long trouble-shooting delays, and in general, increase the wear and tear on devices in frequent use.

## Nursing/ Technician Assistance

The conscious sedation policy of most endoscopy units and national GI societies mandates that one endoscopy assistant be dedicated solely to monitoring the patient's vital functions and comfort. This is no different for EUS procedures. An additional technical assistant may be employed to help with all other aspects of the EUS. The unique aspects of EUS studies can be learned easily by most experienced endoscopy assistants. Several points need emphasis. In general, because EUS procedures take longer than conventional endoscopy, longer and deeper periods of intravenous sedation are required. An assistant should be comfortable in the management of patients under these conditions. The experienced EUS assistant will also be especially cognizant of the risk of pulmonary aspiration and fluid expulsion, because large amounts of water are sometimes instilled into the GI tract during the study. These events are less frequent after the members of the EUS team have successfully progressed through the initial phases of the learning curve. The recovery of patients after an EUS exam is essentially the same as for similar endoscopic procedures.

As is true of conventional endoscopic procedures, the EUS assistant should be able to anticipate the needs of the endoscopist and patient. The assistant must have a fundamental understanding of EUS as well as a good working relationship with the endosonographer. The optimal way of achieving these related goals is simply to expose the assistant to as many EUS procedures as possible. For this reason, it is usually best to select one or a few assistants to take part in all of the EUS exams rather than having all of the endoscopy assistants participate on a rotating basis. Reducing the number of potential assistants also enables the endosonographer to focus his or her teaching efforts. Explaining EUS images to the assistants, as well as emphasizing how the results of each exam will influence patient care, is extremely important. Understandably, most endoscopy assistants will perceive EUS procedures as long, unexciting exams (compared to conventional endoscopy) until they gain an appreciation of the particular benefits of EUS in patient management.

### References

1. Prat F, Chapelon JY, Arefiev A, Cathignol D, Souchon R, Theilliere Y. High-intensity focused ultrasound transducers suitable for endoscopy: feasibility study in rabbits. Gastrointest Endosc 1997;46:348–351.

2. Hendee WR. Reflection imaging. In: Putman CE, Ravin CE, eds. Textbook of diagnostic imaging. Vol I. Philadelphia: WB Saunders, 1994.

3. Krenkau FW. Doppler ultrasound: principles and instruments. Philadelphia: WB Saunders, 1990.

4. Goldstein A. Physics of ultrasound. In: Rumack CM, Wilson SR, Charboneau JW, eds. Diagnostic ultrasound. Vol. 1. St. Louis: Mosby Yearbook, 1991: 2–18.

5. Gress FG, Hawes RH, Savides TJ, Ikenberry SO, Lehman GA. Endoscopic ultrasound-guided fine-needle aspiration biopsy using linear array and radial scanning endosonography. Gastrointest Endosc 1997;45: 243–250.

6. Furukawa T, Naitoh Y, Tsukamoto Y, et al. New technique using intraductal ultrasonography for the diagnosis of diseases of the pancreatobiliary system. J of Ultrasound Med 1992;11:607–612.

7. Deviere J. Primary achalasia: analysis of endoscopic ultrasonography features with different instruments. Gastrointest Endosc Clin North Am 1995;5:631–634.

8. Wiersema MJ, Wiersema LM. Endosonography-guided celiac plexus neurolysis. Gastrointest Endosc 1996;44: 656–662.

9. Cotton PB. Practical gastrointestinal endoscopy. Oxford: Blackwell Science, 1990; 16–22.

# 4

# Endoscopic Ultrasound: The Procedure

**Brian R. Stotland**
**Michael L. Kochman**

The successful performance of a safe and useful endosonographic examination requires a thorough knowledge of anatomy, endoscopic procedural skills, and ultrasound principles. Mastery of these diverse talents is a time-consuming, laborious process, and ideally occurs under the tutelage of an experienced mentor. However, once mastered, expertise in endosonography can provide rapid, clinically important and valuable information for the management of a variety of medical conditions. This chapter will review the basic "nuts and bolts" needed to successfully perform endoscopic ultrasound procedures.

## Physician Preparation

Endoscopic ultrasound exams are usually performed to evaluate lesions or stage tumors identified by other means. The patient's past medical history, laboratory results, and prior radiological and endoscopic studies should be carefully reviewed. Once these studies are reviewed the examiner should be able to determine whether or not the exam will be useful for the purpose of clinical decision-making. The endosonographer can then anticipate what equipment is likely to become necessary during the exam, and should have these instruments and accessories available and in working order. If EUS-guided fine-needle aspiration is a consideration, a decision should be made prior to the procedure regarding what specific findings would prompt a biopsy attempt. Proper preparation will minimize the duration of the procedure, decrease patient discomfort and anxiety, and may help decrease the risks associated with a prolonged procedure requiring additional sedation.

There are no formal guidelines regarding the number of procedures one must perform under supervision before becoming proficient. However, as a means of comparison, most physicians who also perform endoscopic retrograde cholangiopancreatography conclude that endosonography is a more difficult procedure to master with a steeper learning curve (1). Although a discussion on training is beyond the scope of this chapter (see Chapter 15), it is understood that an endosonographer should obtain levels of accuracy comparable to published series prior to making recommendations on clinical management based on EUS exam results.

## Patient Preparation

It is important that the patient referred or scheduled for an EUS exam understand the nature of the procedure. Many patients have never had an endoscopic procedure and have anxiety associated with the concept of conscious sedation and the invasive nature of the procedure. In addition, some patients do not understand, or were not told, that the EUS exam is unlike prior extracorporeal ultrasound exams that they may have undergone. We have found that a discussion with the referring physician to ensure that the physician's expectations of the procedure match that of the endosonographer and that the patient also understands these expectations is key to reducing the patient's anxiety.

## Equipment Preparation

Prior to commencing an EUS exam, it is important to properly prepare the equipment. The radial scanning instruments are the most widely used of the currently available devices. For the Olympus EUM-20/130 systems, proper preparation includes placement of a condom-like balloon on the tip of the echoendoscope. When filled with water, the balloon will serve to improve coupling of the ultrasound waves to the gastrointestinal wall by producing a fluid interface and displacing intraluminal air. The balloon is filled with deaerated water injected through the echoendoscope. The image obtained varies with the quantity of air in the water, so the water should be gently poured from a sitting container and should not be from a tap or mixed with simethicone or other compounds. The balloon's integrity should be confirmed prior to starting the exam, and any air bubbles within the balloon should be flushed and removed. The drive motor should be tested, and the image quality assessed. For the Pentax echoendoscopes, the coupling balloon must also be manually affixed to the end of the echoscope prior to each case. In our unit we wrap the end of the Pentax balloon several times with dental floss to reduce the likelihood of a water leak and dislodgment; this maneuver is not needed with the Olympus radial equipment. As with the Olympus system, the integrity of the Pentax balloon should be confirmed and evacuation of air bubbles completed prior to the procedure. Care must be taken to avoid having any of the balloons contact the bite block or the patient's teeth during intubation because the balloons are fragile and are easily torn or displaced. After finishing the procedure, the balloon must be removed gently, with the assistance of an additional person if needed, to avoid damaging the expensive ultrasound transducer.

Finally, image recording devices should be routinely checked prior to the first case of the day. We strongly feel that all procedures should have both hard copy and video images preserved. These serve many purposes, including documentation for the referring physician and medical record, and for training and quality assurance. If the procedure is to be video recorded, generous numbers of blank videocassette tapes should be available to minimize procedure delays.

## General Concepts

The examination usually begins after the patient has been placed in the left-lateral position and has received conscious sedation. We utilize the same standard medications that are available in our unit for other endoscopic procedures: a topical anesthetic, meperidine, midazolam, and droperidol as indicated. Intubation of the esophagus is performed in a blind fashion similar to when using a side viewing duodenoscope. The echoendoscope is advanced into the patient's mouth, deflected caudally into the hypopharynx, and then posteriorly into the upper esophageal sphincter. By applying gentle pressure and asking the patient to swallow, esophageal intubation can usually

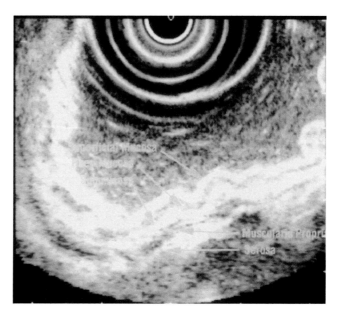

**Figure 4-1.** View of the gastric wall demonstrating the typical appearance of the five-layer wall pattern in the gastric fundus. This is the same pattern that is typically seen through the luminal gastrointestinal tract.

be achieved without difficulty. Upon entering the esophagus, the instrument is gently advanced into the gastric antrum. As with the passage of a side viewing duodenoscope, the pylorus is identified, and the echoendoscope tip deflected up as it is advanced, so that the pylorus will drop out of the field of view (the setting sun maneuver) (2). The scope is then advanced into the third part of the duodenum. Shortening the echoendoscope by reducing the gastric loop once the tip has entered the duodenal sweep will enable the instrument to be advanced beyond the major papilla. In cases where the entry into the duodenal sweep is narrow or compressed, it may help to partially inflate the balloon with water to allow the echoscope to "swim" downstream (3). Echoendoscope placement in the rectum is simpler, but when advancing the scope the oblique viewing angle must be kept in mind. Advancing the upper echoscope proximal to the rectal valves is often difficult and, in any case, is rarely indicated for the management of most common lesions. Dedicated colonic echoendoscopes are available for easier passage to the cecum.

A detailed understanding of the endoscopic ultrasound imaging correlation with the wall layers of the organ being studied is essential for accurate staging (Figure 4-1). In patients with active intestinal peristalsis, constant motion may impair the sonographic exam of small mucosal and polypoid lesions. In such cases it is reasonable to administer glucagon intravenously to temporarily inhibit peristalsis, though this is an infrequent occurrence. Air bubbles within the lumen may deflect ultrasound waves, and in some cases instillation

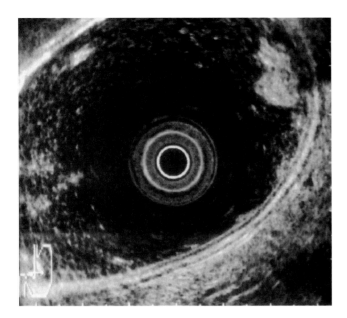

**Figure 4-2.** Water-filling technique demonstrating the five-layer wall pattern of the gastric lumen. Note the seven-layer pattern in the lower right portion of the field. This splitting of the inner and outer layer of the muscularis propria may be seen under optimal circumstances.

of a mucolytic or simethicone may help (4). Because sound waves do not penetrate well through air and contact with air causes reverberation artifacts, attempts to remove and displace luminal air should be made. The copious use of suction to decompress the gastrointestinal lumen coupled with judicious use of water insufflation will allow optimal imaging.

Each echoendoscope and frequency has an optimal focal length that allows for maximal resolution. When imaging retroperitoneal or mediastinal structures, it is useful to press the transducer with its balloon against the gut wall to minimize air artifacts. In contrast, when evaluating a mucosal lesion or polypoid structure, it is best to avoid applying pressure with the echoendoscope balloon, because this may obscure the lesion and its adjacent wall-layer pattern and be too close to the transducer to allow for optimal resolution. When characterizing intramural or submucosal lesions, filling the lumen with deaerated water is often the best way to highlight the target and its wall layer of origin (Figure 4-2). This may be difficult in the esophagus, but elsewhere it is generally easy to accomplish. Depending on the location of the lesion, the patient may need to be turned, placed flat, or tilted into position to allow the water to flow over the desired area. If the patient's head is put into a level or dependent position, great care must be taken to avoid aspiration of instilled water. Water insufflation may be accomplished with a mechanical pump and coupler attached to the echoendoscope, or simply by injecting water (roughly 250 to 500 ml) through the biopsy channel.

EUS is generally performed to evaluate abnormalities suspected by history or other imaging modalities, or previously identified on prior imaging studies. EUS exams are typically begun distal to the targeted lesion. As the echoscope is withdrawn, the lesion and surrounding structures are carefully studied. For mucosal or intramural lesions, it is best to first identify the lesion endoscopically to facilitate transducer placement. With small lesions, identifying the target on ultrasound may be easier with ultrasound probes placed through the channel of an end-viewing endoscope. It is particularly important to try to obtain a view of the lesion from a perpendicular axis. Imaging a lesion obliquely will produce a tangential image and cause errors in staging or assessing lesion size.

The echoendoscope should be passed back and forth across the lesion several times. Viewing adjacent, normal wall-layer patterns and extraluminal landmarks will help to achieve proper orientation and ensure accurate imaging. Ultrasound physics dictate that a higher frequency corresponds not only to greater tissue resolution but also to less depth penetration. Most currently available echoendoscopes can scan at dual frequencies of either 7.5 and 12 MHz, or 5 and 7.5 MHz. Choice of frequency should be dependent on the distance to the target being scanned; however, it is useful to try both frequencies to help decide which provides more useful information.

## Retroperitoneum and Mediastinum

For viewing the retroperitoneum, six standard positions are described. The *station pull-through technique* refers to identification of major retroperitoneal structures on "pull back" from the descending duodenum at each of these positions (5) (Table 4-1). There are an additional six positions for imaging the mediastinum from within the esophagus (Table 4-2). When attempting to identify these structures, it quickly becomes evident that a thorough understanding of cross-sectional anatomy is necessary. As experience is gained, the strict reliance on the standard positions may actually make imaging of some lesions more difficult and may even delay completion of the exam. Several additional helpful concepts are outlined in the following paragraphs.

As the echoendoscope is withdrawn or rotated, the imaging plane is continuously changing such that the section may be transverse, sagittal, or coronal. The transducer balloon should be inflated and intraluminal air evacuated. With the echoscope shortened, small, subtle movements along the long axis and in angulation will make significant changes in the image. Most observers tend to make large movements at first and may miss even large lesions.

**Table 4-1.** Standard positions for examination of the retroperitoneum

| Position | Location | Structure Images |
|---|---|---|
| 1 | 3rd part of duodenum | panc head, aorta, IVC |
| 2 | 2nd part of duodenum | panc head, CBD, IVC, PV, C, SMA |
| 3 | Duodenal bulb | panc head, SV, C, CBD, GB, liver, HA |
| 4 | Gastric antrum | panc body, GB, liver, SV, C |
| 5 | Gastric body | panc body, SV, SA, CA, HA, RV |
| 6 | Gastric fundus | panc tail, spleen, SA, SV, LK |

CBD = common bile duct; panc = pancreas; RK = right kidney; IVC = inferior vena cava; PV = portal vein; C = confluence of superior mesenteric vein and splenic vein; GB = gall bladder; SV = splenic vein; SMA = superior mesenteric vein; SA = splenic artery; CA = celiac axis; HA = hepatic artery; RV = renal vessels; LK = left kidney.

**Table 4-2.** Standard positions for examination of the mediastinum

| Position | Location | Structures Images |
|---|---|---|
| 1 | Cervical esophagus | spine, trachea, L SCA, carotid |
| 2 | Prox esophagus | aortic arch, trachea, spine |
| 3 | Prox-mid esophagus | trachea, spine, desc aorta, SVC, AZV, TD |
| 4 | Midesophagus | main bronchi, spine, desc aorta, AZV, TD |
| 5 | Prox-distal esophagus | L atrium, L PV, spine, AZV |
| 6 | Distal esophagus | LV, liver, IVC, HV, spine, aorta |

L = left; SCA = subclavian artery; desc = descending; SVC = superior vena cava; AZV = azygous vein; TD = thoracic duct; PV = pulmonary vein; LV = left ventricle; IVC = inferior vena cava; HV = hepatic veins.

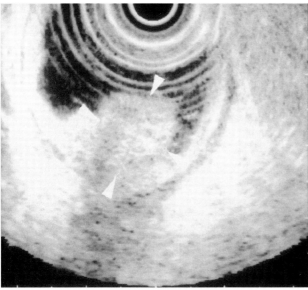
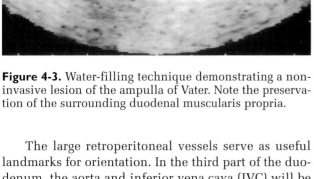

**Figure 4-3.** Water-filling technique demonstrating a noninvasive lesion of the ampulla of Vater. Note the preservation of the surrounding duodenal muscularis propria.

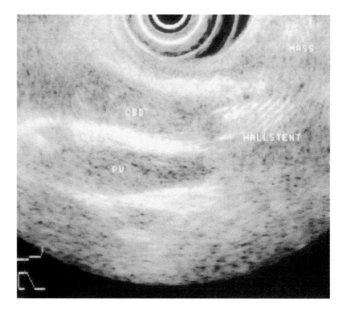

**Figure 4-4.** The common bile duct (containing a deployed metal stent) and the portal vein as they course near a mass in the head of the pancreas.

The large retroperitoneal vessels serve as useful landmarks for orientation. In the third part of the duodenum, the aorta and inferior vena cava (IVC) will be seen in longitudinal section with a radially scanning echoendoscope, and these vessels will be seen in cross-section as the echoscope is withdrawn into the second part of the duodenum. In the third part of the duodenum, the inferior portion of the pancreatic head (uncinate process) and left renal vessels may be seen. The

aorta serves as a good reference point to reorient oneself should there be any confusion.

In the descending portion of the duodenum, the right kidney can be identified. The kidneys are easy to recognize due to their doughnut-shaped appearance. Tumors of the papilla will naturally be identified from this level as well (Figure 4-3). Another important landmark at this level is the superior mesenteric vein, which rises from roughly the five-o'clock position. It

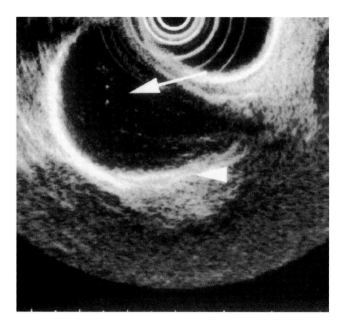

**Figure 4-5.** Typical appearance of the gallbladder wall. The arrowhead demonstrates the three-layer wall pattern. The arrow points out microlithiasis in a "starry-sky" pattern.

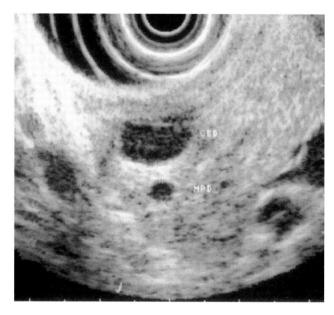

**Figure 4-7.** Typical endosonographic appearance of the head of the pancreas. The common bile duct and pancreatic ducts are shown. They measure 6 mm and 3 mm respectively.

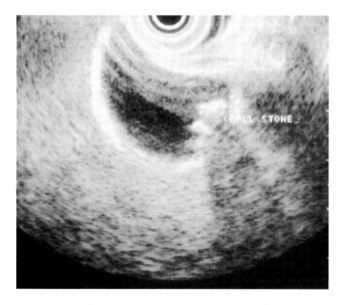

**Figure 4-6.** Endosonographic appearance of gallstones demonstrating the echogenicity of the stones coupled with the image attenuation on the distal side of the stone.

can frequently be traced as it joins with the splenic vein to form the portal vein posterior to the pancreatic head (Figure 4-4). This is an important location for staging pancreatic head carcinomas. The superior mesenteric artery (SMA) is also seen at this level. Because the SMA may be difficult to trace, care must be taken to avoid confusing it with a pancreatic mass. The portal vein can be followed as the echoendoscope is withdrawn into the duodenal bulb.

From the duodenal bulb, the hepatic artery, splenic and portal veins, common bile duct (CBD), and gall-

bladder are identifiable. The gallbladder is seen as an elliptical hypoechoic structure with a three-layer wall pattern (Figure 4-5). Identification of stones (bright hyperechoic mobile structures with acoustic shadowing) can be achieved from the duodenal bulb or the distal gastric antrum (Figure 4-6). The CBD runs parallel to the portal vein into the liver. From this location the distal CBD may be measured to determine if it is dilated. The normal duct measures 4 mm, but this may increase up to 10 mm in the normal CBD after cholecystectomy or with advancing age. The pancreatic head may be seen in multiple orientations as the echoendoscope is withdrawn from the third part of the duodenum into the gastric antrum. The normal pancreatic parenchyma has a homogeneous, fine "salt and pepper" appearance. The splenic vein and portal confluence are helpful in locating the pancreas. The pancreatic duct will usually be identified, and normally measures 3 mm in the head, tapering to 1 mm in the tail (Figure 4-7). Major side branches will often be seen in the normal pancreas as well. Criteria have been published to aid in differentiating normal pancreatic parenchyma from chronic pancreatitis (6). In many patients the dorsal pancreas is slightly more echogenic than the ventral pancreas. The ventral pancreas will often appear as a triangular-shaped mildly hypoechoic area, and care must be taken to avoid confusing it with a neoplasm (7) (Figure 4-8).

From the gastric antrum, the portal confluence, superior mesenteric artery, gallbladder, and head and neck of the pancreas may be identified. The antrum and duodenal bulb are also good locations for evaluating the left lobe of the liver for unsuspected metastatic

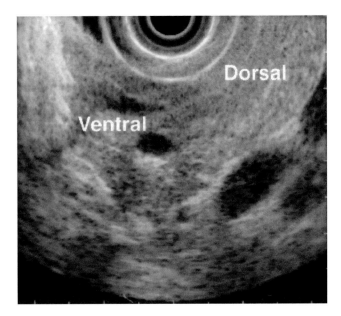

**Figure 4-8.** The ventral/dorsal split. The ventral portion of the pancreatic head is relatively hypoechoic, contains the pancreatic duct, and may appear similar to a mass. The dorsal pancreas is relatively hyperechoic in comparison.

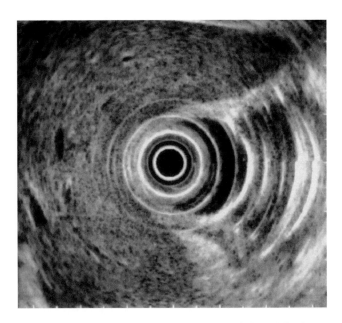

**Figure 4-9.** Trans-antral view of the left lobe of the liver demonstrating the wide views that may be obtained. The liver should routinely be scanned during staging of malignancies, as unsuspected metastatic disease may be detected.

disease and other abnormalities (Figure 4-9). However, with EUS, complete evaluation of liver parenchyma is not possible.

From the gastric body, the pancreatic body, splenic vein, splenic artery, celiac axis, and hepatic artery will be identified. Due to the tortuous nature of the splenic artery, the vessel will be seen to come in and out of the

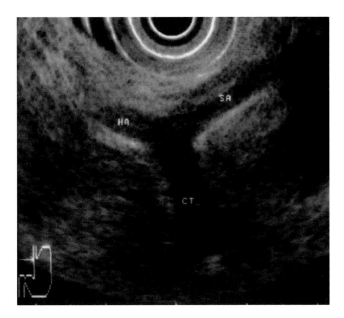

**Figure 4-10.** The typical appearance of the celiac axis as it arises from the aorta. The celiac take-off is typically identified upon withdrawal of the instrument from the stomach toward the gastro-esophageal junction. The splenic artery is on the right and the hepatic artery is on the left in this view.

image as the echoendoscope is passed slowly back and forth in this location. The celiac axis is an important landmark for locating malignant adenopathy. As the echoscope is withdrawn from the antrum, the abdominal aorta will be seen in cross-section, and by slowly moving the scope up towards the gastroesophageal junction, the take-off of the celiac trunk will usually be located (Figure 4-10). The hepatic and splenic arteries are often identified branching off to the right and left in a "whale's tail" configuration (the left gastric artery is more difficult to locate).

From the gastric antrum and body, the aorta, left kidney, body and tail of the pancreas, splenic artery, and splenic hilum can be identified. It is useful to follow the pancreas laterally into the splenic hilum to confirm that a complete EUS study of the pancreas has been performed. The splenic parenchyma has a homogeneous echo pattern similar to that of the liver except for the notable absence of bile ducts.

As the echoscope is withdrawn into the distal esophagus, the left lobe of the liver, left ventricle of the heart, spine, inferior vena cava, and aorta can be located. The aorta is posterior and the IVC passes through the parenchyma of the liver on the right. In a slightly more proximal position the left atrium is seen anteriorly, the left aorta has moved toward the left, and the spine and azygous vein are seen in the posterior. The spine is a useful landmark because it consistently appears as a hyperechoic structure located posteriorly throughout the chest.

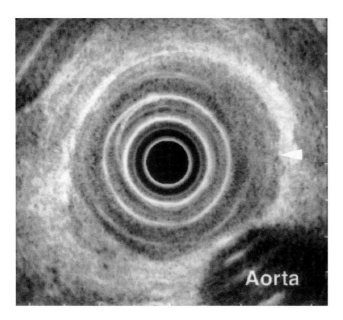

**Figure 4-11.** Staging examination of an esophageal carcinoma demonstrating a tight stenosis. Note that the balloon is not inflated and that water filling is not used. The arrowhead at the three-o'clock position demonstrates invasion into the peri-esophageal fat, making this a T3 lesion.

In the midesophagus, the right and left bronchi are easily identified by the echogenic air located within them. As the echoendoscope is withdrawn, the two main bronchi can be followed as they join together to form the trachea. Also noted in the midesophagus is the azygous vein, which is found adjacent and to the left of the aorta. In some patients, especially those with portal hypertension, the thoracic duct will also be identified adjacent to the aorta. In addition, it is not uncommon to identify triangular, homogeneous, isoechoic benign lymph nodes adjacent to the mid- and proximal esophagus. These nodes are particularly common in patients with a history of cigarette smoking as well as in inner-city dwellers, and typically are less than 10 mm in greatest diameter (8). In the proximal esophagus, the aortic arch can be identified. In the cervical esophagus, above the level of the aortic arch, the carotid and left subclavian arteries may be identified, although the ability to image well in this area is often compromised by patient intolerance of balloon insufflation near the upper esophageal sphincter.

## Esophagus, Stomach, Duodenum, and Rectum

The esophagus and rectum are usually easy to image and are prime locations for the novice to practice technique and gain experience. However, because of the narrow lumen and proximity of the transducer to the wall, a suboptimal focal length may result and yield only a three-

layer wall pattern. It is important to avoid overinflation of the balloon, as this may compress and distort the normal anatomy. The normal mucosal thickness in these organs is 2 to 3 mm. The water-filling techniques described previously are useful to obtain optimal images.

When staging esophageal tumors, the lumen may be stenotic and not permit passage of the echoendoscope (Figure 4-11). Under these circumstances the accuracy of staging declines because the region of interest cannot be examined and more distal abnormalities cannot be assessed (9). Options to increase the accuracy of staging when stenosis is present include the use of small endosonographic probes, if available, or dilation of the malignant stricture. Earlier studies yielded conflicting results regarding the safety of esophageal dilation for endoscopic ultrasound. In a retrospective survey of 42,105 EUS exams (all types), Rösch et al. reported 10 perforations occurring after combined stricture dilation and EUS. However, the perforation rate in patients with stenosing esophageal carcinoma strictures was not specifically noted. Van Dam et al. reported a 24% perforation rate (5/21) after dilation and EUS using the Olympus GF-UM2 or GF-UM3 echoendoscopes in esophageal cancer. Based in part on these studies, the Working Party for the Tenth World Congress of Gastroenterology has stated that "dilation of stenotic tumors to allow passage of the echoendoscope is not generally recommended because of a considerably increased risk of perforation" (10). The American Society for Gastrointestinal Endoscopy issued a Technology Assessment Status Evaluation that included this statement regarding EUS: "the risk of perforation may be reduced by avoiding dilation of malignant stricture" (11). However, recent prospective series from our institution and elsewhere have suggested that malignant strictures may be safely dilated to allow echoendoscope passage (12,13). We feel that dilation of malignant strictures for performance of EUS is not absolutely contraindicated and that the information obtained can be useful in clinical management.

The gastric wall, including intramural and submucosal lesions, is best visualized with water filling the stomach. A five-layer wall pattern will usually be seen. The normal thickness is 3 to 4 mm. The antrum may be thicker than the body or fundus (Figure 4-12). In some patients, the muscularis propria will have a thin hyperechoic line running through it, corresponding to the separation of muscular layers. The duodenum also has a five-layer wall pattern. The ampulla of Vater and major papilla are identified on the medial aspect of the second part of the duodenum. With patience, the common bile duct and main pancreatic duct can be traced into the papilla. Staging of tumors of the papilla can be difficult; the papilla should first be identified endoscopically, and water filling of the duodenum may facilitate obtaining high-quality images (14).

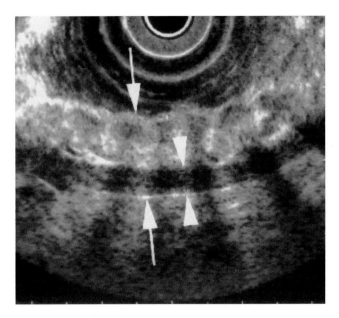

**Figure 4-12** Typical appearance of a gastric linitis plastica. The arrows demonstrate the thickening of the entire gastric wall, which measures 11 mm in total. The muscularis propria is delineated by the arrowheads and measures 3 mm by itself. This pattern is nearly pathognomonic for malignancy and should be thoroughly investigated if found.

EUS examination of the rectum is usually performed for staging of rectal carcinoma. Other indications include evaluation of the anal sphincters and for identification of perirectal abscesses, particularly in patients with Crohn's disease. Prior to the exam the bowel should be prepped in a fashion similar to the prep for a flexible sigmoidoscopy—typically with enemas. As in the stomach, the colonic wall has five layers. The fluid-filled bladder is easily identified anteriorly. In male patients, as the echoscope is withdrawn, the seminal vesicles will be identified just superior and lateral to the prostate. The normal prostate appears as a homogeneous isoechoic structure. The spongy urethra will frequently be seen within the prostate parenchyma. In women, the vagina will be identified. As the echoscope is withdrawn further, the internal and external anal sphincters will be seen in detail. The internal sphincter is a hypoechoic layer that extends into the anal verge. The external sphincter is slightly more heterogeneous in echotexture and extends to the pelvic floor. Rectal EUS is discussed in more detail in chapter 12.

## Endoscopic Ultrasound-Guided Aspiration

Prior to the development of real-time EUS-guided FNA, EUS-assisted FNA was performed as a two-step procedure (15). First, a lesion was identified via EUS.

After careful characterization of the size and location of the lesion, the echoendoscope was withdrawn and FNA or core biopsies were obtained through a conventional endoscope. This method was cumbersome and of limited value because it could only be applied to lesions that were visible on conventional endoscopy. For these reasons, this technique has been largely replaced by real-time EUS-guided FNA.

EUS-guided FNA may be performed with either a radial scanning or curved linear array echoendoscope (16–18). There are two reported series on FNA biopsies using the radial scanning Olympus GF-UM20 instrument (19,20). The advantage of using a radial scanning echoendoscope is that, as it is the preferred choice for cancer staging in most centers, it is the more widely-available echoendoscope system. The biopsy can be obtained without exchanging the echoscope, saving time and potentially reducing cost, as well. However, because the image produced is oriented perpendicular to the axis of the echoscope, during FNA the needle tip will pass into and then out of the ultrasound field and will not be visible during the actual aspiration of the lesion. Despite this limitation, FNA using the radial scanning echoscope has been performed using a 4 cm-long Wilson-Cook biopsy needle (Wilson-Cook Medical, Winston-Salem, North Carolina). In a study that compared the radial scanning and curved linear array echoendoscopes, no difference was noted in accuracy when an adequate aspirate was obtained. However, it was not clear from the study which of the two echoendoscope systems was more likely to be successful in obtaining sufficient tissue for diagnosis.

In contrast to the radial scanning instrument, the curved linear array echoendoscopes (from Pentax/Hitachi, Orangeburg, NY and Olympia, Melville, NY) provide images parallel to the long axis of the echoscope. This is advantageous because it allows for continuous visualization of the needle tip as it passes into the target of interest (Figure 4-13). This echoendoscope also has Doppler ultrasound capability, which may be beneficial in helping to identify vessels. For these reasons, it has become the instrument of choice for EUS-guided FNA. Recently, both mechanical and electronic echoendoscopes with dedicated biopsy capability have been developed (Olympus Corporation, Melville, NY). We have utilized the latest electronic curved array release of this instrument (GF-UCLA30P) and have not only found its image resolution to be superior to earlier versions but also that the needle is easily visualized along its entire path.

For cancer staging, the radial scanning echoendoscope remains the better choice. Therefore, many endosonographers first perform staging with a radial scanning echoendoscope, and then switch to a dedicated biopsy echoendoscope if FNA is to be per-

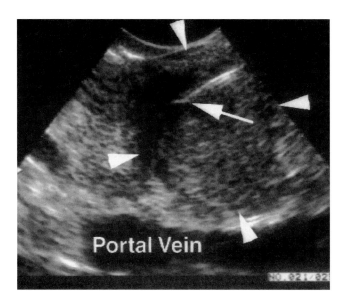

**Figure 4-13.** Typical appearance of a pancreatic head mass during biopsy with the Pentax system. The arrowheads define the limits of the pancreatic mass. The arrow demonstrates the tip of the GIP needle well within the mass. Note that both walls of the needle may be visualized.

formed. The 160 cm-long 22-gauge GIP needle (GIP Medizin Technik GMBH, Grassau, Germany) is most often used. Wilson-Cook, Inc. has recently released a disposable device and Olympus has a dedicated needle that accompanies their biopsy echoendoscope. The needles can penetrate up to 6 cm, and have sufficient tensile strength to puncture most lesions. Limitations of the needles include cost, kinking, and dulling of the tip, which may require it to be discarded after three or four passes. A prototype mechanical echoendoscope (GFUM-30P Olympus America Corp., Melville, NY) uses a rotatable mirror at the tip of the transducer to create a linear scanning image to facilitate aspiration biopsy. Although experience with this unit is limited, a recent report suggested that it is effective for biopsy of adenopathy, but less so for biopsy of pancreatic masses.

Using electronic array scanning echoendoscopes, FNA is performed by first maneuvering the target into the center of the imaging field. The tip of the echoscope should be pressed firmly against the mucosa to prevent the advancing needle from significantly altering the echoscope position. Inflation of the echoendoscope balloon may help lodge the tip of the scope in position (21). This technique is particularly helpful when sampling paraesophageal nodes from within the esophagus and when aspirating the pancreas from within the duodenum. Doppler ultrasound may be helpful to ensure that there are no blood vessels coursing through the anticipated path of the needle. The needle and its sheath are advanced through the biopsy

channel of the echoscope into the gastrointestinal lumen. Small adjustments with the elevator and sheath placement will allow precise localization of the needle. The needle stylet is then retracted 1 to 2 cm to allow the needle to puncture through the wall without sliding, and advanced into the target under direct ultrasound guidance. As the needle is advanced, small readjustments of the echoendoscope position may be necessary to ensure that the needle follows the desired path. Once within the targeted lesion, the stylet is advanced to the tip of the needle to remove from the needle tip any unwanted cells that may have been captured while the needle traversed through the gut wall. The stylet is then removed. The tip of the needle is easy to identify as a bright echo that moves across the image as the needle is advanced. A syringe is then applied to the hub of the needle. In cases where the precise location of the tip of the needle is momentarily unclear, a small whiff of air (0.5 ml or less) can be injected. This generates a bright echo that should be easily identifiable. Suction is then applied as the needle is advanced back and forth in 3 to 5 mm to-and-fro movements with careful maneuvering of the echoendoscope to slightly alter the needle track with each needle advancement. Great care must be taken to avoid pushing through the lesion into adjacent structures. The suction is then gently released and the needle is withdrawn.

Finally, the contents of the needle are expressed onto slides for cytologic preparation. The stylet is used to ensure complete and controlled clearance of the needle sheath. In general, the yield of the procedure is improved when a cytologist can immediately evaluate the adequacy of the specimen at the time of the procedure. We repeat needle passes for cytology until an adequate specimen is obtained for analysis. In most cases, six passes are sufficient. EUS-guided FNA biopsy is discussed in more detail in chapter 13.

## Pulsed or Color Doppler

Doppler technology uses the concept that movements between a reflector and a sound source result in changes in wavelength, and thus sound frequency. By detecting changes in frequency, velocity of flow can be determined. The currently-available electronic array endoscopic ultrasound units are equipped with Doppler capability, and can be used to detect blood flow. This is particularly useful when planning the trajectory of an EUS-guided FNA needle. In some patients, a low-lying splenic artery or superior mesenteric artery may be confused with a mass, and Doppler examination of the area is quite helpful in these settings.

## Artifacts

Errors that occur in the interpretation of endoscopic ultrasound images include the misidentification of normal structures, often due to incomplete appreciation of the principles of ultrasound. Standard extracorporeal ultrasound texts should be studied prior to commencing performance of the procedures. Obtaining a proper, perpendicular orientation to the target of interest is of vital importance. Failure to do so will lead to an oblique, tangential image with an accompanying distortion of size and/or depth of penetration of the lesion under study. For malignant neoplasms, these errors will artificially "upstage" the tumor.

When imaging the pancreas, care must be taken to avoid mistaking bowel loops for a pancreatic mass. Loops of bowel are mobile and have a wall-layer pattern; even so, without careful study, the endosonographer can be easily confused. Also, the reverberation of sound waves within bowel loops may produce a mirror-image artifact. Occasionally, an overinflated transducer balloon may cause an intussusception of bowel as the echoscope is withdrawn. This can be identified as a double wall-layer pattern, but the unsuspecting endosonographer may confuse this for a hypoechoic mass. Similarly, differences in echodensity between the ventral and dorsal pancreas, felt to be due to uneven lipomatosis, can be confused for a hypoechoic mass lesion, as described above. It should also be noted that pancreatic parenchyma normally becomes more echogenic with advancing age. However, there is a lack of the other EUS criteria (such as ductal changes) associated with chronic pancreatitis in older patients.

Reverberation artifacts occur when there is repeated reflection of the ultrasound beam by two highly reflective surfaces. This anomaly produces false echoes that appear as equally-spaced parallel reflectors. Although this artifact has been observed within a simple cyst, it most often occurs with an air interface. When this phenomenon occurs distal to a very strongly reflective surface, such as a metallic clip, it is referred to as a *ring-down* or *comet-tail artifact*.

Other artifacts in ultrasound occur due to refraction. Refraction develops when the sound beam interacts at an oblique angle with an interface. If there are significant differences in sound conductivity on either side of the surface, a shadow is produced as the beam converges or diverges and the shadow may obscure deeper structures. When ultrasound passes through dense tissue, such as fat, loss of penetration into deeper structures due to attenuation of the sound waves may simulate an underlying mass. Through transmission, artifact occurs when fluid overlies part of a solid structure. Because sound travels more quickly through fluid, the tissue on the distal side of the fluid will appear more echogenic than the same tissue without overlying fluid (which will be more attenuated).

Even in experienced hands, the correct diagnosis of adenopathy as malignant or benign by EUS examination is difficult. As mentioned previously, benign mediastinal adenopathy is not uncommon in the general population. Benign inflammatory nodes that simulate the appearance of malignant adenopathy are particularly problematic. In contrast, small nodes with microscopic metastases may appear completely normal. These observations point to an important concept in interpretation of diagnostic data from EUS in general. Conclusions and clinical decisions based on results must be made within the context of the known sensitivity, specificity, and accuracy of a given test. While EUS-guided FNA has improved the accuracy of nodal staging, one should not assume 100% accuracy, and so the limitations of EUS discussed throughout this text must be borne in mind when making critical clinical decisions.

## Complications

Endoscopic ultrasound has proven to be a safe procedure. The most common complications are cardiopulmonary and are related to the use of conscious sedation. There is now a sufficient body of published literature confirming that the risks associated with EUS are no greater than with regular endoscopy, with some important caveats. Because of oblique-viewing optics, passage of the scope must be done gently and with great care to avoid perforation. As noted, it remains controversial whether malignant esophageal strictures should be dilated to allow scope passage. Rarely, an inflated echoendoscope balloon may dislodge a biliary plastic stent during scope pull-back, but this can usually be easily avoided.

EUS-guided fine-needle aspiration has also proven to be safe. Reported complications have related to biopsy of pancreatic cystic lesions (infection and bleeding) and pancreatitis (in patients with a prior history of pancreatitis). In a multicenter review, the overall complication rate in 457 patient examinations was 1.1%, or 0.5% if complications related to investigations of cystic lesions are excluded (22).

## Conclusion

Performing clinically-relevant endosonographic procedures requires not only a thorough understanding of the anatomic, endoscopic, and radiologic principles alluded to in this chapter, but an awareness of the indications and clinical implications of the procedure as well.

Mastery of these diverse skills can be readily accomplished provided sufficient time is devoted to the task. Available tutorials are helpful but are no substitute for hands-on experience and a patient, experienced mentor in this endeavor. In order to develop and maintain standards of accuracy, it is advisable to continually compare EUS findings to pathology specimens in patients who subsequently undergo surgery. Periodic assessment of the impact of EUS on one's own clinical practice is also important. The continued expansion in EUS indications, tissue sampling capability, and therapeutics, as outlined elsewhere in this text, should ensure that proficiency in endosonography will continue to result in improved patient care.

### References

1. Hoffman B, Hawes R. Endoscopic ultrasound and clinical competence. Gastrointest Endosc Clinics of North Am 1995;5:879–884.
2. Cotton PB, Williams CB. Practical gastrointestinal endoscopy. 3rd ed. Cambridge, MA: Blackwell Scientific, 1990:40.
3. Kadish SL, Ginsberg GG, Kochman ML. Safe maneuvering of echoendoscopes in patients with distorted duodenal anatomy. Gastrointest Endosc 1995;42:278.
4. Yiengrukawan A, Lightdale CJ. Mucolytic-antifoam solution for reduction of artifacts during endoscopic ultrasonography: a randomized controlled trial. Gastrointest Endosc 1991;37:543–546.
5. Yasuda K, Nakajima M, Kawai K. Technical aspects of endoscopic ultrasonography of the biliary system. Scand J Gastro 1986;21(Suppl 123):143–150.
6. Wiersema MJ, Hawes RH, Lehman GA, et al. Prospective evaluation of endoscopic ultrasonography and endoscopic retrograde cholangiopancreatography in patients with suspected abdominal pain of pancreatic origin. Endoscopy 1993;25:555–564.
7. Savides TJ, Gress FG, Zaidi SA, et al. Detection of embryologic ventral pancreatic parenchyma with endoscopic ultrasound. Gastrointest Endosc 1996;43:14–19.
8. Hawes RH, Gress F, Kesler KA, et al. Endoscopic ultrasound versus computed tomography in the evaluation of the mediastinum in patients with non-small cell lung cancer. Endoscopy 1994;9:784–787.
9. Catalano MF, Van Dam J, Sivak MV Jr. Malignant esophageal strictures: staging accuracy of endoscopic ultrasonography. Gastrointest Endosc 1995;41:575–579.
10. Working Party for the Tenth World Congress of Gastroenterology. Am J Gastroenterology. 1994;89:S138–S143.
11. ASGE Technology Assessment Status Evaluation. Gastrointest Endosc 1994;40:796–797.
12. Stotland BR, Ginsberg GG, Faigel DO, et al. Efficacy and safety of esophageal dilation for EUS evaluation of malignant strictures. Gastrointest Endosc 1997;45:A625.
13. Ciaccia D, Ikenberry SO, Gress FG. Staging esophageal carcinoma with endoscopic ultrasound (EUS): a prospective evaluation in patients with high grade malignant strictures requiring dilation. Gastrointest Endosc 1997;45:A585.
14. Cannon ME, Carpenter SL, Elta GH, et al. EUS compared with CT, MRI and angiography and the influence of biliary stenting on staging accuracy of ampullary neoplasms. Submitted to Gastrointest Endosc.
15. Wiersema MS, Wiersema LM, Khusro Q, et al. Combined endosonography and fine-needle aspiration cytology in the evaluation of gastrointestinal lesions. Gastrointest Endosc 1994;40:199–206.
16. Wiersema MJ, Kochman ML, Cramer HM, et al. Endosonography-guided real-time fine-needle aspiration biopsy. Gastrointest Endosc 1994;40:700–707.
17. Vilmann P, Jacobsen GK, Henriksen FW, et al. Endoscopic ultrasonography with guided fine needle aspiration biopsy in pancreatic disease. Gastrointest Endosc 1992;38:172–173.
18. Chang KJ, Karz KD, Durbin TE, et al. Endoscopic ultrasound-guided fine-needle aspiration. Gastrointest Endosc 1994;40:694–699.
19. Ikenberry SO, Gress F, Savides T, Hawes R. Fine-needle aspiration of posterior mediastinal lesions guided by radial scanning endosonography. Gastrointest Endosc 1996;43:605–610.
20. Gress F, Savides T, Cummings O, et al. Radial scanning and linear array endosonography for staging pancreatic cancer: a prospective randomized comparison. Gastrointest Endosc 1997;45:138–142.
21. Faigel DO, Ginsberg GG, Bentz JS, et al. Endoscopic ultrasound-guided real-time fine-needle aspiration biopsy of the pancreas in cancer patients with pancreatic lesions. J Clin Oncology 1997;15:1439–1443.
22. Wiersema MJ, Vilmann P, Giovannini M, et al. Endosonography-guided fine-needle aspiration biopsy: diagnostic accuracy and complication assessment. Gastroenterology 1997;112:1087–1095.

# 5

# Radial Imaging of the Upper Gastrointestinal Tract

**Bonnie J. Pollack**

**Harry Snady**

Endoscopic ultrasonography provides high-contrast resolution of the upper gastrointestinal (UGI) tract. It is unsurpassed by any other imaging technique, including transcutaneous ultrasonography (US), computed tomography (CT), and nuclear magnetic resonance imaging (MRI) (1–6). The mechanical rotating radial scanning EUS instruments have been shown to be particularly useful for imaging the upper gastrointestinal (UGI) tract, including the retroperitoneum (7–17). Although the transducer can be maneuvered only within the confines of the gastrointestinal lumen, the echoendoscope provides excellent imaging of luminal and many paraluminal structures. Frequencies of 7.5 and 12 MHz are used for the echoendoscopes and up to 20 MHz for echoprobes.

Interpretation of EUS images relies heavily on an understanding of the anatomic relationships of the various organs and blood vessels of the UGI tract and retroperitoneum. An understanding of the normal anatomic relationships can be obtained from standard anatomy, CT, US, and angiography texts (18–21). Knowledge of sonographic principles is also important in order to obtain clear, accurate images. Equally important is the ability to maneuver the echoendoscope to and around the target area while limiting artifacts (22,23). Many UGI tract and retroperitoneal structures are in close proximity and overlap, which can make interpretation complex. By placing the echoendoscope in certain standard locations, landmark structures can be identified. Then, by maneuvering the transducer, the target area can be accurately evaluated.

This chapter is devoted to radial endosonographic imaging of the normal anatomy of the UGI tract. Mediastinal, esophageal, gastric, paragastric, and retroperitoneal organs will be reviewed, as well as the techniques used to find various EUS landmarks (Table 5-1). The UGI tract structures are organized into three groups: 1) esophageal and mediastinal structures, 2) gastric and paragastric structures, 3) the duodenal sweep and retroperitoneal structures.

Unless otherwise specified, "right" will refer to the patient's right and "left" will refer to the patient's left. This can be confusing, as the patient's right is often on the left-hand side of the screen while the patient's left is often on the right side of the image.

## General Technique

Standard endoscopy is usually performed prior to endosonography to assess the contour of the lumen and detect any abnormality. Intubation of the echoendoscope is performed in a manner similar to the passage of a duodenoscope. A very thin film of lubricant can be placed on the tip of the echoendoscope with care taken not to obscure the optics or to contaminate the balloon. Alternatively, the tip of the scope can be dipped into water just prior to intubation. The scope is held in a relatively neutral position while it is inserted into the mouth. As it is gently advanced into the posterior pharynx, the tip is deflected downward. Care should be taken not to over-deflect the scope—let the natural scope curvature serve as a guide. Often a very slight 1-mm torque of the scope, as translated from the right hand, which rests on the shaft of the scope, is required for passage as the patient swallows.

At all times, the operator should hold the echoendoscope in a comfortable position. This is best achieved with the motor unit held by the left hand and the shaft of the scope held in the right hand. The cradle of the fairly weighty control head and motor unit rests on the thenar aspect of the palm between the thumb and the remaining digits. This frees up the index and middle fingers to operate the suction and water con-

**Table 5-1.** Major structures, vessels, and organs visualized with EUS from different station/locations within the upper gastrointestinal tract.

| | |
|---|---|
| Horizontal Duodenum | Left renal vessels<br>Descending aorta<br>Inferior vena cava |
| Descending Duodenum | Inferior vena cava<br>Right kidney and renal vessels<br>Uncinate process<br>Superior mesenteric vein and artery<br>Ampulla of Vater<br>Right adrenal gland<br>Pancreatic head<br>Common bile duct<br>Portal confluence |
| Duodenal Bulb | Pancreatic head*<br>Bile duct*<br>Portal vein*<br>Hepatic artery*<br>Splenic vein*<br>Gallbladder |
| Antrum | Inferior vena cava<br>Portal confluence*<br>Superior mesenteric artery<br>Head and neck of pancreas*<br>Gallbladder |
| Gastric Body and Fundus | Celiac and hepatic arteries*<br>Descending aorta<br>Splenic vein and artery<br>Spleen<br>Liver, hepatic veins, IVC<br>Body and tail of the pancreas<br>Left kidney and renal vessels<br>Left adrenal gland |
| Distal Esophagus | Liver, hepatic veins, IVC<br>Descending aorta<br>Spine<br>Left atrium and other cardiac chambers<br>Pulmonary vasculature<br>Ascending aorta<br>Right and left lung |
| Midesophagus | Thoracic duct<br>Descending aorta<br>Spine<br>Azygos vein<br>Aortic arch<br>Right and left bronchi<br>SVC<br>Carina<br>Ascending aorta<br>Trachea |
| Proximal Esophagus | Trachea<br>Spine<br>Great vessels of the neck<br>Thyroid and thymus |

Vessels and organs seen from each location are listed in order of appearance as the echoendoscope is withdrawn proximally from the horizontal duodenum.
*Structures usually seen well from the "withdrawn-wedged" position.

trols. This also gives the thumb the mobility to turn the up/down deflection control knob to and fro to bring the transducer closer to or further away from the gastrointestinal tract wall.

The balloon surrounding the ultrasound transducer housing is inflated with 5 to 15 mL of water. Intraluminal air is evacuated to maximize the contact between the intestinal wall surface and the 360 degrees of the transducer. Throughout much of the exam, the suction port is depressed to maintain optimal imaging by minimizing intraluminal air. As the scope is withdrawn, various organs and vessels are brought into the field of view. Small movements of the scope are used to obtain the optimal angle and focus of each specific target area. Patience and persistence is often what makes the difference between average and superior imaging.

Radial instruments utilize a mechanically rotating transducer that produces a 360-degree circular image in a plane perpendicular to the axis of the tip of the echoendoscope. EUS is not, however, restricted to uniplanar imaging as the EUS scanning plane can be turned in almost any direction. At certain locations in the stomach and duodenal bulb, the transducer can be rotated or even inverted to point cephalad. Initially, EUS imaging can be quite disorienting. The easiest images to comprehend are obtained when the scope points caudally along the long axis of the body, such as in the esophagus and upper portions of the body of the stomach. Images obtained will be in horizontal or transverse planes, and comparable to conventional CT transverse sections. *In these more familiar images, the echoendoscope is torqued so that the patient's left is on the right of the EUS image, and the patient's right is on the left of the screen. The lower part of the EUS image is the patient's posterior and the upper part of the image is anterior.* As the transducer passes initially into the antrum and then into the duodenal sweep, the image will rotate clockwise. Using tip deflection and other scope manipulations, the EUS scanning plane can be oriented into sagittal (longitudinal) and even coronal planes. Knowledge of standard CT images and US helps in understanding the relationships of various structures in different horizontal or sagittal sections. However, it is unusual to obtain the best views with EUS when the transducer is exactly in a horizontal or longitudinal plane. This is especially true while scanning the retroperitoneum. When performing EUS, the transducer is commonly placed in the same locations with different orientations to scan various structures.

## Gastrointestinal Tract Wall

The unique advantage of EUS is its ability to interrogate histologic layers of the GI tract wall. The relationship between the ultrasonographic layers and histologic structures has been confirmed in studies that correlate EUS layers with corresponding histologic sections (5,24–26). The wall is displayed as five ultrasonographic layers. By convention, these are numbered from innermost (luminal) to outermost (serosal) layers. The first or innermost layer, which appears bright (echogenic, hyperechoic), is due to the interface echo of the mucosa and surrounding fluid. This corresponds to the superficial mucosa. The second (dark, hypoechoic) layer corresponds to the remaining mucosa, or the deep mucosa. The third (hyperechoic) layer corresponds to the submucosa and the acoustic interface between the submucosa and the muscularis propria. The fourth (hypoechoic) layer represents the muscularis propria minus the acoustic interface. Occasionally, the fourth layer is split by a fine hyperechoic layer that corresponds to a fibrous band that separates the inner circular and outer longitudinal muscles. The fifth layer (hyperechoic) is interpreted as the serosa in the stomach and small bowel or adventitial tissue in the esophagus and portions of the stomach where the serosa is absent (Figure 5-1).

## Mediastinal and Esophageal Anatomy

The esophagus is the easiest of the organs in the UGI tract to scan, as very little manipulation of the transducer is required to maintain proper orientation. However, a thorough understanding of mediastinal anatomy relative to the esophagus is essential to perform a complete examination. Scanning should begin distally at the GE junction while withdrawing the scope proximally so as to limit scanning artifacts. As the endosonographer withdraws the echoendoscope, the aorta should be maintained in the five-o'clock position, which generally allows proper orientation of the paraesophageal structures. If the main interest is the esophageal wall, care must be taken not to inflate the balloon excessively because this will flatten the wall. Overinflation of the balloon can cause artifacts and must be avoided if the wall itself is the area of interest. Overinflation of the balloon is not as critical if imaging of paraluminal structures is the main point of the study. In fact, it can often serve to anchor the transducer, making scanning easier for certain locations.

The normal thickness of the esophageal wall is only approximately 3 mm. Often this is difficult to visualize and the esophageal wall may appear as a three-layer structure rather than a five-layer structure. This can be avoided with the 20 MHz echoprobes, which provide the greatest resolution (a nine-layer structure can be seen) but they do not penetrate more than 1 cm, thus limiting their utility for lesions larger than 1 cm. On the other hand, if the area of interest is the paraesophageal structures, then more liberal use of water instillation in the balloon may be required.

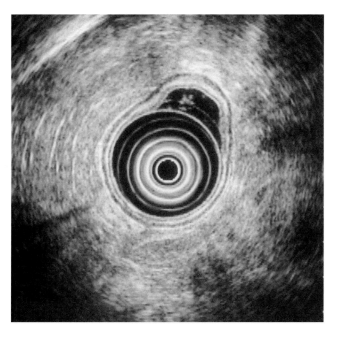

**Figure 5-1.** EUS image from the antrum showing a normal five-layer wall. The liver is in the upper portion of the image.

### Distal Esophagus from the Cardia to the Subcarina

In the distal esophagus, the major landmark for orientation is the descending aorta, which is placed at five to six o'clock in the ultrasound field. This structure can easily be recognized as the circular anechoic structure, approximately 1.5 to 2 cm in diameter, with a relatively bright border due to back wall enhancement (a normal artifact seen in vessels). Occasionally atherosclerotic plaques can be seen along the wall and appear as hyperechoic solid stranding. The spine is also easily identified in the seven-o'clock position next to the aorta. It has irregular echo features with artifacts produced by the poor penetration of echoes through bony structures. The left lobe of the liver appears at the six- to twelve-o'clock position. Often the hepatic veins and inferior vena cava can be appreciated as they course through the liver. The stomach is often seen from the one- to four-o'clock positions with the rugae usually well defined within the fundus (Figures 5-2.A, 5-2.B).

As the scope is withdrawn, the beating of the heart is appreciated as the left atrium comes into view at the twelve-o'clock position. In certain patients, the mitral valve leaflets can be distinctly seen as the valve opens from the left atrium into the left ventricle. The pulmonary veins can also be seen entering the left atrium. The left pulmonary artery arches posteriorly to the left of the ascending aorta and tends to be easier to view than the right pulmonary artery, which can be seen just below the carina. Because the left ventricle, right atrium, and right ventricle lie deep to the left atrium, it can be more difficult to visualize these structures com-

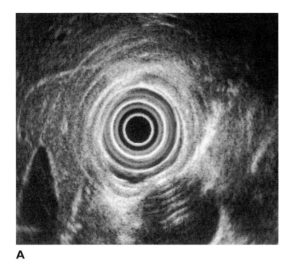

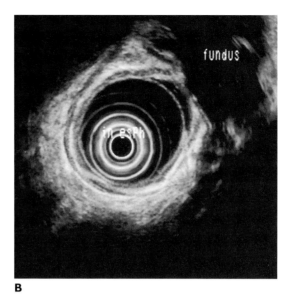

**Figure 5-2.** (A) EUS image from the gastroesophageal junction. The liver is visualized from the seven-o'clock position to the twelve-o'clock position. The IVC is seen at the lower left coursing through the liver. The aorta is seen at the five-o'clock position. The fundus is faintly seen at the two-o'clock position. (B) Angling the transducer brings the fundus into clearer view.

pletely. The aortic outflow tract can be appreciated as the scope is withdrawn further. It can, however, be difficult to trace the complete path of the ascending aorta. This structure runs deep to the hilar structures (pulmonary vessels) and, due to air within the bronchi and trachea, the ascending aorta is often not fully imaged. Small pericardial effusions may be seen adjacent to the cardiac chambers. The right lung appears as hyperechoic rings emanating from the nine-o'clock position while the left lung appears at the two-o'clock position. The spine will continue to be seen at the six- to seven-o'clock positions if the descending aorta is maintained at the five-o'clock position (Figures 5-3.A, 5-3.B, 5-3.C).

### *Midesophagus from the Carina to the Aortic Arch*

As the scope is withdrawn further, the azygos vein can be seen coming into position to the right of the aorta. The azygos vein will move anterior to the spine and then toward the right lung. Occasionally lymph nodes can be seen at this level; these tend to be hyperechoic, with ill-defined borders and an oblong, rectangular, or triangular shape. On further withdrawal of the scope, the left and right main stem bronchi come into view. These structures can easily be demarcated as the hyperechoic rings seen at eleven and one o'clock. As one further withdraws the scope, the left and right bronchi come together to form the trachea—this normally occurs at 27 to 28 cm from the incisors. On the right, the azygos can be seen to move forward and extend anteriorly into the superior vena cava. On the left, the arch of the aorta can be seen arising from the descending aorta. As the aortic arch moves anteriorly across the screen, it

curves right. Careful inspection of this area may reveal the thoracic duct adjacent to the aorta and spine (Figures 5-4.A, 5-4.B, 5-4.C, 5.4.D).

### *Proximal Esophagus from the Aortic Arch and Its Branches*

Above the level of the aortic arch lies the base of the great vessels of the neck. The left subclavian artery lies more posterior in the image and the base of the left common carotid artery and brachiocephalic trunk can be found anteriorly. The left subclavian artery tends to be the easiest to view. The venous system is more lateral and can appear slightly larger as compared to the arterial system. The thyroid gland is visible at the center of the image from the eleven-o'clock to the one-o'clock position. The thymus lies distal to the thyroid at the level of the clavicle and can be challenging to view.

The cervical spine remains at the posterior aspect of the image. The trachea will remain in the twelve-o'clock position and lies adjacent to and slightly to the right of the esophagus. On the screen, the trachea will appear slightly to the left of the transducer within the esophagus. There is little or no intervening fat plane between the esophagus and the trachea. The air-filled trachea severely limits or totally prevents sound wave penetration, and therefore essentially blocks visualization of more anterior structures. As one approaches the upper esophageal sphincter (UES), which is typically located at 17 to 18 cm, the patient will become more intolerant of the exam. Images just below the UES are somewhat difficult to obtain due to air within the trachea and within the apices of the lung (Figures 5-5.A, 5-5.B, 5-5.C). When the scope can be held in

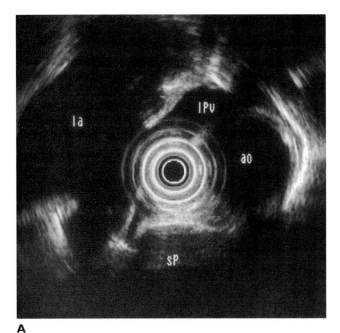

**A**

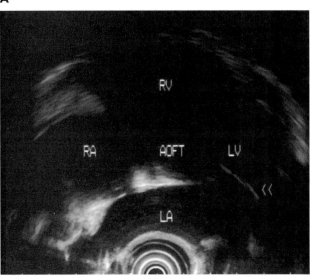

**B**

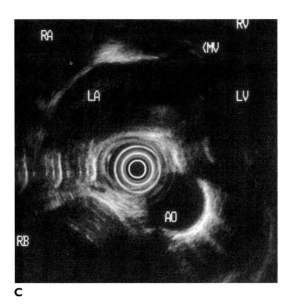

**C**

**Figure 5-3.** (A) EUS image higher up in the distal esophagus. The left atrium (*la*) occupies the majority of the image with the left pulmonary vein (*lPV*) entering the atria. The aorta (*ao*) is shifted slightly anterior in this particular image. The spine (*sP*) remains at six o'clock. (B) The right atrium (*RA*) is seen adjacent to the left atrium (*LA*) with the right ventricle (*RV*) and left ventricle (*LV*) lying posterior. The base of the aortic outflow tract (*AOFT*) can be seen, as well as the leaflets of the mitral valve (*double arrowhead*). (C) Full view of similar structures to Figure 5-3B. The right bronchi (*RB*) and lung are seen at the nine- to seven-o'clock position and the aorta is seen at the four-o'clock position with the cardiac chambers seen at the top of the image.

this position, the proximal aspect of the common carotid arteries and internal jugular veins can be imaged. When the patient lies on his or her left side, the left system is easier to visualize than the right system.

## Gastric and Paragastric Structures

The gastric wall is generally quite easy to image. Using the water-filled balloon technique and the instillation of water (100 to 600 ml) within the lumen, excellent images of the wall layers can be obtained. The optimal focal point is 1.5 to 2.5 cm with the 7.5 MHz transducer. Radial scanning of the stomach and paragastric organs should begin distally in the antrum and proceed proximally, similar to the scanning technique for the esophagus. The target area should always be imaged

by withdrawal of the scope, using tip deflection and torque to focus the image. Ideally, the probe is placed perpendicular to the lesion or area of interest to obtain the proper focal point. Occasionally, it is necessary to change the position of the patient to obtain optimal images (27).

As previously described, the gastric wall is displayed as five ultrasonographic layers with an aggregate thickness of 3 to 4 mm, with slightly greater thickness in the antrum (28). The width of the first two layers is approximately 1.2 mm. The third layer is approximately 1.4 mm in width, and the fourth layer is approximately 0.8 mm in width.

Because the stomach is large and easy to distend, the endosonographer may become disoriented. The descending aorta serves as an easy landmark in the proximal half of the stomach. The portal vein, splenic vein, left kidney, and liver serve as the easiest landmarks to locate in the mid-to-distal portions of the stomach.

### Antrum

In the antrum (Figure 5-1), the anterior wall of the stomach is generally seen on the left side of the EUS image and the posterior wall on the right side of the screen. The scanning plane is perpendicular to the greater curvature. The gallbladder can be visualized from the

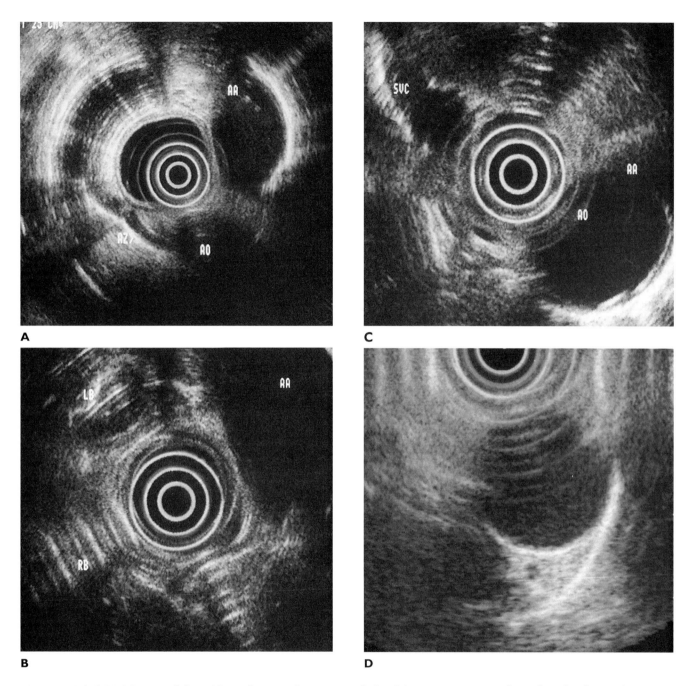

**Figure 5-4.** (A) EUS image of the midesophagus. The aortic arch (*AA*) is crossing over to the right. The descending aorta (*AO*) remains at five o'clock. The right lung is at the left of the image. The azygos vein is seen at the lower left of the image next to the spine. (B) The EUS image from the level of the carina. The aortic arch (*AA*) is located from one o'clock to three o'clock. The spine is at five o'clock. The air-filled right bronchus and left bronchus are seen as concentric bright rings. (C) The superior vena cava (*SVC*), where it joins the azygos vein, is seen at the upper left of the image with the top of aorta (*AO*) and aortic arch (*AA*) at the lower right. (D) Adjacent to and beneath the aorta, the thoracic duct is visualized as a very small, well-circumscribed hypoechoic area.

antrum (Figure 5-6.A) and in the first to second portions of the duodenum (Figure 5-6.B). The wall is usually 1 to 2 mm thick, and three distinct echo layers can be seen. It is relatively easy in most cases to discern stones that appear as hyperechoic structures with posterior shadowing (Figure 5-7). A maneuver often used to image para-antral structures is anchorage of the scope tip in the antrum. This is accomplished by ex-

panding the balloon with more water to keep the transducer in place. Then by pushing the scope further in, a loop forms in the scope, pivoting the transducer and causing an angle change in the scanning plane. From the antrum and/or body, the liver, porta hepatis, gastrohepatic ligament, hepatic artery, pancreas, and confluence of the superior mesenteric vein and splenic vein can be seen.

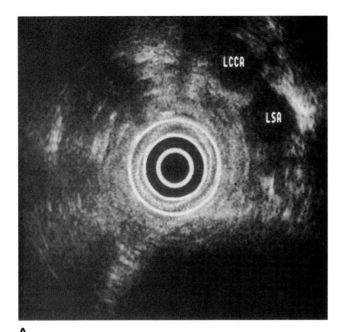

**A**

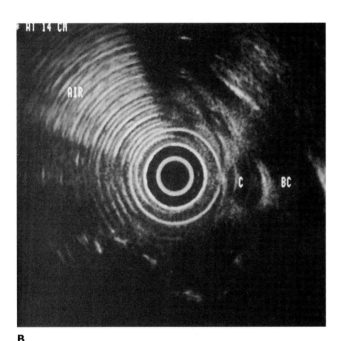

**B**

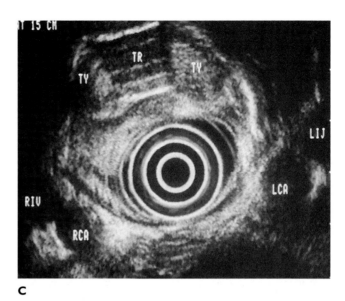

**C**

**Figure 5-5.** (A) EUS image of the proximal esophagus. The left common carotid artery (*LCCA*) is seen adjacent to the left subclavian artery (*LSA*). (B) The left brachiocephalic (innominate) vein (*BC*) is seen in longitudinal section adjacent to the carotid artery (*C*). Air artifact obscures imaging in the upper left. (C) EUS image of the most proximal aspect of the esophagus at 15 cm from the incisors. The thyroid gland (*TY*) is seen on either side of the trachea (*TR*). The spine is seen in the bottom of the image. The left internal jugular vein (*LIJ*) is seen beside the left common carotid artery (*LCA*). On the left side of the screen, the right internal jugular vein (*RIV*) and right common carotid artery (*RCA*) are seen.

### Body and Fundus

As the scope is withdrawn further proximally, the lesser curve comes into view at the bottom of the screen with the shaft of the scope positioned along the greater curve. As the tip is directed upward, the lesser curve can be seen to change from the normal five-layer wall pattern to a nine- to ten-layered structure at the angularis, with the innermost layers being a "double serosa" formed from the antrum and body portions of the stomach (Figures 5-8.A, 5-8.B, 5-8.C). The body is easily distinguished from the antrum by the presence of rugal folds.

In the midportion of the stomach, the body of the pancreas can be imaged (Figure 5-9.A). More proximally, the tail of the pancreas is visualized (Figure 5-9.B). The splenic artery and vein, the splenic hilum, the gastrohepatic ligament, and parts of the right and left lobes of the liver can also be evaluated from the body of the stomach (Figures 5-10.A, 5-10.B, 5-10.C). The splenic artery is smaller and more difficult to define than the splenic vein (Figure 5-11). The lesser sac area between the stomach and the liver is a good place to look for ascites and lymph nodes (Figures 5-12, 5-13). For complete imaging of the surrounding struc-

In the antrum, the head and genu of the pancreas are seen but may not yield images that are any more valuable than those obtained while scanning the pancreas from the bulb position. Posterior to the pancreas lies the peripancreatic vasculature, including the portal vein, splenic vein, and the superior mesenteric artery (SMA) and vein. However, it may take substantial manipulation of the scope to view the SMA. This is often best accomplished by tilting the up/down deflection control knob toward the up position, bringing the posterior wall closer to the tip of the scope while withdrawing the scope in a slight rightward-torque (clockwise) position. Further review of pancreatic and retroperitoneal structures is found in the next section.

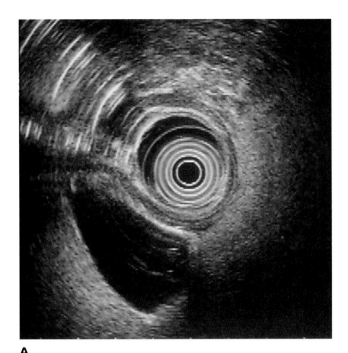

**A**

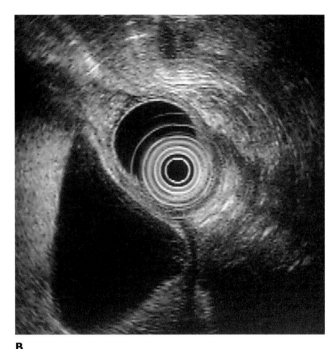

**B**

**Figure 5-6.** (A) EUS image from the antrum showing the gallbladder at 85 cm. (B) With the transducer in the bulb showing the gallbladder from a different angle.

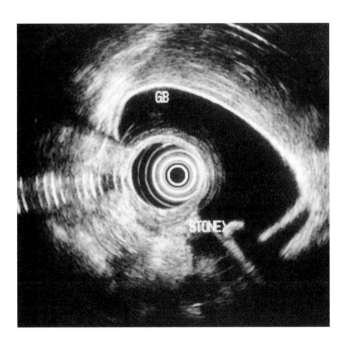

**Figure 5-7.** Gallbladder with a stone.

tures, the scope tip must be directed in all four directions: from the posterior wall to the lesser curvature to the anterior wall to the greater curvature.

The proximal lesser curve and the fundus are often not adequately visualized, in part due to difficulty in placing the probe at the proper focal point, as well as difficulty with sufficient removal of luminal air (1,29). Despite these limitations, the left lobe of the liver, the spleen, the aorta, the spine, and the celiac axis can be

seen. The spleen appears most often at the three- to five-o'clock positions (Figures 5-10, 5-11). Although often described as being isodense with the liver, this organ more often appears slightly hyperchoic than the liver. With some clockwise torque and withdrawal of the scope, the splenic hilum can be delineated (Figure 5-14).

On the left side of the screen, the left lobe of the liver can be examined. The left adrenal gland can be seen just proximal to the celiac axis. The adrenal gland is viewed as a thin triangular strip situated between the left kidney and the descending aorta. This gland, when imaged, has been said to resemble a seagull (Figure 5-15).

The celiac axis, which is discussed more extensively in the following section, can be easily located by placing the scope just below the GE junction. The scanning plane now lies parallel to the greater curvature. When the aorta is located at the five- to six-o'clock position, the scope is advanced straight into the gastric lumen until the Y-shaped celiac branches, the hepatic artery, and the splenic artery, are seen (Figure 5-16). In most patients, as the scope enters the esophagus, the cardia of the stomach and the distal esophagus can be seen simultaneously. Sometimes this occurs as the water-filled balloon pulls the cardia into the distal esophagus. Therefore, as the scope moves from the cardia into the distal esophagus it is important to deflate the balloon to facilitate scope passage. The same is true of passage of the scope from the bulb into the pylorus. Lastly, the crura of the diaphragm can be seen as the probe is withdrawn from the cardia into the distal

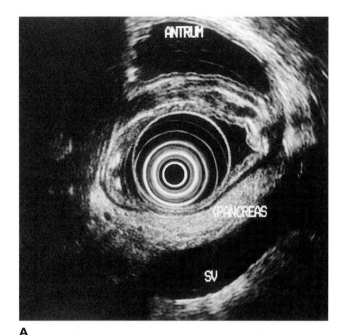

A

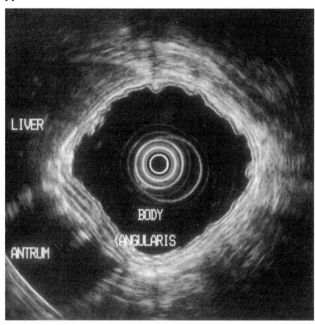

B

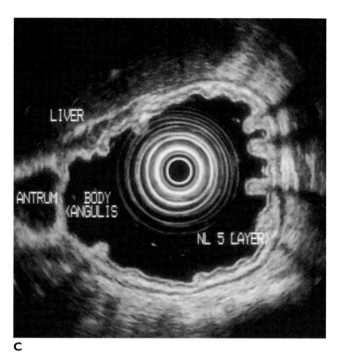

C

**Figure 5-8.** (A) EUS image from the gastric body showing the double five-layer pattern of the angulus as well as the body of the pancreas and splenic vein (*SV*). (B) EUS image that is more proximal, with liver in view to the left. (C) As the echoendoscope is withdrawn further, less of the antrum is seen and more of the liver is visualized. The rugal folds of the gastric wall are seen with the normal five-layer pattern nicely demonstrated.

esophagus. The gastroesophageal junction can be identified when the diaphragm disappears and the circumferential three- to five-layered wall characteristic of the esophagus is visualized.

## The Retroperitoneum

In performing EUS of the retroperitoneum, the transducer is endoscopically placed in one of several easily identified locations in the upper intestinal tract (Table 5-1). Then the area is scanned until an EUS landmark is located. From this reference point, the area immedi-

ately around that landmark can be evaluated. The oblique plane, which results in the best view of landmark structures, will vary somewhat according to each patient's anatomy. Several diagrams of these locations are available and invaluable to understanding EUS of the retroperitoneum (10,11,15,17). The vessels and organs are listed in Table 5-1 in order of appearance as the scope is withdrawn proximally from the horizontal duodenum. Anchoring the transducer with the water-filled balloon is particularly useful in the mobile duodenal bulb. By withdrawing the scope while it is anchored in the bulb, a "withdrawn-wedged" position is obtained, shortening the lesser curvature of the stomach. With this position, different and sometimes better angles of scanning can be achieved.

## Vasculature of the Retroperitoneum

Blood vessels are the most important EUS landmarks used to evaluate retroperitoneal disease. Vessels imaged from each of six locations are consistent for patients with normal anatomy (Table 5-2). The difficulty lies not in identifying an anechoic structure as a vessel, but in ascertaining which vessel that structure repre-

**Table 5-2.** EUS locations of major vessels of the retroperitoneum.

| LOCATIONS | Duodenum | | Gastric Posterior Wall | | | |
| --- | --- | --- | --- | --- | --- | --- |
| | Horizontal | Descending | Bulb | Antrum | Body | Fundus |
| **ARTERIES** | | | | | | |
| Aorta | A | - | - | - | S | A |
| Celiac* | - | - | WW | S | A | S |
| Hepatic* | - | - | WW | S | A | - |
| Splenic* | - | - | WW | S | A | S |
| Superior mesenteric | R | M | WW | S | A | S |
| Inferior mesenteric | - | - | - | - | - | - |
| Pancreaticoduodenal | - | S | - | - | - | - |
| Gastroduodenal | - | S | S | - | - | - |
| Gastroepiploic | - | - | - | R | R | - |
| Left renal | R | - | - | - | S | - |
| Right renal | - | M | - | - | - | - |
| **VEINS** | | | | | | |
| Inferior vena cava | A | A | - | S | - | - |
| Left renal | S | - | - | - | A | - |
| Right renal | - | M | - | - | - | - |
| Portal confluence | - | S | - | - | A | - |
| Portal* | - | - | WW | R | - | - |
| Splenic* | - | - | WW | A | A | S |
| Super mesenteric | S | A | - | - | S | - |
| Inferior mesenteric | - | - | - | S | S | - |
| Gastroepiploic | - | - | - | S | S | - |

Locations from which vessels can be imaged are shown. A = Always; M = Most of the time; S = Sometimes; R = Rarely; WW = Withdrawn-wedge
*Structures usually seen well from the withdrawn-wedged position.

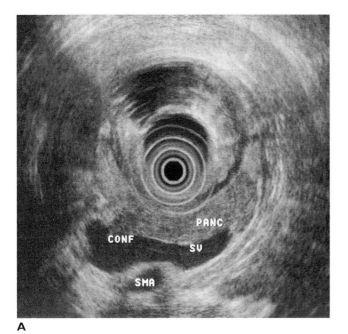

A

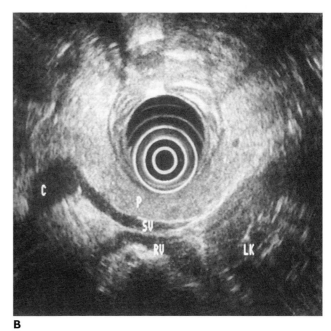

B

**Figure 5-9.** (A) EUS image from the body of the stomach showing the body of the pancreas, splenic vein (*SV*) joining the portal confluence (*CONF*), and the superior mesenteric artery (*SMA*). (B) More proximally in the body, the tail of the pancreas is seen with the confluence (*C*), splenic vein (*SV*), renal vein (*RV*), and left kidney (*LK*).

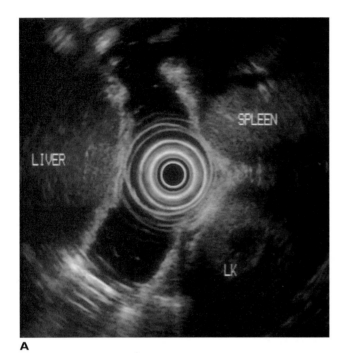

A

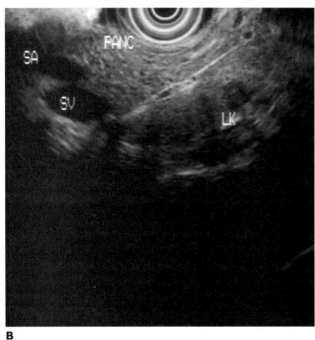

B

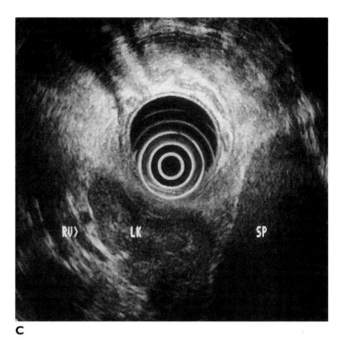

C

**Figure 5-10.** (A) Different angle in the proximal body showing the liver, spleen, and left kidney (*LK*). (B) EUS image from the proximal body showing the tail of the pancreas (*PANC*), left kidney (*LK*), splenic artery (*SA*), and splenic vein (*SV*). (C) Imaging more proximally in the body of the stomach, the tail of the pancreas is seen between the left kidney (*LK*) and spleen (*SP*). The renal vessels (*RV*) are also visualized.

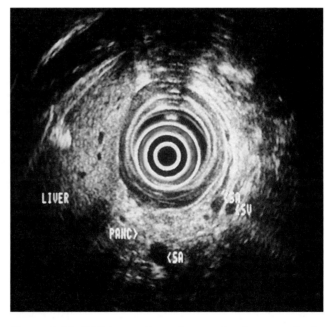

**Figure 5-11.** EUS image from the proximal antrum/body junction showing the left lobe of the liver, pancreas (*PANC*), two segments of the tortuous splenic artery (*SA*), and splenic vein (*SV*). The hyperechoic band representing the diaphragm lies between the liver and the anechoic ventricle.

sents (20,23,30,31). An understanding of the normal vasculature is essential. By manipulation of the scope, the scanning plane is oriented to bring each vessel into optimal focus.

## Aorta, Inferior Vena Cava, and Renal Vessels

The aorta and inferior vena cava are the first major vessels to be visualized from the horizontal duodenum. Depending on the exact position of the scanning plane, these vessels will be recognized either in cross section or longitudinal section. In a 360-degree sector scan, the

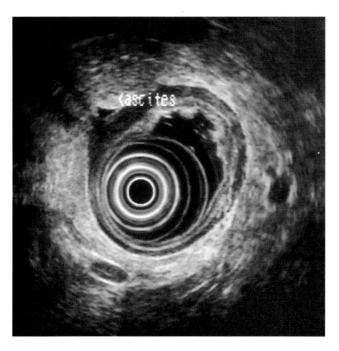

**Figure 5-12.** Trace amount of ascites between the liver and gastric wall.

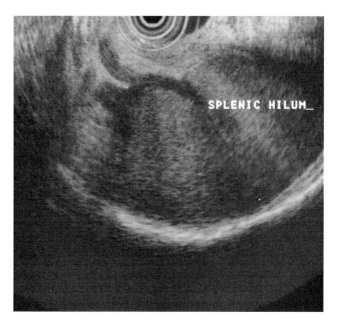

**Figure 5-14.** EUS image from the proximal body showing the splenic hilum.

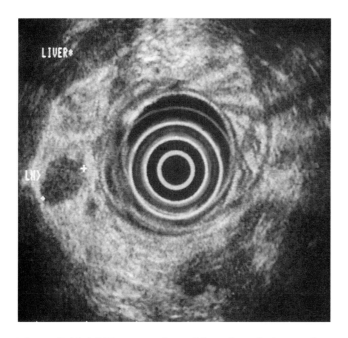

**Figure 5-13.** Malignant, enlarged lymph node is seen between the liver and lesser curve of the stomach. The gastric folds are collapsed but still discernible as such.

aorta and inferior vena cava tend to be seen in cross section, side by side, adjacent to the transducer with the vena cava closest to the duodenum. Pulsations of the inferior vena cava, but not the aorta, can be seen. Longitudinal images are slightly more difficult to obtain, and require the instrument to be positioned deeper within the duodenum. Confirmation that the transducer is in the horizontal duodenum is obtained when two large blood vessels, the aorta and inferior vena cava, are visualized. As the echoendoscope is pulled back, longitudinal sections of these blood vessels transmute to horizontal sections. The vessels at this point appear more circular (Figure 5-17.A), similar to standard axial transverse planes of CT. The aorta and inferior vena cava can also be seen from the stomach (Figure 5-17.B). The orientation of each vessel in the scanning image will depend on the position and shape of the patient's stomach.

With deep insertion of the echoendoscope, parts of the left renal vein and artery can be seen on occasion from the horizontal duodenum. However, the left renal vein is best seen from the posterior gastric wall (Figure 5-18.A). Withdrawal of the transducer toward the descending duodenum will bring the right renal vein and artery into view. Images of the right kidney and renal vein will generally appear in the lower half of a 360-degree sector EUS scan adjacent to the inferior vena cava and spine (Figure 5-19).

## Portal Confluence Vessels

As the transducer is withdrawn from the horizontal to the descending duodenum, the mesenteric vessels come into view. Because both vessels are anterior to the duodenum, the superior mesenteric vein, which generally appears near the five-o'clock position on a sector scan, will be counterclockwise to the superior mesenteric artery, which generally appears near the six-o'clock position (Figure 5-20). From this location, the superior mesenteric vein lies to the right and

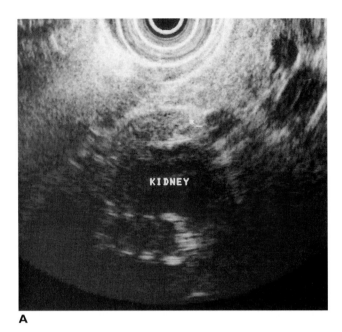

**A**

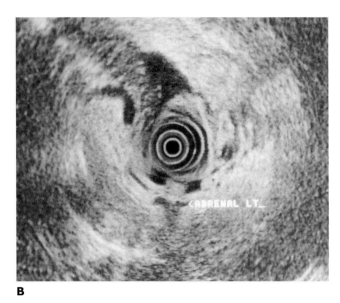

**B**

**Figure 5-15.** (A) EUS image from the body showing the left adrenal (marked at cursor) adjacent to the left kidney. (B) More magnified view of adrenal gland displaying a seagull-like appearance.

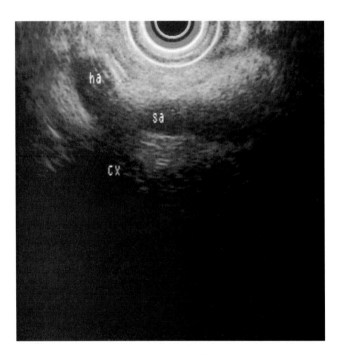

**Figure 5-16.** Celiac axis (*CX*) with hepatic artery (*ha*) and splenic artery (*sa)* branches as viewed from the gastric body.

slightly posterior to the superior mesenteric artery. In some cases, with slow withdrawal of the scope the superior mesenteric vein can be traced into the portal confluence. However, in many patients the duodenal anatomy is such that the required acoustic window to see this junction cannot be maintained.

The mesenteric vessels can also be seen from the body of the stomach or the duodenal bulb "withdrawn-

wedged" position. An image similar to a conventional transcutaneous ultrasound view can be obtained, with the superior mesenteric artery appearing as a circular structure beneath the splenic vein and to the left of the portal-splenic-superior mesenteric vein confluence (Figure 5-21). This has been referred to by some as the *bullet sign* because the fat and mesentery that surround the superior mesenteric artery produces a corresponding hyperechoic ring. Often only the first segments at the origin of the superior mesenteric artery and vein are seen.

The junction of the splenic vein into the portal confluence (Figure 5-22) is generally best visualized from the posterior wall of the body of the stomach. At times, this image is best obtained using the withdrawn-wedged position to shorten the lesser curvature. The course of the splenic vein can be followed to the spleen by tracking the probe proximally and to the patient's left, and across the gastric body. The inferior mesenteric vein can be seen during this maneuver where it joins the splenic vein. Finally, additional images of the portal confluence and superior mesenteric artery can be obtained with further scope withdrawal as the dorsal pancreas comes into view.

## Portal Vein

The duodenal bulb is the best position from which to visualize the portal vein, which appears as a hypoechoic structure, posterior to the bulb. Both the portal vein and common bile duct are visualized along their longitudinal axis with the bile duct being closest to the duodenal wall (Figures 5-23 and 5-24). With the

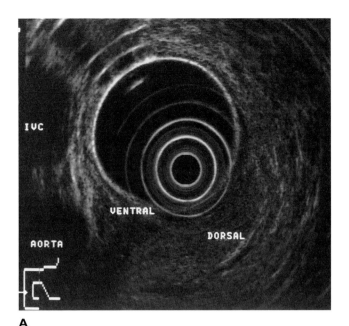

**A**

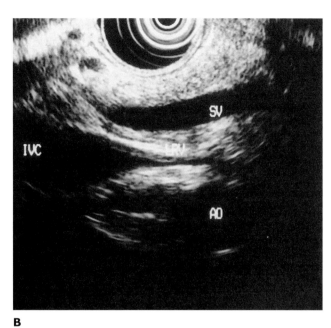

**B**

**Figure 5-17.** (A) In the horizontal duodenum, the aorta and inferior vena cava (*IVC*) appear in transverse section. The dorsal portion of the pancreas is more echogenic than the ventral pancreas. (B) The aorta (*AO*) and inferior vena cava (*IVC*) as seen from the body of the stomach with the left renal vein (*LRV*) and splenic vein (*SV*) in view.

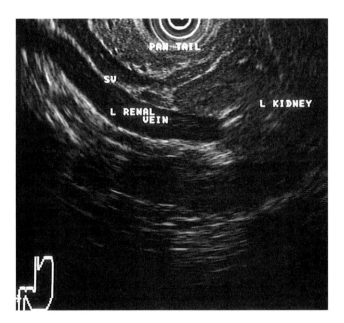

**Figure 5-18.** EUS image from the body of the stomach with transducer against the posterior gastric wall. The left renal vein entering the left kidney, the splenic vein (*SV*), and the tail of the pancreas (*PAN TAIL*) are well visualized.

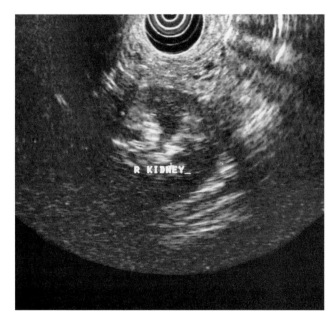

**Figure 5-19.** Imaging from the descending duodenum, the right kidney is seen.

sector scan instrument, the portal vein can be traced up into the liver to the bifurcation of the right and left branches. Obtaining these images of the portal vein in relation to the common bile duct is considerably more difficult than most maneuvers, because some degree of torque is needed simultaneously with insertion or slight withdrawal of the scope.

When the bile duct and portal vein are viewed on the left side of the screen, the pancreas is generally maintained in the lower half of the image. The distal bile duct can be traced into the head of the pancreas. The so-called *stack sign* refers to the simultaneous view of the pancreatic duct, bile duct, and portal vein while imaging in the apex of the bulb (Figure 5-25)

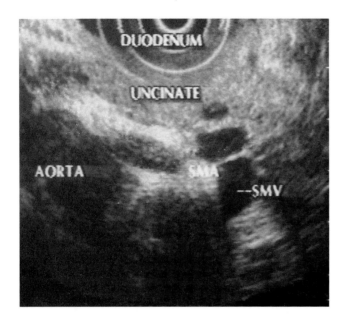

**Figure 5-20.** Imaging from the descending duodenum, the uncinate process, the aorta, the superior mesenteric artery (*SMA*), and the superior mesenteric vein (*SMV*) are seen.

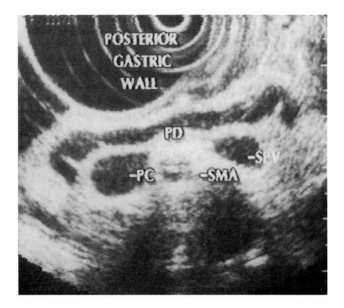

**Figure 5-21.** Imaging from the posterior gastric wall, the superior mesenteric artery (*SMA*) appears below the splenic vein (*SPV*) and portal confluence (*PC*). A slightly dilated pancreatic duct (*PD*) is also seen.

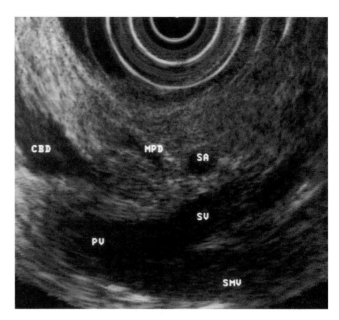

**Figure 5-22.** From the posterior gastric wall, the confluence of the portal vein (*PV*), splenic vein (*SV*), and superior mesenteric vein (*SMV*) is seen. In this image the common bile duct (*CBD*), main pancreatic duct (*MPD*), and splenic artery (*SA*) are also visualized.

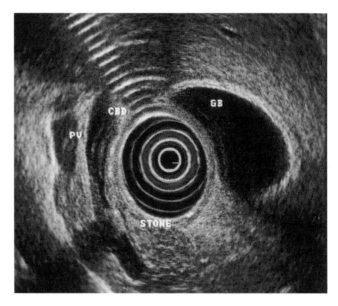

**Figure 5-23.** The common bile duct (*CBD*) with a stone in the distal duct is visualized against the duodenal wall. The portal vein (*PV*) is seen more laterally. Additionally, in this image the gallbladder (*GB*) is seen.

(32). The hepatic artery can, at times, be seen between the bile duct and portal vein. The gastroduodenal artery (GDA) may appear between the bile duct and duodenal wall; it is important to keep this in mind when the exam is being performed to evaluate the CBD, because the GDA can be mistaken for the CBD. The IVC remains deep to the portal vein and can be visualized in longitudinal section.

## Celiac and Splenic Vessels

The celiac axis is an important landmark to visualize because it is a common site for lymph node metastases from various upper gastrointestinal tumors. The celiac axis is best imaged from the posterior wall of the body of the stomach, orienting the sonographic plane horizontally. It is located by first obtaining a longitudinal

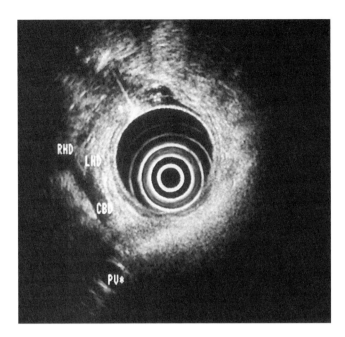

**Figure 5-24.** EUS image of the common bile duct (*CBD*) and the bifurcation into the right hepatic duct (*RHD*) and left hepatic duct (*LHD*).

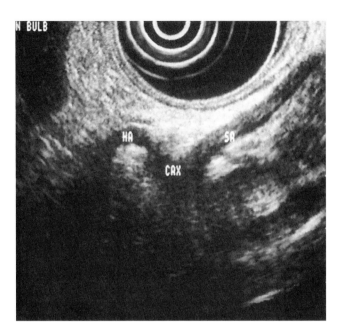

**Figure 5-26.** Imaging the celiac axis (*CAX*), hepatic artery (*ha*), and splenic artery (*sa*) from the withdrawn-wedge position in the duodenal bulb.

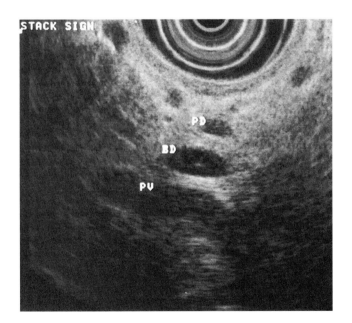

**Figure 5-25.** EUS image showing the "stack sign": a vertical line-up of the pancreatic duct (*PD*), bile duct (*BD*), and portal vein (*PV*).

view of the splenic vein. Then, by tracking the probe distally toward the portal confluence, the splenic artery can generally be seen taking a sharp posterior (downward on the screen) course toward the aorta. Alternatively, the splenic artery can be traced from the region of the pancreatic tail up to the celiac axis. Another technique used to identify the axis is to withdraw the scope until the aorta is seen in cross section (at about

45 cm from the incisors); then, with mild upward tip deflection and simultaneous advancing of the scope, the axis will be visualized.

By small manipulations of the transducer, a section through the celiac axis will bring into view the hepatic and splenic artery joining into the celiac artery (Figure 5-16). This "Y" configuration of arteries is another EUS landmark. The right branch of the celiac axis is the hepatic artery, which can be traced into the hepatic hilum. The splenic artery forms the left branch and courses to the left to enter the splenic hilum. Occasionally the left gastric artery can be seen but, because it is smaller than the hepatic and splenic arteries, it can be more difficult to image. The celiac area should be examined for lymph nodes by following the course of each vessel. In some patients these images are best obtained from the duodenal bulb withdrawn-wedged position (Figure 5-26).

## Secondary Branches of Vessels

In the area between the first and second part of the duodenum, various blood vessels lying close to the duodenal wall between the pancreas and duodenum can be found. These include the pancreaticoduodenal artery, gastroepiploic artery, gastric vein, and prepyloric vein. These small veins, as well as the gastroepiploic vein, are not readily visualized except where a major vessel obstruction renders them visible through dilation. An enlarged gastroepiploic vein may be mistaken for a normal splenic vein if the splenic vein is occluded. The pancreaticoduodenal artery and vein may be seen adjacent to the left inferior duodenal wall when the gallbladder is in the 360-degree field near the opposite duodenal wall.

## Retroperitoneal Organs

The sizes of organs on EUS are within the range of those reported in texts describing other imaging methods (18,19,33). The dimensions of an organ image will depend on the level and angle of the scanning plane as it slices through that organ.

### Pancreas

The pancreatic parenchyma has a finely granular, homogeneous echogenicity, sometimes referred to as a "salt and pepper" appearance. The body, which is the easiest part of the pancreas to visualize, is best seen from the posterior wall of the stomach or from a withdrawn-wedged position in the duodenal bulb. The splenic vein is the most useful landmark for finding the pancreas, because it is mostly posterior and slightly superior to the pancreas. Medially, the pancreas is therefore between the splenic vein and the transducer, where the splenic vessels are posterior to the neck and body of the pancreas. The position of the splenic artery is generally superior to the pancreas and splenic vein, but varies depending on its tortuosity (Figure 5-27). As the splenic vessels are followed to the spleen, they may cross the tail of the pancreas, becoming anterior. The tail of the pancreas is located by tip deflection and slight scope withdrawal as one follows this organ toward the patient's left side. The tail of the pancreas generally takes a downward turn on the EUS screen to lie between the left kidney and spleen (Figure 5-28). As the scope is withdrawn into the proximal body and fundus, while maintaining a clockwise torque, the renal and splenic vessels can be brought into view surrounding the distal-most aspect of the pancreatic tail.

Although superior parts of the head of the pancreas can be visualized from the stomach, the head of the pancreas is generally best seen from the first and second parts of the duodenum, in the five- to ten-o'clock position (Figure 5-29). At some point between the bulb and second part of the duodenum, as the pancreatic head is scanned, the liver will be seen in the upper part of the screen with the right kidney slightly counterclockwise. The inferior vena cava will be on the left part of the screen behind the pancreas and next to the aorta. Not all of these organs and large vessels are likely to be seen simultaneously on the same sonographic plane.

The uncinate process can be seen only from the second and third parts of the duodenum. The uncinate is about 1 cm in diameter and will generally appear in

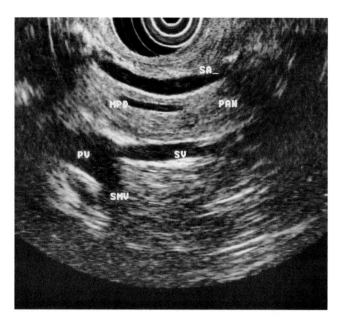

**Figure 5-27.** EUS image from the body of the stomach with the splenic artery (*SA*) seen superior to the pancreas (*PAN*), portal vein (*PV*), superior mesenteric vein (*SMV*), and splenic vein (*SV*). The main pancreatic duct (*MPD*) is well visualized.

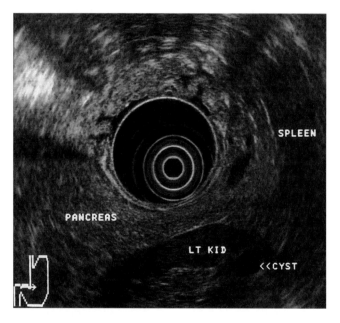

**Figure 5-28.** EUS image of the tail of the pancreas, which lies between the left kidney (*LT KID*) and spleen. A renal cyst is seen.

the six- to eight-o'clock position; a cross-sectional image of the aorta may also appear on the left of the screen. The SMV lies just below the pancreas, and a circular view of the SMA is seen between the SMV and the aorta (Figure 5-29). In the area of the ampulla of Vater, the pancreas will appear somewhat circular because the orientation of the probe is axial. As the probe is withdrawn above the ampulla and into the apex of the bulb, the sonographic plane rotates toward a coronal orientation. From this angle the shape of the pancreas becomes elliptical. The pancreas will be in the five- to nine-o'clock position on the screen, adjacent to the transducer. Slight torquing and tip deflection of the scope will allow scanning of the entire head. In the great majority of individuals, the dorsal pancreas has been reported to be slightly more echogenic than the ventral pancreas due to the presence of more fat in this part of the gland (22) (Figure 5-17.A).

As the scope is withdrawn into the pyloric channel, resistance will be felt. At this point it can be extremely useful to deflate the balloon, re-advance the scope into the apex of the bulb and re-inflate the balloon. This maneuver provides optimal imaging of the bile duct, portal vein, and proximal pancreatic duct as it courses through the head of the pancreas. The bile duct and pancreatic duct appear as hypoechoic structures within the homogeneous, finely granular pancreatic parenchyma.

The pancreatic duct can be traced along the course of the pancreas into the tail (Figure 5-30). Major branches of the duct can be seen in most patients. A normal pancreatic duct tapers in diameter from a maximum of 4 mm (depending on the patient's age) in the head to 1 mm in the tail. These measurements are less than the accepted normals for the dye-injected duct seen in ERCP (33,34). If the pancreatic duct is dilated, care must be taken not to confuse it with the splenic artery.

The echoendoscope can be advanced to the ampulla more than 99% of the time except when duodenal stenosis is present. Approximately 10% of patients with tumors of the pancreas have some duodenal stenosis, which prevents optimal visualization of the region around the uncinate and ampulla (4,23). The entire pancreas can be imaged in at least 95% of patients; however, a complete examination of the whole organ can be time consuming.

### Extra Hepatic Biliary Tract

The distal common bile duct and, at times, the cystic duct are generally best seen from the first and second part of the duodenum (1,8). Pancreatic parenchyma surrounds the distal common bile duct. As the scope is maneuvered around the ampulla, the common bile duct can be traced to its origin where it joins the pancreatic duct. As the scope is withdrawn into the sharp angle of the duodenal sweep just beyond the duodenal bulb, a longitudinal view of the common bile duct is obtained where it passes through the pancreas toward the liver. Practice is required to hold the transducer steady long enough for optimal focus in this part of the duodenum. Because the normal common bile duct diameter is generally no larger than 5 mm, it is easier to

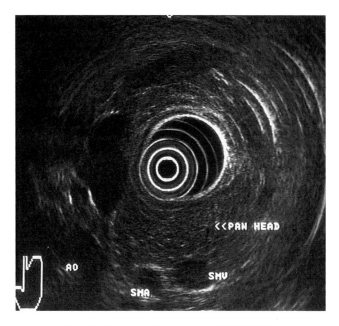

**Figure 5-29.** The head of the pancreas (*PAN HEAD*) is seen from the second portion of the duodenum. The superior mesenteric artery (*SMA*), superior mesenteric vein (*SMV*), and aorta (*AO)* are also visualized.

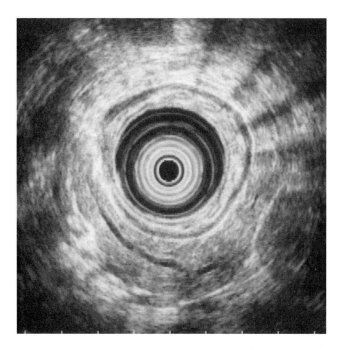

**Figure 5-30.** EUS image from midbody of the stomach with the main pancreatic duct in full view.

find when dilated due to a tumor or stone. Care should be taken to avoid confusing the gastroduodenal artery (GDA) for the common bile duct; the GDA is closer to the duodenal wall.

When a longitudinal plane is obtained through the common bile duct, the portal vein is generally seen more posterior, slightly further from the probe (Figure

5-23). By pulling back on the scope to the withdrawn-wedged position, the bile duct often can be followed into the liver to its bifurcation into right and left hepatic branches. In some patients a longitudinal view of the cystic duct and hepatic artery can be obtained, but not all of these structures (i.e., the common bile duct, common hepatic duct, cystic duct, portal vein, and hepatic artery) will be seen in longitudinal axis simultaneously. When the bile duct is seen in its longitudinal axis, the hepatic artery may be seen as a circular structure between the bile duct and the portal vein.

### Kidneys and Adrenal Glands

The kidneys are generally among the easiest of the retroperitoneal organs to recognize, although the lower poles of these hypolucent, doughnut-shaped structures are rarely seen. Depending on the transducer orientation, the kidney will be seen in coronal, sagittal, or horizontal planes. Up to 50% of the right kidney can be seen from the duodenum. On occasion the sonographic plane can be angled to bring the adrenal gland into view. The right adrenal gland is difficult to see because the upper pole of the right kidney generally lies at the level of the duodenal bulb and the distal lesser curvature. When the transducer is positioned in the bulb, it points toward the porta hepatis and cannot readily be turned to visualize the gland.

The left kidney and renal vein can be visualized from the posterior wall of the stomach when the probe is pushed down as far as possible along the greater curvature without causing the scope to loop toward the lesser curve (Figure 5-10.C). The left renal vein runs just inferior to the splenic vein. The left adrenal can at times be seen as a thin hypoechoic structure, contiguous with the upper pole of the kidney. Its visualization, however, is usually difficult (see Figure 5-15).

### Lymph Nodes

Small (<3 mm), benign, noninflamed lymph nodes are generally somewhat difficult to visualize, because normal nodes tend to be echogenic with irregular shapes and indistinct margins (Figure 5-13). Lymph nodes, when visualized, are generally easiest to find around the pancreatic head and celiac axis, or along the portal venous system, bile duct, or lesser curve of the stomach (35,36).

### Duodenum

The wall of the duodenal sweep has the typical five-layer architecture recognized in EUS images of other parts of the gastrointestinal tract (3,24,35,37). Although no specific in vitro studies of the duodenal wall have been reported, the five layers undoubtedly correspond to the superficial mucosa, deep mucosa, submucosa, muscularis propria, and serosa with adventitia, as previously de-

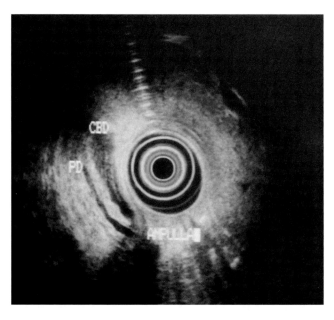

**Figure 5-31.** The common bile duct (*CBD*) and pancreatic duct (*PD*) course through the head of the pancreas and enter the ampulla. From 6 to 7 o'clock air artifact is present.

scribed. The aggregate thickness is approximately 3 mm. The EUS appearances of the ampulla of Vater and adjacent duodenal wall have been described (38). The normal papilla will appear as a slight protuberance unless the balloon surrounding the transducer compresses it. When imaging the ampulla, it can be helpful if water is instilled into the lumen. This helps to displace any air not removed by suctioning and also opens up the duodenal folds to help identify the ampulla (Figure 5-31).

## Summary

The high-frequency sound waves used in EUS provide soft-tissue resolution that is unsurpassed by any other imaging technique. An understanding of the normal anatomic relationships of the various organs and blood vessels of the upper gastrointestinal tract and retroperitoneum is essential for accurately performing EUS. This knowledge can be obtained from standard anatomy, CT, abdominal ultrasound, and angiography texts. With a good three-dimensional mental image of these structures, the echoendoscope can be guided in various directions from specific EUS landmarks to image most gastrointestinal organs and the retroperitoneum.

### References

1. Caletti G, Ferrari A, Barbara L. Normal endosonographic anatomy of the esophagus and stomach. Gastrointest Endosc Clin North Am 1992;2:601–614.
2. Tytgat GN. Transintestinal ultrasonography—present and future [editorial]. Endoscopy 1987;19:241–242.

3. Lees WR. Future perspectives in endoscopic ultrasound. In: K. Kawai, ed. Endoscopic ultrasonography in gastroenterology. Igaku-Shoin, Ltd. Tokyo 1988: 132–137.

4. Shorvon PJ, et al. Upper gastrointestinal endoscopic ultrasonography in gastroenterology. British J Radiol 1987;60:429–438.

5. Kimmey MB, et al. Histologic correlates of gastrointestinal ultrasound images. Gastroenterology 1989; 96:433–441.

6. Snady H. The role of endoscopic ultrasonography in diagnosis, staging, and outcomes of gastrointestinal diseases. Gastroenterologist 1994;2:91–110.

7. Kawai KE. Endoscopic ultrasonography in gastroenterology. Tokyo: Igaku-Shoin, Ltd., 1988.

8. Tio TL, Tytgat GNJ. Atlas of transintestinal ultrasonography. Aalsmeer, The Netherlands: Smith, Kline & French b.v. /Gegenens Koninkligke Bibliotheek Den Haag, 1986.

9. Colin-Jones DG, Rosch T, Dittler HJ. Staging of gastric cancer by endoscopy. Endoscopy 1993;25:34–38.

10. Caletti GC, et al. Technique of endoscopic ultrasonography investigation: esophagus, stomach and duodenum. Scand J Gastroenterol Suppl 1986;123:1–5.

11. Lux G, Heyder N. Endoscopic ultrasonography of the pancreas. Technical aspects. Scand J Gastroenterol Suppl 1986;123:112–118.

12. Rosch T, et al. Endoscopic ultrasound in pancreatic tumor diagnosis. Gastrointestinal Endosc 1991;37: 347–352.

13. Snady H, Cooperman A, Siegel J. Endoscopic ultrasonography compared to computerized tomography for pre-operative staging and assessment of resectability of a pancreatic adenocarcinoma or mass. Am J Gastroenterol 1989;84:A1210.

14. Snady H, Cooperman A, Siegel J. Endoscopic ultrasonography compared with computed tomography with ERCP in patients with obstructive jaundice or small peri-pancreatic mass. Gastrointest Endosc 1992; 38:27–34.

15. Strohm WD, Classen M. Endoscopic ultrasonography. In: Sivak M, ed. Gastroenterologic endoscopy. Philadelphia: WB Saunders, 1987:182–202.

16. Tio TL, et al. Ampullopancreatic carcinoma: preoperative TNM classification with endosonography. Radiology 1990; 175:455–461.

17. Yasuda K, et al. The diagnosis of pancreatic cancer by endoscopic ultrasonography. Gastrointest Endosc 1988;34:1–8.

18. Haaga JR, Alfidi RJE. Computed tomography of the whole body: vol. II. St. Louis, MO: CV Mosby, 1988.

19. Han MC, Kim CW. Sectional human anatomy. Seoul, Korea: Pyung Hwa Dang Printing, 1989.

20. Reuter SR, Redman HC, Cho KJ. Gastrointestinal angiography. Philadelphia, PA: WB Saunders, 1986.

21. Zirinsky K, Markisz JA. Cross-sectional abdominal anatomy: CT, MRI, and ultrasound: a programmed atlas. New York, NY: Igaku-Shoin, 1992.

22. Kremkau FW, Taylor KJ. Artifacts in ultrasound imaging. J Ultrasound in Med 1986;5:227–237.

23. Snady H. Artifacts and techniques of endoscopic ultrasonography in investigating gastrointestinal pathologies and therapeutic options. In: Preedy V, Watson R, eds. Methods in disease: investigating the gastrointestinal tract. London: Greenwich Med. Media, 1998:141–155.

24. Tio TL, Tytgat GN. Endoscopic ultrasonography of normal and pathologic upper gastrointestinal wall structure. Comparison of studies in vivo and in vitro with histology. Scand J Gastroenterol Suppl 1986; 123:27–33.

25. Bolondi L, et al. The sonographic appearance of the normal gastric wall: an in vitro study. Ultrasound Med Biol 1986;12:991–998.

26. Heyder N. Endoscopic ultrasonography of tumours of the esophagus and the stomach. Surg Endosc 1987;1: 17–23.

27. Boyce H, Boyce G. Endoscopic ultrasonography: instruments and techniques. Gastrointest Endosc Clin North Am 1992;2:575–599.

28. Songur Y, et al. Endosonographic evaluation of giant gastric folds. Gastrointest Endosc 1995;41:468–474.

29. Vilmann P, et al. Endoscopic ultrasonography-guided fine-needle aspiration biopsy of lesions in the upper gastrointestinal tract. Gastrointest Endosc 1995;41: 230–235.

30. Snady H, Bruckner H, Siegel J, Cooperman A, Neff R, Kiefer L. Endoscopic ultrasonographic criteria of vascular invasion by potentially resectable pancreatic tumor. Gastrointest Endosc 1994;40:326–333.

31. Rosch T, et al. Staging of pancreatic and ampullary carcinoma by endoscopic ultrasonography. Comparison with conventional sonography, computed tomography, and angiography. Gastroenterology 1992;102: 188–199.

32. Bhutani MS, Hoffman BJ, Van Velse A. Diagnosis of pancreas divisum by endoscopic ultrasound (EUS). In: 10th International Symposium on Endoscopic Ultrasonography. Cleveland, OH, 1995.

33. Rosch T, et al. The normal pancreas in endoscopic ultrasound. Gastrointest Endoscopy 1991;37:A255.

34. Ansel H. Normal pancreatic duct. In: Stewart E, Vennes J, Greenen J, eds. Atlas of endoscopic retrograde cholangiopancreatography. St. Louis, MO, CV Mosby, 1977:43–47.

35. Aibe T, et al. Endoscopic ultrasonography of lymph nodes surrounding the upper GI tract. Scand J Gastroenterol Suppl 1986;123:164–169.

36. Tio TL, Tytgat GN. Endoscopic ultrasonography in analyzing peri-intestinal lymph node abnormality. Preliminary results of studies in vitro and in vivo. Scand J Gastroenterol Suppl 1986;123:158–163.

37. Bolondi L, et al. Problems and variations in the interpretation of the ultrasound feature of the normal upper and lower GI tract wall. Scand J Gastroenterol Suppl 1986;123:16–26.

38. Fujino M, et al. Diagnosis of carcinoma of the major duodenal papilla by endoscopic ultrasonography. Gastroenterology 1991;100:A316.

# 6

# Linear Array Endosonography: Normal EUS Anatomy

## Richard A. Erickson

The first commercially-available echoendoscopes were introduced in the United States in the mid-1980s. These instruments produced radially oriented, 360-degree images perpendicular to the shaft of the echoendoscope. The advantage of this type of orientation is that it is ideally suited to the rapid survey of the perilumenal structures of the longitudinally-oriented gastrointestinal tract. Additionally, the anatomic view of many of the organs visualized by radial endosonography is similar to the familiar images produced by computerized tomography. As endosonography matured, the benefits of obtaining needle-aspiration cytologic samples from the pathologic lesions identified by radial endosonography became evident. However, an aspiration needle passing out of the biopsy channel of a radial echoendoscope produces only an echogenic dot in the ultrasonographic image (1). Thus, the tip of the needle is very difficult to follow into the lesion being biopsied. Interest then arose in producing echoendoscopes with a linear beam orientation in which the endosonographic image was oriented parallel to the shaft of the echoendoscope. With this design, the whole path of an aspiration needle passed through the ultrasonic field of view, allowing the tip to be followed as it exited the biopsy channel and entered a lesion. In the early 1990s, convex linear array echoendoscopes became commercially available, resulting in the rapid development of endoscopic ultrasound-guided fine-needle aspiration, therapeutic EUS, and a concomitant rise in interest in learning linear EUS anatomy.

Linear endosonographic anatomy is oriented 90° from the more familiar radial anatomy. Thus, one of the challenges endosonographers who want to perform EUS-guided fine-needle aspiration must meet is learning linear endosonographic anatomy both to examine normal structures as well as to locate pathologic lesions seen by a previous radial EUS examination. Al-

though most active EUS centers use both radial and linear EUS, many endosonographers have successfully used only linear instrumentation for both diagnostic and therapeutic endosonography (2). Comparative studies suggest that diagnostic linear and radial endosonography are similar in their detection rates for most lesions (3,4).

There are currently two basic types of linear echoendoscopes commercially available. The curved linear array echoendoscope uses a series of electronically coupled solid state ultrasound transducers to produce a 100-degree or 180-degree linear view. When coupled to the appropriate ultrasonic base unit, curved linear array echoendoscopes can also have Doppler and color-flow capabilities. The second type of linear echoendoscope uses a rotating acoustical mirror or transducer to produce a 270-degree linearly oriented image and is designated as a linear mechanical echoendoscope. This engineering design does not allow for color flow or Doppler. The ultrasonographic anatomy with these linear instruments is similar, with the only major difference being the field of view (100 degrees, 180 degrees or 270 degrees) available to the endosonographer.

As with radial endosonographic anatomy, two key principles guide the linear endosonographic examination. First, the EUS exam must be performed systematically such that all pertinent anatomic structures are identified and examined. This will accelerate learning the many variations in normal anatomy and avoid missing pathology in areas outside the primary organ of interest. The second principle is to identify "home-base" structures in each major anatomic region to allow the endosonographer to maintain proper orientation and perspective during an endosonographic examination. For EUS of the upper gastrointestinal tract, some endosonographers prefer performing an examination by advancing the echoendoscope deep into

58

the second or third portion of the duodenum and then withdrawing systematically from that point. Other endosonographers prefer completing the examination of each anatomic region (the mediastinum, the perigastric region, and the periduodenal region) as the echoendoscope passes through it. Still others first focus on the organ of interest, and then examine other anatomic regions. There are advantages to each approach, and as long as the endosonographic examination is done systematically, all of these techniques are acceptable.

## The Mediastinum

As in radial endosonography, the esophagus and peri-esophageal structures probably represent the simplest area of the gastrointestinal tract to examine by linear EUS because the relationships between the esophagus and surrounding structures are fairly constant. A thorough evaluation of the mediastinum, using a linear echoendoscope, requires rotating the echoendoscope 360 degrees (180 degrees with the linear mechanical instrument) at intervals of a few centimeters as the echoendoscope is passed down the esophagus. In general, vascular structures provide the major orienting landmarks for each endosonographic view. The home-base structure in the mediastinum is the easily located descending aorta (Figure 6-1.A). The descending aorta is identified by initially advancing the linear echoendoscope some 30 to 35 cm into the esophagus. At that location, the echoendoscope is rotated right or left until the descending aorta comes into view as a large longitudinal echolucent structure with posterior acoustic enhancement (Figure 6-2). With the descending aorta in view and the patient lying on his or her left side, rotating the shaft of the echoendoscope clockwise will bring the structures anterior to the esophagus (e.g., the heart) into view and rotating counterclockwise will bring the structures posterior to the esophagus (e.g., the spine) into view. After finding the descending aorta at 30 to 35 cm, the next most easily identifiable structure is the left atrium, which is revealed by rotating the echoendoscope shaft clockwise about 90 degrees. With some minor fine adjustments of the echoendoscope, the left atrium is seen as a large, pulsating, echolucent structure within which the mitral valve can be easily seen opening into the more distal and deep left ventricle (Figure 6-3). From the left atrium, slightly more clockwise rotation and withdrawal of the echoendoscope by a few centimeters will bring into view the left ventricular outflow tract with its tricuspid aortic valve (Figure 6-4). From that point onward, the echoendoscope can be withdrawn with only minor rotation to the left or right to keep the ascending aorta in view. As the superior portion of the left atrium is encountered, another round echolucent pulsating structure will be seen just

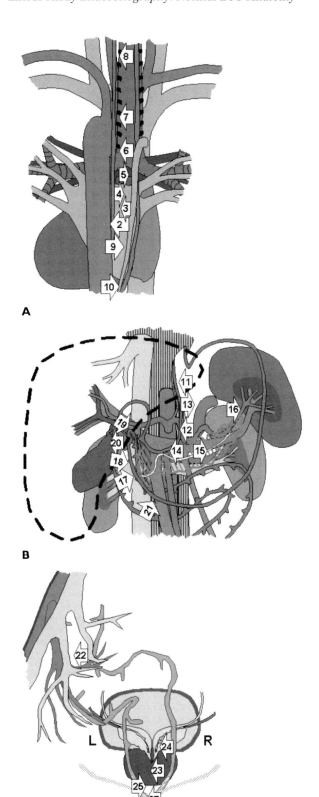

**A**

**B**

**C**

**Figure 6-1.** (A) Posterior view of peri-esophageal mediastinal anatomy. (B) Anterior view of perigastroduodenal anatomy. (C) Posterior view of the male perirectal anatomy. Endosonographic station numbers *(number arrows)* are discussed in the body of the text and the corresponding figures.

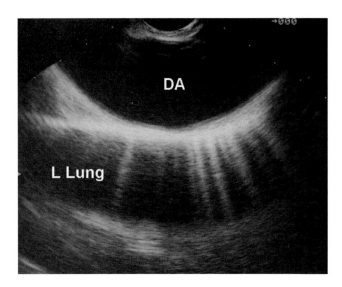

**Figure 6-2.** Curved linear array view through the mid-distal esophagus of the descending aorta (*DA*) with the left lung deep to it. This is "home base" for the mediastinum. (Unless otherwise designated, the linear endosonographic views in Figures 6-2 through 6-27 were produced using the Pentax FG 32UA echoendoscope at 7.5 MHz. All views are oriented with the control end of the echoendoscope toward the right.)

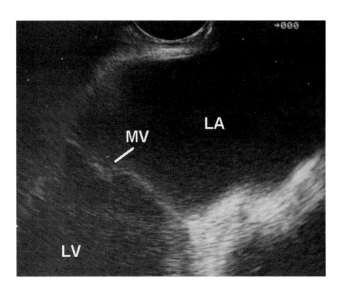

**Figure 6-3.** Curved linear array view through the mid-distal esophagus of the left atrium (*LA*) with the left ventricle (*LV*) and mitral valve (*MV*) deep to it.

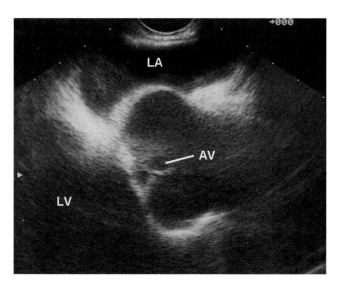

**Figure 6-4.** Curved linear array view through the mid-esophagus of the left atrium (*LA*) with the left ventricle (*LV*) outflow tract leading to the aortic valve (*AV*) and ascending aorta.

proximal to the left atrium. This represents the cross-sectional image of the right pulmonary artery (Figure 6-5.A). The space between the left atrium and the right pulmonary artery is the subcarinal region. There are often benign triangular-shaped subcarinal lymph nodes seen in this area (Figure 6-5.B). It is a vital region to examine when looking for pathologic adenopathy in the setting of pulmonary or esophageal malignancies. Further clockwise rotation from the view of the ascending

aorta may bring the superior vena cava into view draining into the right atrium (Figures 6-5.B, 6-5.C). Further withdrawal of the echoendoscope from the subcarinal region (25 to 30 cm) will meet with an endosonographic blind spot as the ultrasound transducer passes over the air-filled (and therefore impenetrable) left mainstem bronchus. After passing the left mainstem bronchus and with a few degrees of counterclockwise rotation, two round echolucent structures should appear (Figure 6-6). The most proximal of these represents the cross-sectional view of the aortic arch, and the more distal structure is the left pulmonary artery. The region between these two structures is the aortopulmonary window; again, an important area for assessing pathologic adenopathy. Withdrawing the echoendoscope a centimeter or two from this level, a small amount of further counterclockwise rotation will reveal the great vessels (left common carotid and left subclavian) coming off of the arch of the aorta (Figure 6-7). The bracheocephalic (innominate) artery is usually hidden behind the trachea. Sometimes the left innominate vein will be seen as an ovoid structure deep to the aortic arch at this level. The left common carotid artery can be followed from the aortic arch into the neck, where the left internal jugular vein may appear as a larger echolucent structure deep to the carotid artery (Figure 6-8). Rotating the echoendoscope approximately 180 degrees at this level will sometimes bring the right common carotid and right internal jugular into view, although the right internal jugular vein is often obscured by the intervening trachea. If the echoendoscope is again reinserted to 30 to 35 cm until the descending aorta is in view and then rotated counter-

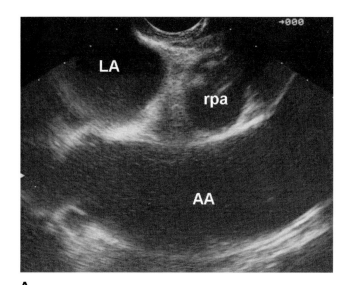

**A**

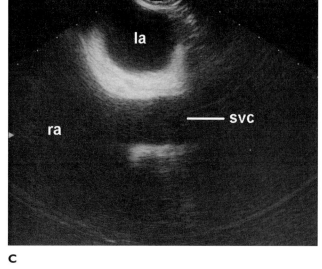

**C**

**Figure 6-5.** Curved linear array view through the mid-esophagus of the subcarinal region. (A) Shows the left atrium (*LA*) next to the right pulmonary artery (*rpa*) with the ascending aorta (*AA*) lying deep to these structures. (B) Further clockwise rotation brings the superior vena cava (*svc*) into view. (C) The superior vena cava can sometimes be followed draining into the right atrium (*ra*).

**B**

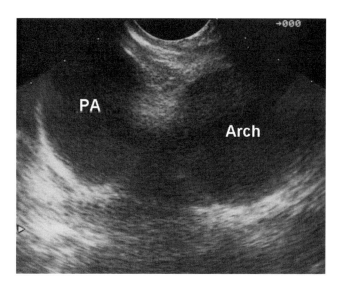

**Figure 6-6.** Curved linear array view through the mid-upper esophagus of the aortic arch (*Arch*) and pulmonary artery (*PA*).

clockwise, the ultrasonically impenetrable spine comes into view. After an approximately 90-degree counterclockwise rotation, the azygos vein is seen as a thin, echolucent structure (Figure 6-9.A). The azygos can usually be followed proximally along its course of drainage to its arch into the superior vena cava by withdrawing the echoendoscope and continuing to gently rotate the echoendoscope a few degrees counterclockwise (Figure 6-9.B). When the echoendoscope is inserted further into the esophagus at the level of the gastroesophageal junction, counterclockwise rotation from the descending aorta will bring the liver into view (Figure 6-10). Again, with some minor right-left rotation of the shaft of the echoendoscope, the hepatic veins can be followed as they drain from the liver into the inferior vena cava, which can then be followed into the right atrium. Portions of the right lung may obscure the view of the inferior vena cava/right atrial junction.

## The Stomach

In the stomach, the abdominal aorta represents the home-base structure for the endosonographer (Figure 6-1.B). After entering into the stomach, the echoendoscope can be pulled up to just below the gastroesophageal junction and rotated right or left until the

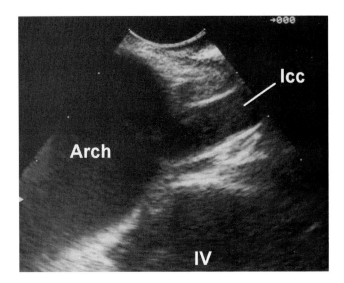

**Figure 6-7.** Curved linear array view through the midupper esophagus of the aortic arch (*Arch*) with the left common carotid (*lcc*) coming out of the arch. The innominate vein (*IV*) is visible deep to the aortic arch.

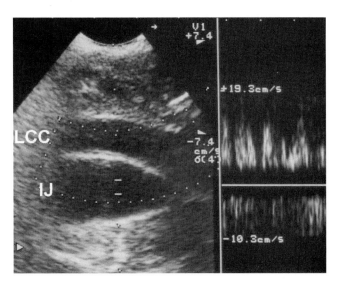

**Figure 6-8.** Curved linear array view through the upper esophagus of the left common carotid (*LCC*) and deeper left jugular vein (*LJ*). Doppler wave form of the internal jugular vein shows the typical sawtooth pattern of a systemic vein.

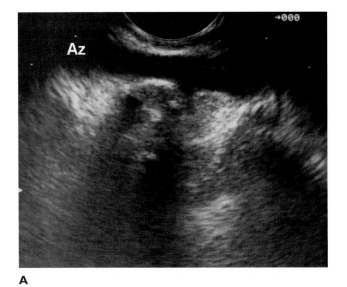

**A**

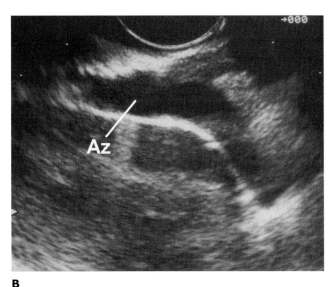

**B**

**Figure 6-9.** (A) Curved linear array view through the midesophagus of the azygous vein (*Az*). (B) Curved linear array view through the upper esophagus of the azygous (*Az*) arch as it sweeps anteriorly toward the superior vena cava.

abdominal aorta comes into view (Figure 6-11). Between the gastric wall and the aorta, the crus of the diaphragm will usually be seen. Depending on the patient's habitus, the crus can be quite subtle or appear very large, resulting in the novice endosonographer confusing it with a mass lesion, lymph node, or the left adrenal gland. This can be avoided by rotating the scope shaft right to left and following the course of the crus proximally across the aorta toward the patient's left. From the upper abdominal aorta, the echoendoscope is then advanced directly into the stomach, while keeping the aorta in view with slight right-left rotations on the shaft of the echoendoscope or the use of the tip

deflection controls. The abdominal aorta will usually appear to be moving away from the wall of the stomach, and after a few centimeters of insertion two major vessels will be seen coming off the abdominal aorta toward the echoendoscope (Figure 6-12). The most proximal vessel is the celiac artery and the more distal represents the superior mesenteric artery. The superior mesenteric branch usually comes off at a more acute angle from the aorta than does the celiac artery. Once the celiac trunk is identified, the echoendoscope can be withdrawn about two centimeters and then rotated clockwise a few degrees to bring the left adrenal gland into view (Figure 6-13). The left adrenal gland can be

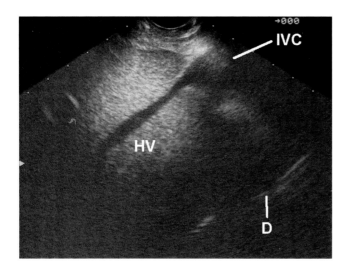

**Figure 6-10.** Curved linear array view through the cardia of the liver with a hepatic vein (*HV*) draining into the inferior vena cava (*IVC*). The diaphragm (*D)* is seen deep to the liver.

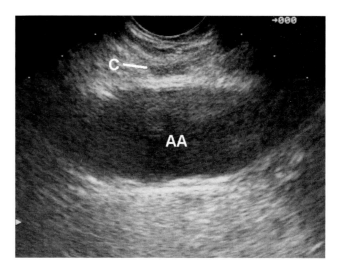

**Figure 6-11.** Curved linear array view through the cardia of the abdominal aorta (*AA*) with the left diaphragmatic crus (*C*) between the lumen and the aorta. This is "home base" for the stomach.

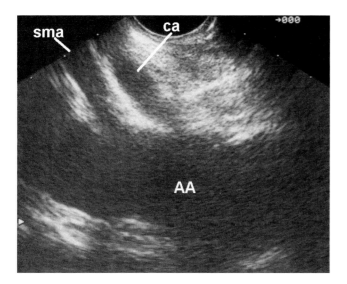

**Figure 6-12.** Curved linear array view through the gastric fundus of the abdominal aorta (*AA*) and the origins of the celiac artery (*ca*) and superior mesenteric artery (*sma*).

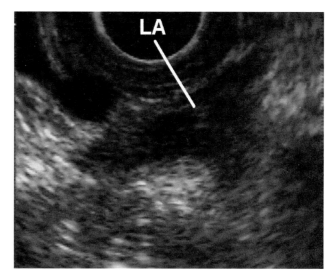

**Figure 6-13.** Curved linear array view of the left adrenal (*LA*). Image was produced using the Olympus curved linear array GF-UC20P echoendoscope at 7.5 MHz (courtesy of Kenneth J. Chang, M.D.).

quite subtle in its appearance and is usually not as prominent on linear endosonography as it is on radial endosonography. Also, it typically appears as a more longitudinal, stripe-like structure rather than the "seagull" shape sometimes seen on radial endosonography (5). After examining the left adrenal gland, the echoendoscope is repositioned over the abdominal aorta and advanced further down the aorta to the celiac artery. At the level of the celiac artery, the shaft of the echoendoscope is rotated at least 90 degrees right and left to look for any celiac adenopathy. From this level, with the patient on his or her left side, rotation of the echoendoscope shaft clockwise will bring the left retroperitoneal structures into view. Rotation of the echoendoscope shaft counterclockwise will demonstrate the left lobe of

the liver adjacent to the lesser curve and anterior wall of the stomach. If the echoendoscope is advanced deeper into the stomach just beyond the level of the celiac artery, the neck of the pancreas will come into view (Figure 6-14). Rotating the shaft of the echoendoscope toward the right and slightly withdrawing the instrument will move the body and tail of the pancreas progressively into view (Figure 6-15). Two or more vessels may be seen running deep to the pancreas in cross section. The smaller, rounder, and most proximal vessel is usually the splenic artery. The larger vessel that runs just below the pancreas is the splenic vein. Depending on the patient's anatomy, the left renal vein and artery may also be seen deep and more distal to the

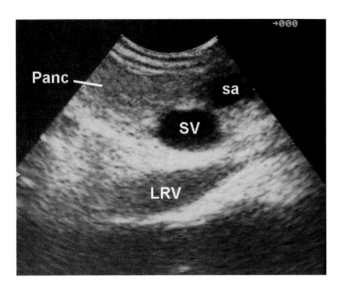

**Figure 6-14.** Curved linear array view through the gastric body of the pancreatic neck (*Panc*). The splenic artery (*sa*) and splenic vein (*SV*) lie deep to the pancreas, and the left renal vein (*LRV*) lies below these.

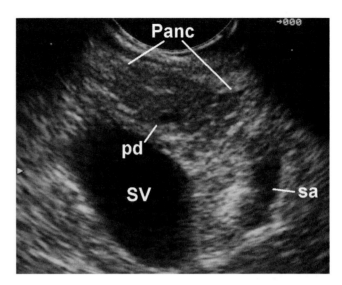

**Figure 6-15.** Curved linear array view of the pancreatic body (*Panc*) with the pancreatic duct (*pd*) seen in cross section above the splenic vein (*SV*) and splenic artery (*sa*).

splenic vein (Figure 6-14). The normal pancreatic duct measures only 1 to 2 mm in diameter and is seen as only an echolucent dot in cross section on linear examination of the pancreatic neck, body, and tail (Figure 6-15). Thus, it can be quite difficult to identify at times. From the level of the pancreatic neck, counterclockwise rotation of the echoendoscope brings the left lobe and part of the portal region of the liver into view. The spleen is typically examined by identifying the pancreas and then rotating the echoendoscope clockwise with continued withdrawal while following the splenic vein. The splenic vein will lead to the splenic hilum (Figure 6-16). Insertion of the echoendoscope deep into the antrum usually does not demonstrate any new organs except for portions of the gallbladder in some patients and more of the liver parenchyma.

## The Duodenum

Linear duodenal anatomy usually presents the beginning endosonographer with the most difficulty because of the variety of anatomic structures seen and the normal variations that commonly exist. Home base in the duodenum is best oriented around the ampulla (Figure 6-1.B). The echoendoscope is inserted deeply into the second portion of the duodenum and the ampullary region located with the partially side-viewing optics of the echoendoscope. Once the ampulla is localized, the echoendoscope transducer is placed directly over the ampulla with some slight right-left rotation of the echoendoscope to bring the origins of the common bile duct and pancreatic duct into view (Figure 6-17). The parenchyma of the pancreatic head and uncinate por-

tion of the pancreas can then be examined by right-left rotation of the shaft, tip deflection, or slight insertion and withdrawal of the echoendoscope. In linear endosonography, the common bile duct and pancreatic ducts usually appear in cross section. The common bile duct is closer to the duodenal wall than the pancreatic duct and, typically being larger than the pancreatic duct, is the more easily followed structure. The relative echolucency of the ventral pancreas seen by radial mechanical endosonography (6) is less apparent on curved linear array endosonography. On withdrawing the echoendoscope toward the first portion of the duodenum, the common bile duct is kept in view by slight, progressive counterclockwise rotation of the shaft of the echoendoscope. Deep to the common bile duct and pancreatic parenchyma, a cross-sectional view of the superior mesenteric vein, which merges into the portal vein, is obtained (Figure 6-18). On reaching the junction between the first and second portion of the duodenum, continued counterclockwise rotation of the echoendoscope will sweep the ultrasonographic view up the porta hepatis toward the hilum of the liver. If the common bile duct has been carefully followed from the ampulla, it is usually fairly simple to identify the other structures of the porta hepatis that appear, such as the hepatic artery, the origins of the gastroduodenal artery, and the much larger and deeper portal vein (Figure 6-19.C). Doppler or color-flow examination can also be used to help differentiate these structures (Figures 6-19.A, 6-19.B). If the echoendoscope is rotated counterclockwise even further, the gallbladder usually comes into view (Figure 6-20); however, its location can be quite variable and the gallbladder may best be seen from deep in the duodenum, duodenal bulb, or antrum.

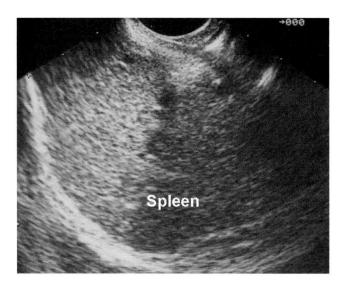

**Figure 6-16.** Curved linear array view through the gastric fundus of the spleen.

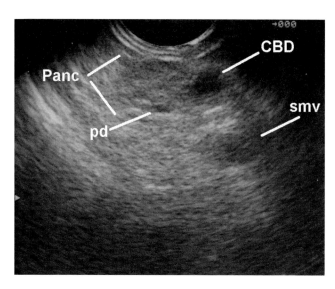

**Figure 6-17.** Curved linear array view through the second portion of the duodenum at the level of the ampulla. The ventral pancreas is in view with cross sections of the pancreatic duct (*pd*), common bile duct (*CBD*), and superior mesenteric vein (*smv*). This is home base for the duodenum.

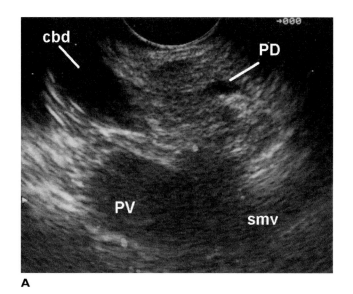

A

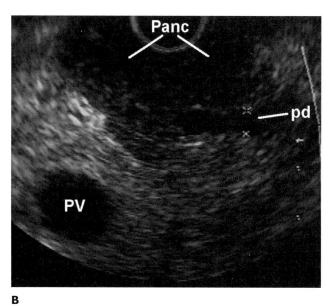

B

**Figure 6-18.** (A) Curved linear array views through the proximal second portion of the duodenum showing common bile duct (*cbd*), pancreatic duct (*PD*), portal vein (*PV*), and superior mesenteric vein (*smv*). (B) Similar view produced with the Olympus curved linear array GF-UC30P echoendoscope (courtesy of Kenneth J. Chang, M.D.).

Rotation of the echoendoscope back toward the right follows the porta hepatis down the distal common bile duct and will bring the head of the pancreas again into view. This is an important maneuver when trying to localize pancreatic carcinomas of the head of the pancreas for endoscopic ultrasound-guided fine-needle aspiration and for assessing the relationship between the pancreatic cancer and the portal and superior mesenteric veins. The echoendoscope sometimes has to be inserted very deep into the second and third portions of

the duodenum with downward deflection of the controls to bring the deep portion of the uncinate pancreas into view (Figure 6-21).

## The Rectum

Linear anatomy in the rectum (Figure 6-1.C) obviously differs between males and females. To start the examination, the echoendoscope is usually inserted to the mid-

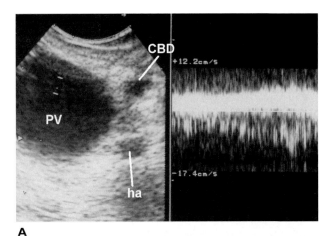

A

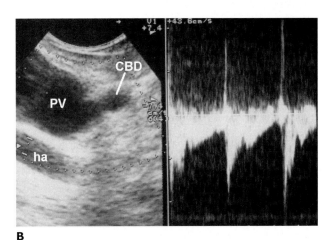

B

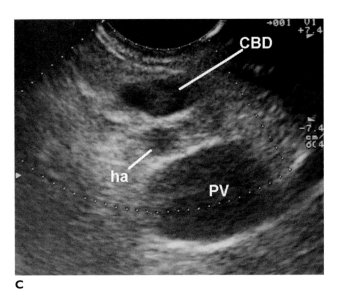

C

**Figure 6-19.** Curved linear array views through the proximal second portion of the duodenum showing the relationship between the common bile duct (*CBD*), hepatic artery (*ha*), and portal vein (*PV*). (A) Shows the Doppler tracing of the portal vein with the typical uniform flow of a splanchnic vein . (B) Shows the Doppler tracing of the hepatic artery. (C) Shows the hepatic artery between the common bile duct and deeper portal vein.

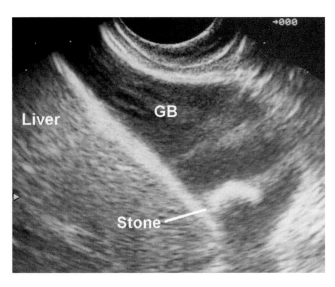

**Figure 6-20.** Curved linear view of the gallbladder (*GB*) with a gallstone in it with posterior shadowing.

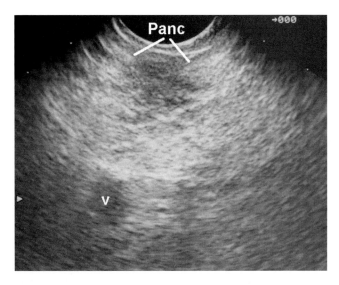

**Figure 6-21.** Curved linear array view of uncinate portion of pancreas (*Panc*) with a mesenteric vessel (*v*) deep to the pancreas.

sigmoid colon and then withdrawn. The first structures to come into view will be cross-sectional images of the iliac vessels (Figure 6-22). These can be seen anywhere from 15 to 25 cm from the anus, depending on the orientation of the sigmoid colon. In males, withdrawal of the echoendoscope to approximately 8 to 10 cm in the rectum, with rotation to the right or left, will bring the easily identified anterior prostate into view anteriorly (Figure 6-23). Withdrawal of the echoendoscope distally from the prostate reveals a short portion of the membranous urethra diving away from the lumen of the rectum toward the base of the penis (Figure 6-24). Proximal to the prostate lie the seminal vesicles arising to the right

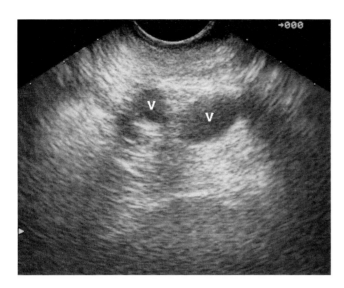

**Figure 6-22.** Curved linear array view of sigmoid colon at pelvic rim. Here internal iliac vessels (*v*) are seen in cross section.

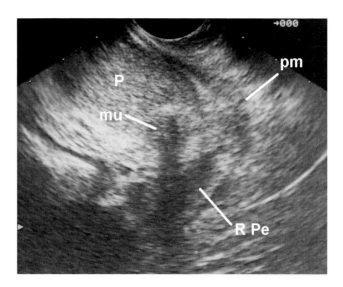

**Figure 6-24.** Curved linear array view of the distal prostate (*P*). The membranous urethra (*mu*) runs from the prostate through the peroneal membrane to the root of the penis (*R Pe*).

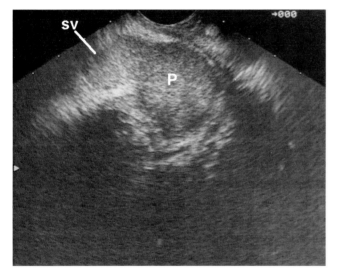

**Figure 6-23.** Curved linear array view of the prostate (*P*) and the more proximal seminal vesicles (*sv*).

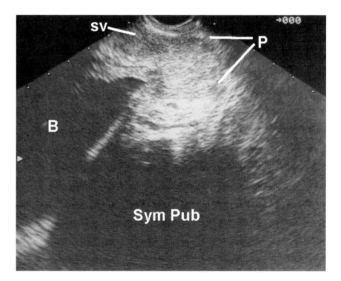

**Figure 6-25.** Curved linear array view of the proximal prostate (*P*) with some echogenic calcifications within it. Proximal to the prostate lies the seminal vesicle (*sv*) with the bladder (*B*) deep to it.

and left of the prostate, with the bladder seen more proximally and deep to the seminal vesicles (Figure 6-25). In older men, the prostate often contains bright echos from small calcifications.

In females, withdrawal of the echoendoscope from the sigmoid colon will bring the uterus into view with the deeper and more proximal bladder (Figure 6-26.A). Sometimes the left or right adnexal structures can also be seen on deep insertion near the pelvic rim vessels. Withdrawal from the level of the uterus will show the subtle stripe of the vagina anteriorly, with the urethra seen deep to the vagina (Figure 6-26.B). The anal

sphincters are more difficult to assess with linear endosonography than by radial endosonography. The internal sphincter is seen as an echolucent layer just deep to the bright anal mucosal layer. Deep to the internal sphincter, the external sphincter blends into the other muscle layers of the levator ani complex (Figure 6-27).

## Conclusion

Because linear endosonography has become the standard format for performing most invasive endosonog-

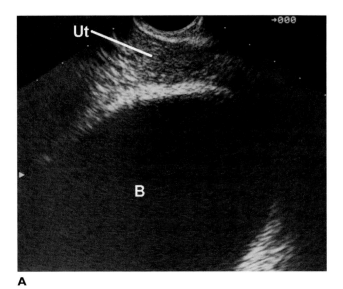

**A**

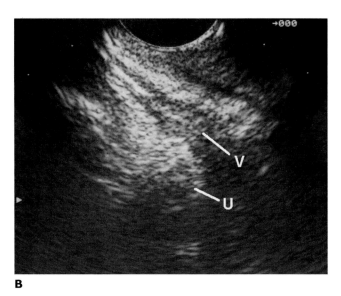

**B**

**Figure 6-26.** Curved linear array views of the female rectum. (A) The uterus (*Ut*) with the deeper bladder (*B*). (B) Distal to the uterus, the vagina (*V*) appears as a longitudinal echolucent stripe with a bright central stripe caused by the air within the vagina. The urethra (*U*) may be seen in longitudinal cross section deep to the vagina.

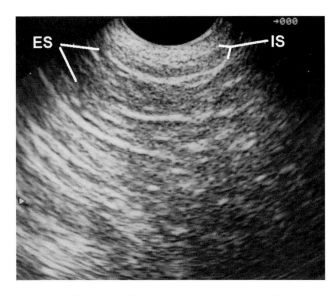

**Figure 6-27.** Curved linear array view of anus. The internal sphincter (*IS*) appears as the first echolucent layer in the anal canal with the thicker and more homogeneous external sphincter (*ES*) visualized deep to the internal sphincter.

**References**
1. Gress FG, Hawes RH, Savides TJ, et al. Endoscopic ultrasound-guided fine-needle aspiration biopsy using linear array and radial scanning endosonography. Gastrointest Endosc 1997;45:243–250.
2. Villman P, Hancke S. Endoscopic ultrasound scanning of the upper gastrointestinal tract using a curved linear array transducer: "the linear anatomy." Gastrointest Endosc Clin North Am 1995;5:507–521.
3. Gress F, Hawes R, Ikenberry S, Savides T, et al. A prospective randomized comparison of radial scanning and linear array endosonography for staging pancreatic cancer. Gastrointest Endosc 1996;43:423.
4. Lachter J, Rubin A, Shiller M, et al. Linear EUS for bile duct stones. Gastrointest Endosc 2000;51:51–54.
5. Chang KJ, Erickson RA, Nguyen P. Endoscopic ultrasound (EUS) and EUS-guided fine needle aspiration of the left adrenal gland. Gastrointest Endosc 1996; 44:568–572.
6. Savides TJ, Gress FG, Zaidi SA, et al. Detection of embryologic ventral pancreatic parenchyma with endoscopic ultrasound. Gastrointest Endosc 1996;43:14–19.

raphy, mastering linear endosonographic anatomy is necessary for the physician interested in advanced endosonography. As with radial endosonography, a consistent and systematic approach to identifying each anatomic structure will make for a rapid and thorough endosonographic examination.

# 7

# Endoscopic Ultrasound of the Esophagus

## Paul Fockens

Locoregional staging of esophageal cancer is the most widely accepted indication for endoscopic ultrasound. As a consequence, esophageal EUS is the most frequently performed EUS examination worldwide. Esophageal EUS is probably also one of the easiest of all EUS examinations. The fact that the esophagus runs down as a straight tube from the upper sphincter to the diaphragm makes positioning of the instrument relatively easy and artifacts due to tangential imaging rare. With a water-filled balloon there is almost always good acoustic coupling between transducer and the esophageal wall. Furthermore, the mediastinal anatomy is relatively simple, especially directly adjacent to the esophagus, with the aorta always clearly visible serving as a landmark for easy orientation.

Although esophageal EUS seems to be the easiest EUS examination, studies suggest that it is necessary to perform more than 100 examinations to become accurate in the staging of esophageal carcinoma (1). This data illustrates the fact that EUS in general is one of the most difficult endoscopic procedures to perform and interpretation of results is equally complex. It is likely that the availability of EUS will remain limited for some time until the necessary skills are more generally available. In this chapter we will discuss the indications for EUS of the esophagus (excluding the topic of submucosal tumors) (see Chapter 9). This chapter will cover the role of EUS in evaluating benign as well as malignant disease of the esophagus and will focus on the clinical impact of EUS for those indications.

## Instruments
### Radial Scanning

In the esophagus the radial scanning instruments are most commonly used. They provide a penetration of 6 cm at 7.5 MHz, which makes the entire posterior mediastinum visible. The current standard is the radial scanning echoendoscope (Olympus GF-UM130), a video instrument with a second frequency of 12 MHz that is especially useful for mural abnormalities. The higher resolution has the disadvantage of providing lower tissue penetration (only 2.5 to 3 cm). A more recent addition to the spectrum of EUS equipment is a video-echoendoscope with switchable 7.5 MHz and 20 MHz frequencies (GF-UMQ130, Olympus America). This ultra-high frequency has even more limited penetration, but the extreme high resolution of the 20 MHz frequency enables visualization of a clear nine-layer esophageal wall structure with separate delineation of the mucosal muscle layer as a fourth, hypoechoic layer (2). This instrument is therefore especially useful for early tumors of the esophageal wall and for evaluating Barrett's esophagus.

Another important instrument for esophageal EUS is the 8 mm blind probe (Olympus MH-908 or esophagoprobe). At the tip of this instrument a small bougie has been attached that allows passage of a guide wire. This instrument has a 7.5 MHz frequency only and is especially useful for stenotic esophageal tumors. It allows clear delineation of the outer border of the tumor. The steerable tip allows for adequate maneuvering in the stomach, which is necessary to image the celiac trunk. Staging accuracy was reported to be similar to that of the standard conventional instrument (3). Before this instrument became available, 25% or more of all esophageal carcinomas did not allow passage of an echoendoscope, resulting in incomplete staging in these patients. Dilatation of a tumor to allow a complete study has been reported to be associated with a high risk of perforation. In one of the published series the perforation rate for diagnostic EUS in this setting was 25%—clearly unacceptable for a diagnostic procedure

(4). With the esophagoprobe, however, almost every tumor can now be staged once a guide wire has been passed through the stricture.

### Curved Linear Array

The curved linear array instruments are not ideal for diagnostic esophageal EUS, and particularly not for esophageal cancer staging. To obtain a thorough exam, it is necessary to stop passage of the curved linear array scope at 3- to 5-cm intervals to rotate the shaft of the instrument 360 degrees to image every part of the mediastinum and every possible lymph node site. As might be expected, this becomes a very time-consuming procedure. The curved linear array instrument is more appropriate for EUS-guided fine-needle aspiration biopsy of the mediastinum. Although EUS-guided FNA has also been recently reported with the rotating sector or radial scanners with equal accuracy, the increased risk of complications makes this instrument less appropriate for fine-needle aspiration biopsy (5). The details of EUS-guided FNA are more thoroughly discussed in Chapter 12.

### Miniprobes

Miniprobes that can be advanced through the working channel of an ordinary endoscope can also be very useful in the esophagus. They can be used with both early and advanced disease. In early disease they often achieve superior resolution due to their high frequencies. In advanced disease they have the advantage of a small diameter, allowing passage through stenotic tumors. In fact, in patients with small lesions and those with esophageal varices the miniprobes may well be the preferred instrument. The balloon-filled tip of a standard echoendoscope stretches the esophageal wall around the instrument and may compress small abnormalities and distort normal anatomy. In contrast, miniprobes allow visualization of the esophageal wall with its normal folds intact. With gentle instillation of some water into the esophagus, miniprobes usually allow generation of an adequate 360-degree image. Care, however, has to be taken to prevent patients from aspirating during miniprobe use, and some investigators have experimented with balloons in the proximal esophagus to reduce aspiration risk. Such systems are still under investigation and are not commercially available. Balloon sheaths for the miniprobes are also available and they provide good acoustic coupling of the transducer with the esophageal wall; however, compression artifacts can be introduced (6). In advanced lesions, the miniprobes can usually be inserted through the tumor stenosis without much difficulty. With the improved resolution and penetration of the 12-MHz miniprobes, it is now usually possible to accurately visualize the outer margins of a tumor. Unfortunately, in terms of tumor staging, the celiac trunk is only rarely visible with the miniprobes because tip deflection is lacking and the high frequencies used limit penetration of the ultrasound waves beyond 2 to 3 cms.

### Three-Dimensional EUS

Three-dimensional reconstruction of EUS images is a new and promising area of research in EUS imaging of the esophagus and mediastinum. In the two commercially-developed systems now available, a miniprobe is automatically pulled back through a shaft that remains in the same position in the esophagus (7). The images that are sequentially collected at intervals of 1 millimeter or less are then reconstructed by the 3D image processor and displayed as a 3D reconstruction. Even after the patient has already left the examination room, the examiner can still look at different slices and different areas of the electronically reconstructed image. The benefits of this 3D technology to the surgeon are obvious, and it is also a useful teaching tool when reviewed in a multidisciplinary setting together with a radiologist. The ability to accurately demonstrate and review the entire EUS examination will markedly accelerate the acceptance of EUS as a necessary imaging modality for esophageal disease.

## Technique

EUS examinations typically start with a patient in the left lateral position. Conscious sedation is commonly used although it may not always be necessary; for staging esophageal cancer, the examination usually does not last longer than 15 minutes in experienced hands. The most difficult part of the examination is insertion of the scope tip into the proximal esophagus. After the instrument has been introduced, the fact that only minimal movement of the instrument is needed and air insufflation is limited makes the procedure more comfortable for a patient than an ordinary endoscopy. In our practice, about half of all esophageal EUS examinations are currently performed with topical pharyngeal anesthesia only. The specific technique used for an EUS study depends on the indication for the examination. EUS of the esophagus is usually a targeted procedure. Often it is being performed on a patient in whom a histological diagnosis is already available or to better delineate a specific area of interest defined by earlier studies. Depending on the indication, only a predetermined number of areas are ultrasonically scanned. For staging esophageal cancer, the endoscope is also introduced into the stomach to visualize the celiac trunk (Figure 7-1). It is uncommon and very time consuming to perform a complete EUS examination of the upper gastrointestinal tract and surrounding organs in most patients.

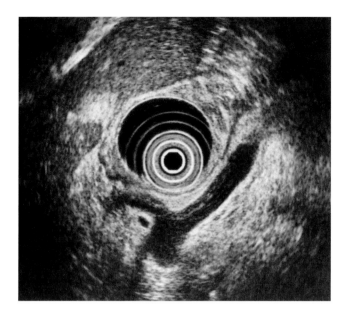

**Figure 7-1.** Typical image of the celiac trunk from which splenic artery and hepatic artery branch off (seagull sign).

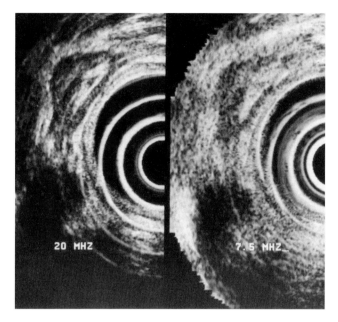

**Figure 7-2.** Two EUS images of the same benign subcarinal lymph node, one taken at 20 MHz, one taken at 7.5 MHz. Note the difference in border, which becomes sharper at higher frequencies.

## Extrinsic Impressions and Mediastinal Tumors

The origin of esophageal impressions caused by extrinsic compression can be difficult to determine on an endoscopic image but relatively simple during an EUS study. In the spectrum of esophageal submucosal lesions, leiomyomas, granular cell tumors, and duplication cysts are among the most common, and these and others are thoroughly discussed in Chapter 9 on submucosal tumors. Extrinsic compression of the esophagus from mediastinal pathology can originate from a wide spectrum of benign or malignant adenopathy, such as primary lung tumors, bronchogenic cysts, and other relatively rare abnormalities. EUS can reliably image the entire posterior mediastinum when the 7.5 MHz frequency is used. It is usually possible to image the mediastinum from the diaphragm proximally to the upper esophageal sphincter. However, patient tolerance of the filled echoendoscope balloon in the esophagus proximal to the aortic arch is a practical limitation.

Lymph nodes in the mediastinum are very common in patients with suspected or known carcinoma as well as in healthy persons. They can be associated with tuberculosis, histoplasmosis, and Hodgkin's or non-Hodgkin's lymphoma (8). The typical image of a benign mediastinal lymph node is that of an oval or crescent-shaped hypoechoic structure, which is rather poorly demarcated at the standard frequency of 7.5 MHz. The center of such nodes is usually hyperechoic and sometimes a small anechoic area can be seen in the very center of the hyperechoic region, representing the hilar part of the node (Figure 7-2) (9). The most frequent location for lymph nodes is the subcarinal area where multiple nodes can be ventrally draping the esophagus. Malignant metastatic lymph nodes are usually hypoechoic and round and only rarely cause an impression on the esophageal lumen. Although differentiation between malignant and benign nodes can be attempted on the basis of the endosonographic image, EUS-guided FNA is necessary in almost all cases for a definitive diagnosis.

When a primary lung mass creates an impression on the esophagus, diagnostic EUS will usually separate benign from malignant disease. In patients with lung cancer, large, hypoechoic, inhomogeneous tumors with irregular margins are usually seen and a biopsy should be performed (Figure 7-3). If an echoendoscope for EUS-guided FNA biopsy is not available, it is also possible to perform an endoscopy-guided biopsy through a standard endoscope after diagnostic EUS with a reported accuracy of 85% (10). Special 19-gauge needles with a needle tip length of 1 cm have been developed for this purpose.

Bronchogenic cysts are usually benign, although malignant degeneration has been described. The EUS image is that of a smooth, clearly delineated, round tumor with a homogeneous echo pattern. Although usually very hypoechoic or even anechoic, a bronchogenic cyst may also show a homogeneous pattern of intermediate echogenicity. This may be the result of bleeding inside the cyst or due to other echogenic features of the cyst fluid.

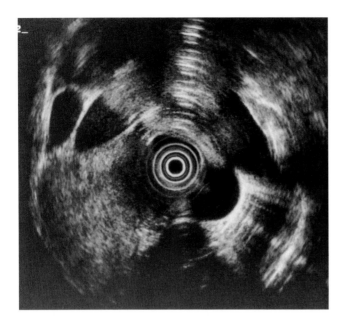

**Figure 7-3.** Large, hypoechoic mediastinal mass (between seven and nine o'clock) which gives an impression in the distal esophagus. After characterization with EUS, FNA biopsy was performed with a standard endoscope showing nonsmall cell lung cancer.

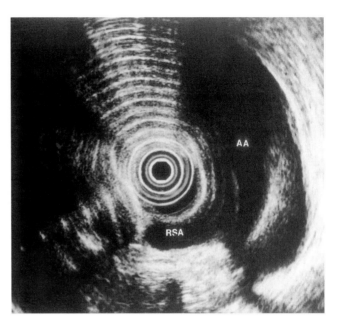

**Figure 7-4.** Aortic arch (*AA*) from which the right subclavian artery (*RSA*) branches off and passage dorsal to the esophagus. This congenital malformation is known as a *lusorian artery.*

When the right subclavian artery crosses behind the esophagus instead of in front it is referred to as a *lusorian artery* (Figure 7-4). This congenital anomaly can sometimes cause symptoms of impaired food passage—*dysphagia lusoria.* This rare diagnosis was made in 6 (0.37%) of 1629 patients who had esophageal EUS when the exam included the region above the aortic arch (11).

## Gastroesophageal Reflux Disease and Barrett's Esophagus

Some studies have been performed investigating the role of EUS in gastroesophageal reflux disease (GERD) (12,13). At this time, it is unclear if there is any need for another imaging modality for reflux disease. Although it is well known that the degree of endoscopic abnormalities does not correlate with symptoms, it is difficult to imagine that EUS will give a better correlation than conventional endoscopy, because EUS findings would be dependent on transmural inflammation. In addition, a 24-hour pH study already offers a method to correlate symptoms with findings. EUS studies performed in patients with GERD have shown that patients with severe esophagitis have a relatively thick esophageal wall. In one study, wall thickening was correlated with decreased lower esophageal sphincter pressure, suggesting that inflammatory damage to the muscle layer of the lower esophagus had impaired sphincter function (12).

Barrett's esophagus is a premalignant condition in which the distal esophagus is lined with metaplastic columnar epithelium. Regular endoscopic surveillance with biopsies is recommended in most patients. When high-grade dysplasia is detected and confirmed by a second pathologist, an esophagectomy is generally recommended because of the high risk of development of an infiltrative malignancy. In fact, in patients who have high-grade dysplasia and undergo resection, up to 50% of resection specimens demonstrate the presence of invasive cancer not detected by endoscopic biopsy.

The clinical role of endosonography in Barrett's esophagus includes the early detection—or exclusion—of invasive carcinomas in patients with high-grade dysplasia. If successful, EUS would allow more accurate patient selection for this major and irreversible surgical procedure (esophageal resection and reconstruction with a gastric pull-up or large bowel interposition).

Two published reports with standard EUS instruments and one with miniprobes have examined the esophageal wall of patients who have Barrett's esophagus with or without dysplasia. These studies showed that in fact it was possible to detect Barrett's esophagus with EUS on the basis of slight wall thickening and a more clearly visible wall layer pattern. Unfortunately, it was not possible to reliably detect or exclude invasive cancer (14–16). Using high-frequency miniprobes (20 MHz or more), it is possible to define the esophageal wall and identify a nine-layer pattern. The fourth layer represents the second mucosal muscle layer, the site of Barrett's and its malignant transformation. The ability to use EUS echoendoscopes or miniprobes to define groups of patients with Barrett's esophagus who are most likely to benefit from surgical resection awaits more experience with high-frequency echoendoscopes and miniprobes as well as more operator experience with interpretation of the complex images that are generated.

## Motility Disorders

EUS has the unique ability to separately image the two layers of the muscularis propria in vivo. At frequencies of 12 MHz and higher, the fourth layer in the five-layer esophageal wall can be seen as two hypoechoic layers separated by a thin hyperechoic layer. When a normal esophageal wall is examined during peristalsis, a relative thickening of the inner (circular) layer of the muscularis propria occurs with resulting narrowing of the esophageal lumen. The outer layer of the muscularis (the longitudinal layer) maintains a more constant diameter. In the early EUS literature conflicting reports appeared about the thickness of the muscularis propria in patients with achalasia. Occasionally, definite thickening of the inner muscle layer was seen but in other patients no specific abnormalities could be detected. In an interesting study from Cleveland, EUS was performed with the radial scanning echoendoscope in 17 patients with manometrically confirmed achalasia and in six healthy volunteers (17). It was shown that there was a slight increase in esophageal wall thickening, especially 3 to 4 cm above the lower esophageal sphincter in patients with achalasia. However, artifacts due to tangential imaging of the esophageal wall in patients with longstanding achalasia were common. Puckering of folds just proximal to an area of stenosis was another source of error. Patients with secondary achalasia were not included in the study.

Another possible use of the echoendoscope in patients with achalasia was described by Hoffman et al. (18). They used a linear array echoendoscope to guide endoscopic injection of botulinum toxin precisely into the circular muscle layer. Their hypothesis was that these EUS-guided injections could be more effective in blocking neural transmission and reducing symptoms than the usual "blind injections" done during routine endoscopy. Though long-term results are not yet available, it is hoped that the effect of such EUS-guided injection therapy will be more durable as well.

Other motility disorders such as nutcracker esophagus have also been studied and muscle layer thickening has been described in different conditions (19,20). In fact, EUS may become a useful adjunct research tool for a variety of poorly characterized esophageal motility disorders. Even at this early stage, it is clear that for this research to succeed, miniprobes—either linear or radial scanning—are needed to minimize any disturbance of normal physiological function during the EUS examination.

## Varices

Endoscopic ultrasonography can visualize a large part of the portal circulation. In most patients the portal vein, splenic vein, spleen, and azygos vein can be accurately delineated. Gastric or esophageal varices, perigastric or peri-esophageal collaterals, and even portal hypertensive gastropathy can be demonstrated with EUS. Using standard echoendoscopes, the sensitivity for detection of esophageal varices seems to be slightly inferior to endoscopy (due to balloon compression of varices), but EUS with miniprobes reduces the false negative rate. Possible clinical indications for EUS in this setting include the confirmation of eradication of varices after sclerotherapy or banding. In a prospective study on this subject, EUS was performed before elective sclerotherapy and after endoscopy had suggested complete variceal obliteration in the esophagus (21). Seventeen percent of patients had esophageal varices identified by EUS even when routine endoscopy was negative. With the help of the Doppler mode available on linear array instruments, studies on the changes in flow and volume of the azygos vein and other vessels can now be performed as a minimally invasive technique (22,23). Aside from such research interests, however, the clinical role for EUS in patients with varices and portal hypertension is as yet unclear.

## Esophageal Carcinoma
### TNM-Staging System

Esophageal carcinoma is usually classified according to the TNM stage. In the TNM classification the T-stage represents the primary tumor, the N-stage the locoregional lymph node status, and the M-stage represents the presence or absence of distant metastases. In 1997, the fifth edition of the TNM classification was published (Table 7-1) (24). The T-stage classification remained unchanged with T1 for mucosal (T1a) or submucosal invasion (T1b) (Figure 7-5). T2 tumors have infiltrated the muscularis propria and T3 tumors have penetrated completely through that muscle layer (Figure 7-6). In stage T4 the tumor extends into an adjacent organ such as the aorta, liver, lung, trachea, pericardium, or diaphragm (Figure 7-7). The N-stage was not changed (N0 designates the absence of regional lymph node metastases, N1 designates the presence of regional lymph node metastases), but in the M-stage the presence of lymph nodes close by or far away from the tumor is now also reported. In patients with a tumor in the distal esophagus, stage M1a represents lymph nodes at the celiac axis, and stage M1b represents all other distant metastases. In patients with a tumor in the proximal esophagus stage M1a is reserved for cervical lymph node metastases and M1b for all other distant

**Table 7.1.** TNM classification system.

| | |
|---|---|
| **T 1 a** | Tumor in mucosal layer only |
| **T 1 b** | Infiltration in submucosa |
| **T 2** | Infiltration in muscularis propria |
| **T 3** | Infiltration through muscularis propria |
| **T 4** | Infiltration in adjacent organ |
| **N 0** | Locoregional lymph node metastases absent |
| **N 1** | Locoregional lymph node metastases present |
| **M 0** | No distant metastases |

**Proximal Esophageal Tumors**

| | |
|---|---|
| **M 1 a** | Lymph node metastases in cervical area |
| **M 1 b** | All other distant metastases |

**Middle Esophageal Tumors**

| | |
|---|---|
| **M 1 b** | All distant metastases |

**Distal Esophageal Tumors**

| | |
|---|---|
| **M 1 a** | Lymph node metastases near celiac trunk |
| **M 1 b** | All other distant metastases |

*Source: TNM Classification of Malignant Tumors,* 5th ed. New York: Wiley-Liss, 1997.

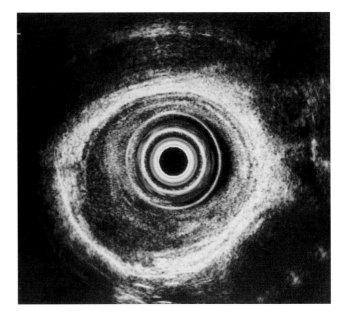

**Figure 7-6.** Esophageal tumor with interrupted muscularis propria and clear, irregular margin between six and nine o'clock. The EUS image suggests stage T3.

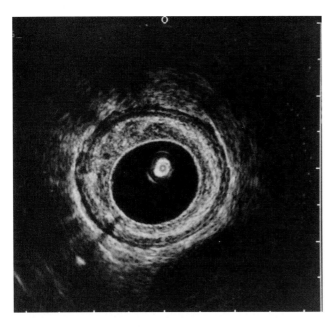

**Figure 7-5.** Balloon-fitted 20 MHz miniprobe image of a T1b Barrett's carcinoma (between eight and one o'clock). The submucosa is thinner in the area of the tumor, suggesting submucosal infiltration. The muscularis propria is seen to consist of three layers with this frequency.

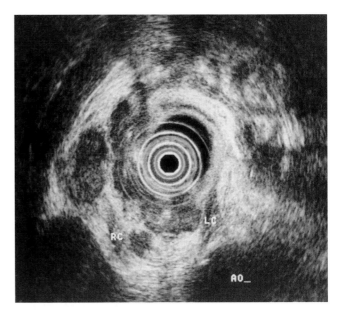

**Figure 7-7.** Cardiacarcinoma with suspicion of infiltration in the right crus of the diaphragm (RC), stage T4. The left crus (LC) and aorta (AO) seem to be free of tumor infiltration.

metastases. Patients with a tumor in the middle part of the esophagus and cervical lymph nodes, celiac trunk nodes, or other distant metastases are all classified as stage M1b, with no stage M1a classification available.

## Preoperative T-Staging

Locoregional staging of esophageal carcinoma has become increasingly important over the past decade as stage-specific treatment protocols combining surgery with neoadjuvant chemotherapy and/or radiotherapy are now routinely used in general practice. As experience with esophageal EUS has grown, it has become clear that locoregional staging can be most accurately performed with endosonography. In the work-up of patients diagnosed with esophageal malignancies, distant metastases are first excluded by CT scanning or transabdominal ultrasound before EUS is performed. EUS staging of esophageal cancer is done by imaging the different layers of the GI tract. Accurate evaluation of the muscularis propria by EUS allows accurate and precise determination of the T-stage of an esophageal cancer. The average accuracy of EUS for T-staging of esophageal carcinoma in more than 1000 patients was 84% (25). In fact, the accuracy of EUS consistently exceeds that observed with CT or MR imaging. All comparative studies between EUS and CT favored EUS, with an average difference in accuracy of more than 20% for both T- and N-stage (26,27).

However, there are some differences in accuracy depending on tumor stage. The accuracy scores for stage T2 esophageal lesions are the lowest (76%), whereas scores for stage T3 reach 92%. The reason for the relatively low accuracy for stage T2 is poorly understood. It may be related to microscopic infiltration of tumors into the muscularis propria that cannot be detected with the current resolution of EUS instruments, resulting in tumor understaging. It may also be caused by peritumorous inflammation leading to overstaging. It is hoped that new instruments operating at a 20-MHz frequency will improve the accuracy in staging T2 tumors through improved resolution with the ability to detect microscopic infiltration. Nevertheless, it might very well be that discrimination of peritumorous inflammation from tumors will always remain difficult, if not impossible, with ultrasound alone.

For T1 esophageal lesions, EUS staging is particularly attractive. As previously noted, with high-frequency miniprobes it is possible to recognize a nine-layer pattern in the normal esophageal wall, with separate delineation of the muscularis mucosae as the fourth layer (2). This fourth layer differentiates between a T1 mucosa (T1a) and T1 submucosa (T1b) tumor. The most important difference between T1a and T1b tumors is the percentage of patients with lymph node metastases. In patients with T1a cancers, lymph node metastases are found in fewer than 10%; the frequency increases to around 50% in T1b tumors (28). For this reason, it is clear that any patient with a T1b tumor will require a surgical resection with lymph node dissection for cure. In T1a tumors local endoscopic mucosal resection (EMR) or other nonsurgical ablative treatments may be considered.

A recent study suggested that the maximal axial diameter of the tumor is one of the most important factors in determining T-stage (29). Differentiation between T1–T2 and T3–T4 was most accurately done by measuring the maximal tumor diameter, which was found to be more accurate than using subjective criteria such as an irregular outer border or interruption of the outer muscle layer (Figure 7-6). A cut-off of 8 mm for overall mass diameter was 89% accurate in differentiation between T1–2 and T3–4 stages. However, differentiation within the T3–4 group was not possible. The staging accuracy of EUS for stage T4 tumors is about 85% in reported series.

The most difficult question—whether endosonographic evidence of unresectability is sufficient to withhold surgery—was addressed in two recent studies. A large retrospective study by Chak et al. looked at a group of 79 patients, endosonographically staged and determined to be unresectable (T4). It was shown that in the entire group the prognosis was very poor, regardless of therapy given (30). The median survival of the entire group was only six months. The surgical group had a similar poor survival (5.2 months) compared to those who underwent nonsurgical therapy (6.6 months). A similar single-center study of 51 patients was recently reported and also did not find a significant difference in survival of surgical verses nonsurgical patients (median survival 9.7 vs. 6.1 months) (31). On the basis of these studies it can be concluded that T-staging by EUS is very helpful in selecting therapy for individual patients with esophageal cancer.

## Preoperative N-Staging

The presence of regional lymph node metastases, (the N-stage of the TNM system), can also be determined with an overall accuracy of 77% (25). The diagnostic interpretation of individual lymph nodes remains difficult, especially because many healthy volunteers have mediastinal lymph nodes identified with EUS (9). A study looking at lymph node characteristics of 100 patients with esophageal carcinoma defined four criteria of importance: size, shape, border demarcation, and a central echo pattern. Of these four EUS features studied, the echo pattern (homogeneous vs. heterogeneous) appeared to be the most sensitive parameter for discriminating malignant from benign nodes. The second most important feature was the lymph node border (sharp vs. fuzzy), followed by shape (round vs. elliptical) and size (greater than 10 mm vs. less than or equal to 10 mm). This study indicates that size alone is a rather insensitive parameter. Malignant lymph nodes were found in 100% of patients studied when all four features were present (Figure 7-8). If mediastinal lymph node status becomes even more important in defining treatment strategies, cytological sampling will also become more important. With the use of a curved array echoendoscope it is possible to sample individual lymph nodes under direct EUS guidance (32). In the mediastinum this technique currently has a sensitivity of more than 90% (33,34). However, there is no reliable method available to sample lymph nodes through a tumor by means of a protected needle (avoiding contamination with known malignant cells). Without such a technique the likelihood of getting false positive results remains unacceptably high.

## Restaging After Neoadjuvant Therapy

It is as yet unclear whether EUS has a role in restaging of patients after neoadjuvant chemo-radiotherapy.

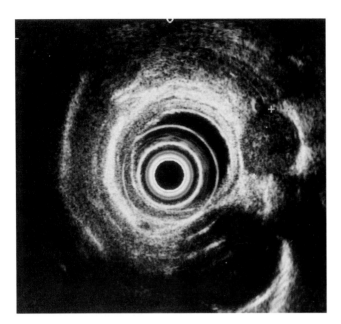

**Figure 7-8.** Patient with a primary esophageal carcinoma who was found to have an enlarged, round, homogeneously hypoechoic, sharply delineated lymph node of 14 mm, suggestive of stage N1.

The side effects of local radiotherapy at the site of the tumor consist of a marked inflammatory reaction that may mimic tumor on EUS. It is not yet possible to distinguish this inflammatory reaction from tumor, and therefore comments can be made only about the tumor volume and not about the individual T-stage after neoadjuvant therapy (35,36). A reduction of the maximal cross-sectional diameter of the tumor of 50% or more can be interpreted as a good response associated with a reasonable probability of downstaging of the tumor. Also, three-dimensional EUS imaging of esophageal tumors is being developed and could be a useful tool for more accurate restaging of esophageal malignancies following neoadjuvant therapy.

### Recurrent Tumors

After surgical resection of an esophageal tumor, continuity is usually reestablished by creation of an anastomosis. Although true anastomotic tumor recurrences are increasingly rare, locoregional recurrences in the mediastinum at the site of the original tumor are common. Whereas CT may have difficulty in detecting such recurrences because of altered postsurgical anatomy, EUS is very accurate in detecting recurrent disease (37). Although early detection is practical, the lack of therapeutic options for these unfortunate patients is usually reason to wait for symptoms before EUS is performed (38).

## Conclusion

The examination and management of esophageal disease has dramatically changed since the introduction of endoscopic ultrasonography. EUS permits accurate imaging of the different layers of the esophageal wall as well as the surrounding mediastinal structures with stunning resolution. Since the introduction of EUS in 1980, it has become possible to investigate patients with esophageal tumors more accurately than ever before. Benign tumors can now be classified and many unnecessary surgical interventions have been prevented. For malignant tumors, EUS has been able to predict prognosis with exceptional reliability and consistency, permitting the design of treatment plans on an individual-patient basis. The lack of effective therapy for advanced tumors has unfortunately not allowed EUS to play a role in improving the prognosis of these patients. In other areas such as motility disorders and portal hypertension, EUS has helped in getting a better understanding of underlying pathophysiology.

Should every gastroenterologist be performing esophageal EUS, the easiest of all EUS examinations? EUS is a difficult procedure that requires extensive training and the answer must be no. As is true for other gastrointestinal procedures, it is necessary to perform a minimum number of EUS examinations annually to maintain competency after completing a formal training program in this area. Thus, esophageal EUS will have to be limited for now to those institutions that have a specific interest and expertise in esophageal disease and also have high patient volume.

Competition for EUS may come from noninvasive imaging with, for example, improved CT or MR technology. Competition can also be expected from invasive methods with an even higher resolution, such as optical coherence tomography. Other imaging methods, such as light-induced fluorescence endoscopy, which may permit tissue recognition without biopsy, can be expected to play an important role in the early detection of malignant degeneration in Barrett's esophagus. Taken together, all of these methodologies already offer physicians and their patients better and safer diagnostic and therapeutic opportunities for patients with esophageal disease.

### References

1. Fockens P, Vandenbrande JHM, Van Dullemen HM, et al. Endosonographic T-staging of esophageal carcinoma: a learning curve. Gastrointest Endosc 1996; 44:58–62.
2. Wiersema MJ, Wiersema LM. High-resolution 25-megahertz ultrasonography of the gastrointestinal wall: histologic correlates. Gastrointest Endosc 1993; 39:499–504.

3. Binmoeller KF, Seifert H, Seitz U, et al. Ultrasonic esophagoprobe for TNM staging of highly stenosing esophageal carcinoma. Gastrointest Endosc 1995; 41:547–552.

4. Catalano MF, Van Dam J, Sivak MV. Malignant esophageal strictures: staging accuracy of endoscopic ultrasonography. Gastrointest Endosc 1995;41:535–539.

5. Gress FG, Hawes RH, Savides TJ, et al. Endoscopic ultrasound-guided fine-needle aspiration biopsy using linear array and radial scanning endosonography. Gastrointest Endosc 1997;45:243–250.

6. Fockens P, Van Dullemen HM, Tytgat GNJ. Endosonography of stenotic esophageal carcinomas: preliminary experience with an ultra-thin, balloon-fitted ultrasound probe in four patients. Gastrointest Endosc 1994;40:226–228.

7. Kallimanis G, Garra B, Tio TL, et al. The feasibility of three-dimensional endoscopic ultrasonography: a preliminary report. Gastrointest Endosc 1995;41:235–239.

8. Wiersema MJ, Chak A, Wiersema LM. Mediastinal histoplasmosis: evaluation with endosonography and endoscopic fine-needle aspiration biopsy. Gastrointest Endosc 1994;40:78–81.

9. Wiersema MJ, Hassig WM, Hawes RH, Wonn MJ. Mediastinal lymph node detection with endosonography. Gastrointest Endosc 1993;39:788–793.

10. Wiersema MJ, Wiersema LM, Khusro Q, et al. Combined endosonography and fine-needle aspiration cytology in the evaluation of gastrointestinal lesions. Gastrointest Endosc 1994;40:199–206.

11. Fockens P, Kisman K, Tytgat GNJ. Endosonographic imaging of an aberrant right subclavian (Lusorian) artery. Gastrointest Endosc 1996;43:419. Abstract.

12. Kawamura O, Sekiguchi T, Kusano M, et al. Endoscopic ultrasonographic abnormalities and lower esophageal sphincter function in reflux esophagitis. Dig Dis Sci 1995;40:598–605.

13. Caletti GC, Ferrari A, Mattioli S, et al. Endoscopy versus endoscopic ultrasonography in staging reflux esophagitis. Endoscopy 1996;26:794–797.

14. Falk GW, Catalano MF, Sivak MV, et al. Endosonography in the evaluation of patients with Barrett's esophagus and high grade dysplasia. Gastrointest Endosc 1994;40:207–212.

15. Srivastava AK, Vanagunas A, Kamel P, Cooper R. Endoscopic ultrasound in the evaluation of Barrett's esophagus: a preliminary report. Am J Gastroenterol 1994;89:2192-2195.

16. Adrain AL, Ter H, Cassidy MJ, et al. High-resolution endoluminal sonography is a sensitive modality for the identification of Barrett's metaplasia. Gastrointest Endosc 1997;46:147–151.

17. Van Dam J, Falk GW, Sivak MV Jr., et al. Endosonographic evaluation of the patient with achalasia: appearance of the esophagus using the echoendoscope. Endoscopy 1995;27:185–190.

18. Hoffman BJ, Knapple WL, Bhutani MS, et al. Treatment of achalasia by injection of botulinum toxin under endoscopic ultrasound guidance. Gastrointest Endosc 1997;45:77–79.

19. Kojima Y, Ikeda M, Nakamura T, Fujino MA. Nonspecific esophageal motor disorder associated with thickened muscularis propria of the esophagus. Gastroenterology 1992;103:333–335.

20. Melzer E, Ron Y, Tiomni E, et al. Assessment of the esophageal wall by endoscopic ultrasonography in patients with nutcracker esophagus. Gastrointest Endosc 1997;46:223–225.

21. Pontes JM, Leitao MC, Portela FA, et al. Endoscopic ultrasonography in the treatment of oesophageal varices by endoscopic sclerotherapy and band ligation: do we need it? Eur J Gastroenterol Hepatol 1995;7:41–46.

22. Iwase H, Suga S, Morise K, et al. Color Doppler endoscopic ultrasonography for the evaluation of gastric varices and endoscopic obliteration with cyanoacrylate glue. Gastrointest Endosc 1995;41:150–154.

23. Sato T, Koito K, Nobuta A, et al. The usefulness of endoscopic color Doppler ultrasonography (ECDUS) for endoscopic injection sclerotherapy (EIS). Dig Endosc 1994;6:39–44.

24. TNM Classification of Malignant Tumors, 5th ed. New York: Wiley-Liss, 1997.

25. Rösch T. Endosonographic staging of esophageal cancer: a review of literature results. Gastrointest Endosc Clin North Am 1995;5:537–547.

26. Botet JF, Lightdale CJ, Zauber AG, et al. Preoperative staging of esophageal cancer: comparison of endoscopic US and dynamic CT. Radiology 1991; 181:419–425.

27. Tio TL, Cohen P, Coene PP, et al. Endosonography and computed tomography of esophageal carcinoma: preoperative classification compared to the new (1987) TNM system. Gastroenterology 1989;96:1478–1486.

28. Kato H, Tachimori Y, Watanabe H, et al. Lymph node metastasis in thoracic esophageal carcinoma. J Surg Oncol 1991;48.100–111.

29. Brugge WR, Lee MJ, Carey RW, Mathisen DJ. Endoscopic ultrasound staging criteria for esophageal cancer. Gastrointest Endosc 1997;45:147–152.

30. Chak A, Canto M, Gerdes H, et al. Prognosis of esophageal cancers preoperatively staged to be locally invasive (T4) by endoscopic ultrasound (EUS): a multicenter retrospective cohort study. Gastrointest Endosc 1995;42:501–506.

31. Fockens P, Kisman K, Merkus MP, et al. The prognosis of esophageal carcinoma staged irresectable (T4) by endosonography. J Am Coll Surg 1998;186:17–23.

32. Wiersema MJ, Kochman ML, Cramer HM, et al. Endosonography-guided real-time fine-needle aspiration biopsy. Gastrointest Endosc 1994;40:700–707.

33. Gress FG, Savides TJ, Sandler A, et al. Endoscopic ultrasonography, fine-needle aspiration biopsy guided by endoscopic ultrasonography, and computed tomography in the preoperative staging on non-small-cell lung cancer: a comparison study. Ann Intern Med 1997;127:604–612.

34. Wiersema MJ, Vilmann P, Giovannini M, et al. Endosonography-guided fine-needle apiration biopsy: diagnostic accuracy and complication assessment. Gastroenterology 1997;112:1087–1095.

35. Hirata N, Kawamoto K, Ueyama T, et al. Using endosonography to assess the effects of neoadjuvant therapy in patients with advanced esophageal cancer. AJR 1997;169:485–491.
36. Isenberg G, Chak A, Canto MI, et al. Endoscopic ultrasound in restaging of esophageal cancer after neoadjuvant chemoradiation. Gastrointest Endosc 1998;48:158–163.
37. Lightdale CJ, Botet JF, Kelsen DP, et al. Diagnosis of recurrent upper gastrointestinal cancer at the surgical anastomosis by endoscopic ultrasound. Gastrointest Endosc 1989;35:407–412.
38. Fockens P, Manshanden CG, Van Lanschot JJB, et al. Prospective study on the value of endosonographic follow-up after surgery for esophageal carcinoma. Gastrointest Endosc 1997;46:487–491.

# 8

# Endoscopic Ultrasound of the Stomach and Duodenum

## Douglas O. Faigel

## Technique

Endoscopic ultrasound (EUS) of the stomach and duodenum is easily performed. The Olympus GFUM20 radial sector scanner is the most useful device for performing EUS in these locations. This instrument has switchable frequencies of 7.5 and 12 MHz. The 7.5-MHz setting is useful for imaging lesions and structures surrounding the stomach and duodenum, and the 12 MHz setting allows high-resolution imaging of the wall. High-frequency through-the-scope probes are sometimes employed when staging early carcinomas or submucosal nodules. There is less history of using curved linear array scopes (such as the Pentax system) in imaging gastric or duodenal lesions, but these systems are useful in obtaining fine-needle aspirations of lymph nodes and extrinsic lesions (see Chapter 12 for a discussion of EUS-guided FNA).

The major challenge in performing EUS in the stomach and duodenum is obtaining adequate acoustic coupling between the transducer and the organ's wall. Filling the balloon with water is often adequate when scanning the duodenum, with its relatively narrow diameter. However, due to the large size of the gastric lumen, this method may be inadequate and leaves a large, air-filled space that creates artifacts. In this situation, filling the stomach with water is the best solution. I employ the Olympus UWS-1 water pump, which is connected by rubber tubing to the Olympus MD-744 valve that inserts through the echoendoscope's rubber biopsy cap to access the working channel. Depressing a foot pedal activates the pump, and pressing the button on the valve begins the flow of water. Once flow has begun, further use of the pump is not necessary; simply pressing the valve button will cause water to flow by a siphon effect.

With the patient in the left lateral decubitus position, water will preferentially fill the dpendent portions of the stomach—the fundus and body. For lesions located in these areas, this provides excellent acoustic coupling and high-quality imaging. The antrum may be more difficult to fill. Usually, suctioning all of the air out of the stomach is all that is needed, but at times changing the patient's position on the exam table is necessary. Raising the head of the bed to put the antrum in a more dependent position may be helpful. Since the antrum lies anterior to the body and fundus, rolling the patient prone (belly down) into a position similar to that for ERCP will allow water to fill the antrum when other maneuvers fail.

Mucosal and intramural lesions of the stomach and duodenum should be scanned at both the 7.5- and 12-MHz frequencies. The 7.5-MHz frequency allows imaging of the full extent of larger lesions, and is used to visualize extrinsic masses, lymph nodes, vascular structures, the liver and spleen, and ascites, if present. The 12-MHz frequency provides detailed, high-resolution images of the wall, and is helpful in discerning which layers are involved by a suspected pathological process or tumor.

## Benign Disorders

In addition to submucosal lesions (see Chapter 9), EUS is useful in the evaluation of several benign lesions.

### Gastric Varices

In evaluating a patient with thickened gastric folds (Table 8-1), the presence (or absence) of gastric varices must be the first item in the differential diagnosis.

**Table 8-1.** EUS in patients with thickened gastric folds.

| Diagnosis | Layer | EUS Findings |
|---|---|---|
| Varices | 3 | Serpiginous hypoechoic structures in the body and fundus. |
| Hypertrophic Gastropathies* | 1,2 ± 3 | Diffuse thickening of mucosal ± submucosal layers with preserved 5-layer pattern |
| Infiltrating Malignancy (Carcinoma, Lymphoma) | 3,4 | Prominently thickened submucosa (3rd) and muscularis propria (4th) layers. Lymphoma may have mucosal thickening with or without deeper involvement. |

*See text for etiologies

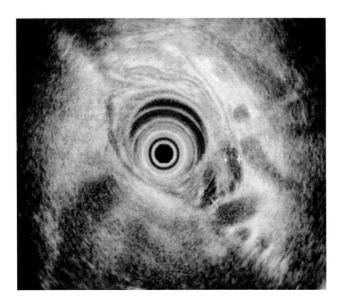

**Figure 8-1.** Gastric varices. These 5-mm gastric varices located in the fundus are visualized as serpiginous anechoic structures in the submucosa. (7.5 MHz)

Aggressive biopsy protocols are often employed in assessing enlarged folds and should not be done if varices may be present! Absence of concomitant esophageal varices is not very helpful because isolated gastric varices may be present, particularly in cases of splenic vein obstruction.

Gastric varices are seen as serpiginous hypoechoic structures within the wall of the stomach, usually in the body and fundus (Figure 8-1) (1). They are generally located in the third (submucosal) layer (2). Varices surrounding the stomach (paragastric varices) are invariably found when submucosal varices are present, and will often be greater than 5 mm in diameter. Sometimes, on careful endosonography, small (2 to 3 mm) collateral vessels near the fundus will be seen in the absence of varices or other evidence of portal hypertension. These are a normal finding (3).

The presence of gastric varices should prompt a search for the cause: either portal hypertension or sinistral hypertension due to splenic vein obstruction.

Findings compatible with the diagnosis of portal hypertension on EUS include the presence of esophageal or paraesophageal varices or ascites (4). Splenic vein obstruction is usually due to a pancreatic process. The pancreas should be imaged for evidence of pancreatitis or tumor (Chapter 11). CT scanning and Doppler ultrasonography may be useful for further evaluation of the pancreas and splenic vein patency.

## Duplication Cysts

Foregut duplications are congenital anomalies rarely encountered in adults. Although two-thirds are discovered in the first year of life, up to 30% present after age 12 and have been found in patients past the seventh decade (5,6). Although the genesis of duplications is unknown, the most commonly accepted theory is an error during recanalization of the embryonic gastrointestinal tract (7). Duplications are located in close proximity to the gastrointestinal tract and are usually cystic without luminal communication. Although they can occur anywhere throughout the alimentary canal, small intestinal (ileal) duplications are the most common and gastric duplications the least common (6,7). Most duplication cysts are discovered incidentally during radiologic examination or during evaluation of a gastric submucosal nodule.

The majority of gastric duplications are found in females (7). The cyst is usually located along the greater curvature of the stomach and shares a common wall and blood supply with the stomach. Symptoms may include abdominal pain, distension, vomiting, hemorrhage, and peritonitis from free perforation (6,8). Relapsing pancreatitis has been reported in patients with antral and duodenal cysts. In these patients, duplication cysts had developed in close association with the pancreas and at resection-contained pancreatic tissue (9,10). Duodenal duplications located in proximity to the ampulla of Vater may also present with recurrent pancreatitis due to pancreatic duct obstruction (11), but more commonly are found incidentally (10) or during investigations of patients with recurrent abdominal pain (12).

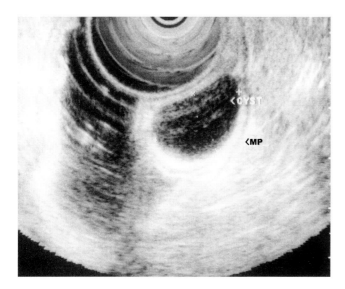

**Figure 8-2.** Gastric duplication cyst. A 1.3-by-2-cm anechoic cyst located in the submucosa. Note the intact muscularis propria (*MP*) coursing behind the cyst. The diagnosis was confirmed using large-capacity forceps and the bite-on-bite technique to puncture the cyst. Biopsies from within the cyst had benign gastric-type mucosa. (7.5 MHz)

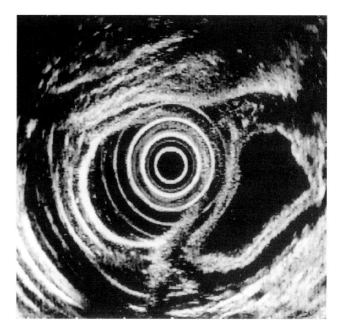

**Figure 8-3.** Gastric duplication cyst. This large gastric duplication cyst was located extrinsic to the antrum. Note the intact five-layer pattern in the cyst wall. A surgical resection was performed confirming a complete duplication of the gastric antrum. (7.5 MHz)

EUS is an important tool in evaluating suspected duplication cysts. It can often distinguish between cystic and solid masses, and define the intramural and extramural relationships of the cyst with the GI tract. Endoscopically, a submucosal bulge associated with a duplication cyst may or may not be evident. On EUS these lesions are imaged as well-circumscribed anechoic structures. They may be located within the submucosa (third layer)(Figure 8-2) or outside the stomach or duodenum (Figure 8-3). Debris and fluid levels may be seen within the cyst. The wall of the cyst is usually thin, although in complete duplication, a five-layer pattern identical to the normal GI tract has been described (see Figure 8-3) (10).

Histological confirmation can often be made endoscopically or with the aid of EUS-guided fine-needle aspiration. Submucosal cysts can sometimes be reached with the jumbo biopsy forceps and the bite-on-bite technique (2). This will puncture the cyst and yield clear fluid. Biopsies within the cavity may identify ectopic gastric mucosa. Needle-knife incision of a bulging duodenal cyst has also been reported (13). Fine-needle aspiration, which may be EUS guided, obtains straw- to yellow-colored viscous fluid containing leukocytes and macrophages (10). Symptomatic cysts should be surgically resected.

## Hypertrophic Gastropathy

The hypertrophic gastropathies are a diverse group of entities that cause giant gastric folds. The etiologies include benign idiopathic conditions (Menetrier's disease, hypertrophic gastritis, Crohn's disease, eosinophilic gastritis, sarcoidosis, amyloidosis, infections (*Helicobacter pylori* gastritis, anisakiasis, cytomegalovirus, herpes simplex, syphilis, tuberculosis, fungal pathogens), Zollinger-Ellison syndrome and hyperrugosity (a normal variant) (14–16). Infiltrating malignancies are an important consideration in the patient with enlarged folds, and are considered later in this chapter. EUS is useful in evaluating patients with enlarged folds by identifying which layers of the stomach wall are thickened. In the benign conditions, the thickening is usually limited to the mucosal layers (first and second) but may sometimes involve the submucosal (third) layer as well. Although this appearance is not specific for any particular entity and can be seen with malignant tumors, it indicates that large-capacity forceps biopsy will be sufficient to sample the affected tissue, provide a diagnosis, and, most importantly, rule out malignancy. Of the benign conditions, there has been particular interest in EUS imaging of Menetrier's disease and *H. pylori* gastritis, because patients with these conditions may have endoscopic findings and clinical presentations that mimic cancer.

Menetrier's disease is defined by the presence of giant folds in the fundus and body (particularly along the greater curvature), protein-losing enteropathy, and hypochlorhydria. Histologically, there is elongation

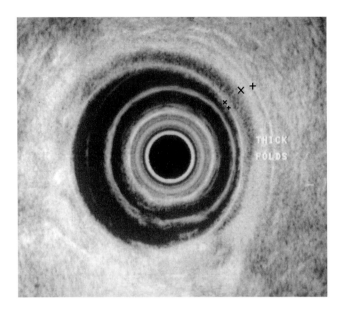

**Figure 8-4.** *Helicobacter pylori gastritis.* This patient underwent EUS evaluation for thickened gastric folds. On EUS the stomach was thickened to 5 mm (+ marks) with a 3 mm mucosa (× marks). Note the thickened deep mucosa (hypoechoic second layer) and submucosa (hyperechoic fourth layer). Biopsies demonstrated inflammatory changes and *H. pylori* organisms. (12 MHz)

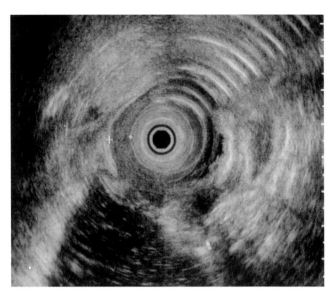

**Figure 8-5.** Refractory antral ulcer. This EUS in a patient with an antral ulcer that failed to heal on medical therapy, demonstrates thickening of the gastric wall to 7 mm with loss of the 5-layer pattern. It is not possible to differentiate a benign from a malignant process on this EUS. The patient underwent a Billroth II gastrectomy and the ulcer was benign. (7.5 MHz)

and tortuosity of the gastric pits (foveolar hyperplasia) with prominent cystic dilations. In adults, the disease is primarily found in men over the age of 50, who have epigastric pain, weight loss, anemia, diarrhea, edema, and hypoalbuminemia. In children, a reversible form of the disease due to CMV infection occurs (17). Menetrier's disease in adults may be associated with an increased risk of gastric carcinoma of 15% (18). The EUS exam in Menetrier's disease demonstrates mucosal thickening primarily of the deep mucosa (second layer). EUS does not demonstrate the the small cystic spaces that are present in these lesions when histologically studied. When an EUS image consistent with Menetrier's disease is obtained, large-capacity forceps biopsies are adequate for histological diagnosis, obviating the need for full-thickness (surgical) biopsy (14,15).

*Helicobacter pylori* infection is the most common cause of chronic gastritis. It is now evident that this infection can cause the formation of enlarged gastric folds. However, the appearance may raise the question of an infiltrating gastric carcinoma or lymphoma, both of which are associated with *H. pylori* infection (19, 20). When EUS is performed in patients with chronic *H. pylori* infection, the mucosal and submucosal layers of the stomach (layers one through three) are thickened (Figure 8-4). Biopsy reveals a chronic active gastritis with typical curved *H. pylori* bacilli present on the luminal surface of the specimen. Successful eradication of the

infection results in regression of the gastric wall thickening and normalization of the EUS appearance (16).

### Refractory Gastric Ulcer

The patient with a nonhealing gastric ulcer presents a difficult clinical problem. Aggressive biopsy protocols will detect the majority of, although not all, gastric malignancies. EUS may be employed to search for and stage an underlying tumor. EUS may detect an obvious tumor mass or evidence for an infiltrating malignant process in the surrounding stomach (see the following sections). The water-fill technique should be used to image the ulcerated area as well as the surrounding uninvolved stomach for evidence of a tumor or wall thickening and infiltration. A 7.5 MHz frequency should be used to examine contiguous organs to rule out extrinsic invasion of the stomach by a nongastric tumor. The presence of enlarged, hypoechoic, round lymph nodes is worrisome for malignancy, particularly if found in the region of the celiac axis or gastrohepatic ligament. However, it is not possible to make a definitive diagnosis of gastric cancer or exclude the diagnosis using EUS alone. The inflammatory process associated with the ulcer may extend into the fourth layer, causing changes on EUS that are indistinguishable from malignancy (Figure 8-5) (21) and enlarged lymph nodes may be benign due to inflammation. Therefore, while EUS may provide a more

**Table 8-2.** Gastric cancer staging.

**T: Primary Tumor**

| | |
|---|---|
| T1: | Tumor limited to mucosa or submucosa |
| T2: | Tumor invades muscularis propria or subserosa |
| T3: | Tumor invades serosa |
| T4: | Tumor invades adjacent structures |
| Tx: | Primary tumor cannot be assessed |

**N: Regional Lymph Nodes**

| | |
|---|---|
| N0: | No regional lymph node metastasis |
| N1: | Metastasis in perigastric lymph nodes within 3 cm of the edge of the tumor |
| N2: | Metastasis in perigastric lymph nodes more than 3 cm from the edge of the primary tumor or in lymph nodes along the left gastric, common hepatic, mesenteric, splenic or celiac arteries |
| Nx: | Regional lymph nodes cannot be assessed |

**M: Distant Metastasis**

| | |
|---|---|
| M0: | No distant metastasis |
| M1: | Distant metastasis present (e.g., hepatic metastases, peritoneal dissemination) |
| Mx: | Distant metastasis cannot be assessed |

**Stage Grouping**

| | |
|---|---|
| Stage IA: | T1 N0 M0 |
| Stage IB: | T1 N1 M0, T2 N0 M0 |
| Stage II: | T1 N2 M0, T2 N1 M0, T3 N0 M0 |
| Stage IIIA: | T2 N2 M0, T3 N1 M0, T4 N0 M0 |
| Stage IIIB: | T3 N2 M0, T4 N1 M0 |
| Stage IV: | T4 N2 M0, or any T, any N, M1 |

accurate preoperative diagnosis, in the absence of a clearly unresectable tumor, it does not make surgical exploration unnecessary.

## Malignant Disorders

The stomach is an important site for the development of primary malignancies. EUS is useful in the staging, management, and follow-up of patients with gastric adenocarcinoma and lymphoma.

### Adenocarcinoma

Gastric adenocarcinoma occurs in two histological types: intestinal and diffuse (signet ring cell). The intestinal type is primarily associated with discrete polypoid fungating or ulcerated tumors, and the diffuse type more commonly infiltrates the wall of the stomach, causing the classic leather-bottle morphology of linitis plastica. While the staging system for the two types is the same, their EUS appearances differ.

### Intestinal Type

Intestinal-type carcinomas are invasive cancers of mucosal origin. The principal objectives when staging these lesions are to determine depth of penetration and assess for local and regional lymph node involvement. In all cases, the TNM staging system should be employed (Table 8-2). The depth of penetration of the tumor into the wall of the stomach determines the tumor stage (or T-stage). This is best accomplished using the water-fill technique to reduce any artifacts produced by intervening air. The majority of smaller to medium-sized lesions are imaged using high-frequency ultrasound (12 MHz with the Olympus GFUM20 or 12 or 20 MHz miniprobe) to provide high-resolution images. Through-the-scope 12 to 20 MHz miniprobes allow for accurate T-staging without the need for a dedicated echoendoscope, but are limited by shallow imaging depth leading to poor N-stage accuracy (21a). With larger lesions, it may not be possible to image the entire thickness of the tumor at high frequency and the 7.5 MHz frequency should be used. In some very thick tumors, it may not be possible to determine the full depth of invasion with EUS.

Gastric carcinomas are generally poorly circumscribed hypoechoic lesions which, at the edges, can be seen to be arising from the mucosal layers. T1 lesions are limited to the mucosa (first and second layers) or may penetrate into the submucosa (third layer). There should be a demonstrable, intact, bright layer of submucosa between the lesion and the dark band of the muscularis propria (fourth layer) (Figure 8-6). T2 lesions extend into but not through the muscularis. Endosonographically, T2 lesions extend through the bright third layer corresponding to where the tumor penetrates through the submucosa into the muscularis. However, the interface at the outer margin of the muscularis where it contacts the serosa (fourth and fifth layers) is smooth and undisturbed by the cancer (Figure 8-7). In T3 lesions the hypoechoic lesion extends completely through the fourth layer, and the serosa (fifth layer), which would otherwise be smooth and uninterrupted, is clearly invaded. Fingerlike projections of tumor, termed *pseudopodia*, may be seen extending into the extragastric space (Figure 8-8). If the lesion extends into a local organ (eg., liver, pancreas, spleen, diaphragm) or large vessel (eg., aorta, celiac axis) it is classified as a T4-stage lesion.

The accuracy of EUS T-staging for gastric cancer ranges from 67% to 92% or about 80% overall (22–30). Sources of error arise from microinfiltration, which may be undetectable by EUS and causes understaging, and peritumoral inflammation, making a tumor appear to be more deeply invasive than it actually is, resulting in overstaging. Inaccuracies in staging T2 versus T3 lesions are a particular problem. The TNM system uses serosal invasion as the main criterion to define a T3 lesion. However, the stomach is not uniformly covered

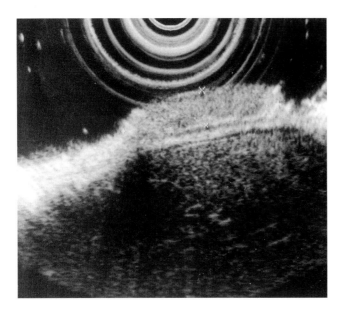

**Figure 8-6.** T1 gastric cancer. A superficial 2.2 cm (+ marks) by 0.5 cm (× marks) tumor. Note the intact-appearing submucosa. (12 MHz)

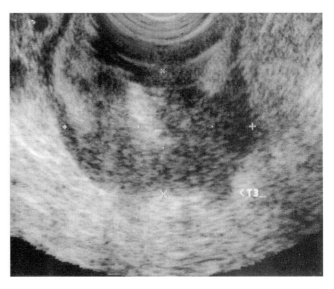

**Figure 8-8.** T3 gastric cancer. This 2.5 cm (+ marks) by 1.6 cm (× marks) tumor invades all layers of the stomach. A pseudopod of tumor extends through the serosa into the perigastric space (<*T3*). (7.5 MHz)

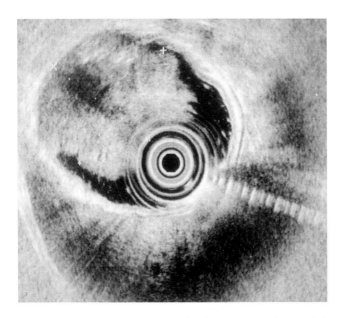

**Figure 8-7.** T2 gastric cancer. This large 4.2 cm (+ marks) by 3.6 cm (× marks) tumor involves the full thickness of the gastric wall. The outer margin of the fifth layer (serosa) is relatively smooth and uninterrupted by pseudopodia. At surgery, T2 staging was confirmed. (12 MHz)

by serosa, being absent in areas of the lesser curvature and anterior wall of the antrum. A tumor that on histological examination completely penetrates the muscularis propria without evidence of serosal invasion would be classified as T2, but when seen on EUS would be indistinguishable from a T3 lesion (31). Nevertheless, despite its limitations, EUS remains the most accurate nonsurgical method for determining depth of invasion and is significantly more accurate than CT, which has a reported accuracy of only 42% (27).

EUS is also used to assess for local or regional lymph node metastasis in patients with cancer. Complete lymph node assessment requires scanning at 7.5 MHz. Attention should be paid to the region surrounding the tumor and to the retroperitoneum, celiac axis, aorta, gastrohepatic ligament, and splenic hilum. With the stomach water-filled and the balloon distended, the entire perigastric region should be imaged at low magnification from the antrum to the gastroesophageal junction. In areas obscured by air, the air should be suctioned out, more water instilled, or the balloon pressed against the gastric wall to ensure complete visualization of all areas. Malignant lymph nodes are usually imaged by EUS as rounded structures that are well circumscribed and uniformly hypoechoic (dark). Abnormal-appearing nodes located within 3 cm of the primary mass are classified as N1 while those more distant or along the large named vessels are classified N2 (see Table 8-2). The liver should also be examined for hypoechoic nodules that may represent metastases. The presence of ascites is a poor prognostic sign and implies the presence of peritoneal metastasis. EUS-guided fine-needle aspiration has been successfully used to detect malignant ascites (32). CT is superior to EUS in the detection of distant metastasis and should also be performed as part of a complete preoperative evaluation.

Much has been written about the inaccuracies of EUS for malignant lymphadenopathy, with values of EUS accuracy varying from 50% to 90% in reported series (24–27,29). This variance is due in part to use of diverse criteria to define a malignant node. Most endosonographers regard rounded, well-demarcated, and homogeneously dark nodes as being malignant without regard to size (33), although ex vivo studies in esophageal and gastric cancer have identified a nodal diameter exceeding 1 cm as the only significant criterion (34). Inaccuracies in EUS assessment also arise from the inability to detect micrometastases and the fact that benign inflammatory lymph nodes may be enlarged and exhibit "malignant" features. Nevertheless, EUS is the single most accurate modality for N-staging, being significantly more accurate than CT (27), and the absence of identifiably enlarged nodes at EUS is fairly specific (85% or more) for predicting the absence of nodal metastasis at surgery (29). The presence of enlarged lymph nodes on EUS, however, is not as helpful in staging these tumors, and histological confirmation (via EUS-guided fine-needle aspiration) is essential if the presence of nodal metastases would alter patient management (35).

The overall utility of EUS depends on the clinical setting. In Western countries, gastric cancer presents late, and gastrectomy is the only option. In these cases, the primary utility of EUS is determining resectability and prognosis. For a gastric primary to be resectable, it must not invade surrounding organs (i.e., be T1–T3). In determining the ability to completely resect a gastric cancer, EUS is at least 85% accurate (28). EUS T-stage is also predictive of the probability of postoperative recurrence. Among patients undergoing attempted curative resections, recurrence occurred in 15% of those with EUS stage T1 or T2 compared with 77% with T3 or T4 (p = 0.0002) (30). Also, the use of EUS in preoperative evaluation alters clinical treatment plans in as many as 30% of cases (36) and may allow selection of patients for more limited resections (36a). Currently, preoperative neoadjuvant therapy is not routinely used in the United States, although small early studies are promising. In the future, EUS may be a useful tool in selecting patients for preoperative neoadjuvant protocols (37).

EUS imaging may be helpful in the follow up of patients after surgery for gastric cancer, as well. This modality has been used to detect anastamotic recurrence with good sensitivity (95%) and specificity (80%) (38). When there is anastamotic recurrence, EUS shows nodularity and irregular hypoechoic thickening of the wall in the region of the anastamosis exceeding 7 mm (thickening to 6 mm with a smooth appearance is normal for an anastamosis). There may be invasion of local organs or the presence of enlarged lymph nodes. Early detection of recurrence may provide prognostic guidance for patient management and improve surgical and oncological outcomes (38).

In terms of natural history, gastric adenocarcinoma can be further divided into early gastric cancer (EGC) and late gastric cancer. EGC comprises the subset of patients with tumors confined to the mucosa or submucosa without invasion of the muscularis propria (T1). Clinically, this is an important lesion carrying a 95% five-year survival following resection (compared to a poor 15% for gastric cancer overall) (39). The majority

of the experience with EGC is from Japan where this particular presentation comprises over 30% of all patients with gastric cancer (40). EGC can be further subdivided into two categories: tumors isolated to the mucosa (T1m) which carry a 5% risk of nodal metastasis, and those that invade through the muscularis mucosae into the submucosa (T1sm) which carry a 10% to 20% risk of metastasis (41,42).

Endoscopic resection can be considered for T1m lesions, but for more deeply invasive tumors (T1sm or higher) surgical resection is preferred. EUS using echoendoscopes at standard frequencies may be incapable of differentiating T1m from T1sm lesions with over- and understaging occurring in about 25% (42). Many endosonographers now feel that catheter-based miniprobes scanning at 20 MHz may be better suited to staging EGC. The 20-MHz frequency resolves the gastric wall into a nine-layer structure, with a fine, hypoechoic line between the conventional second (deep mucosa) and third (submucosa) layers, which is felt to represent the muscularis mucosae (43). Unfortunately, overstaging of EGC with the 20-MHz probe occurs in 19% to 24% of patients due to peritumoral fibrosis mimicking deeper invasion (44,45). Accuracy appears to be better for the small elevated type than the depressed type of EGC (45a). In a recent large series of 104 patients, when both the endoscopic appearance and the 20-MHz EUS findings were applied together for tumor classification, a 92% overall accuracy rate was achieved (45). Thus, when done carefully and consistently, it is possible to use high-frequency EUS to select patients for endoscopic resection of T1m EGC, although long-term outcome studies are needed to verify the clinical advantages of this approach.

**Diffuse Type (Linitis Plastica)**

Linitis plastica carcinomas are poorly differentiated tumors that diffusely infiltrate the stomach wall. Histologically, they consist of single cells or small clusters of cells that contain large mucin vacuoles pushing the nucleus to one side to produce a signet ring appearance. The result of the diffuse infiltration by the cancer cells is a thickened, rigid stomach that has been likened to a leather bottle. Diffuse type cancers carry a much poorer prognosis than the intestinal type due to their propensity for deep invasion and early metastasis (39).

Clinically, patients complain of abdominal discomfort, early satiety, nausea, and weight loss. At endoscopy, thickened, poorly distensible folds may be found without an identifiable mass. Biopsies obtained with standard forceps may be unable to define cancer in up to half of all cases (46,47). More aggressive endoscopic biopsy techniques employing a diathermic snare to obtain a deeper sample carry an increased risk of hemorrhage and perforation (48–50). As previously noted, there are diverse causes of enlarged gastric folds, including malignancies (adenocarcinoma and lymphoma)

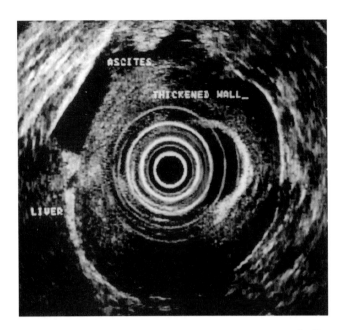

**Figure 8-9.** Linitis plastica. The stomach wall is markedly thickened with a complete absence of the five-layer pattern. The abnormal stomach abuts the liver but there is no apparent direct invasion. Ascites is present, which raises the concern of peritoneal metastasis. Biopsies confirmed a signet ring carcinoma. Surgery was not performed. (12 MHz)

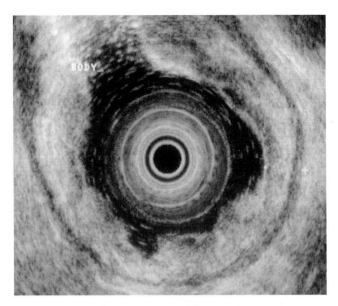

**Figure 8-10.** Linitis plastica. This patient, with a remote history of a Billroth II gastrectomy, developed abdominal pain, satiety, and weight loss. CT and endoscopy showed a thickened stomach, but forceps biopsies were nondiagnostic. This EUS shows gastric wall thickening to 8 mm, with a prominent muscularis propria (dark fourth layer) and thickened submucosa (bright third layer). A complete gastrectomy was performed confirming a signet ring cell carcinoma. (7.5 MHz)

and a variety of benign conditions. Because it can be difficult to rule out an infiltrating malignancy with standard endoscopy, laparotomy with full-thickness biopsy has frequently been necessary (48).

EUS examination has been found to be exceptionally helpful in evaluating the patient with a suspected infiltrating malignancy. The normal stomach is 3 mm in thickness. When an infiltrating cancer is present, the stomach is thickened to greater than 4 mm, and one of two EUS patterns may be seen. In the first, there is complete loss of the normal five-layer pattern, with the markedly thickened wall assuming a homogeneously dark appearance. All layers of the stomach are generally involved and these tumors are stage T3 (Figure 8-9). It has been my experience that endoscopic biopsies are usually positive in these cases. In the second EUS pattern, the thickened stomach maintains its five-layer pattern, but the fourth layer (muscularis propria) is a prominent, thick, dark band beneath a thickened, bright, third layer (submucosa) (Figure 8-10) (14,15). In these cases, forceps biopsies are often negative due to the fact that most of the tumor cells are in the deeper layers. Deep endoscopic or surgical full-thickness biopsy should be performed when forceps biopsies are negative. When the thickening is limited to the mucosal layers (first and second layers), a benign condition is usually present and large-capacity endoscopic forceps biopsies are sufficient for diagnosis, making surgical biopsy unnecessary (14). When performing EUS in pa-

tients with thickened folds, it is important to water-fill the stomach to distend the folds as much as possible. Pressing the transducer against poorly distended areas also smooths out folds and allows a more accurate assessment of stomach wall thickness. Although the presence of a thickened muscularis propria is a sensitive sign for malignancy, care must be taken when scanning in the regions of the cardia and pylorus (Figure 8-11). In these areas, the muscularis propria has a thickened or prominent appearance due to normal physiologic thickening caused by the gastroesophageal and pyloric sphincters (51). Artifactual EUS thickening of gastric layers can also mislead the endosonographer if the scanning plane is tangential to the wall, rather than perpendicular to it. This is a particular problem in the cardia and pylorus where the walls normally come together in a sloping fashion, making it difficult to consistently obtain EUS images in a perpendicular plane. Pressing the water-inflated balloon against the wall while imaging can minimize this latter artifact. When there is doubt as to the cause of the thickening, it is prudent to proceed with a surgical full-thickness biopsy.

## Lymphoma

The stomach is the most common site for primary extranodal lymphoma, comprising one-fourth of all extranodal cases and at least half of all primary gastrointestinal lymphomas. Primary gastric lymphoma

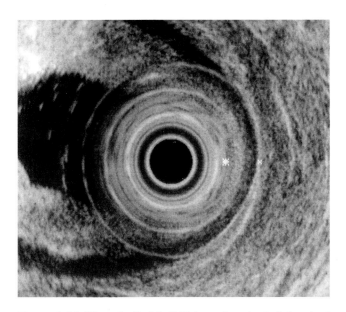

**Figure 8-11.** "Pseudo-linitis." This patient had abdominal pain and nonhealing superficial antral erosions, biopsy benign. EUS in the distal antrum shows wall thickening to 5 mm with a prominent muscularis propria (fourth) layer. The more proximal stomach was EUS normal. A Billroth II gastrectomy was performed, but only benign inflammation was found. Care must be taken when imaging the distal antrum/pylorus because a thickened-appearing muscularis may be normal. (7.5 MHz)

**Table 8-3.** Musshoff staging system for GI lymphomas.

| Stage | Sites of Involvement |
| --- | --- |
| IE | Tumor confined to GI tract |
| IIE$_1$ | Tumor with regional nodal involvement |
| IIE$_2$ | Tumor with extraregional subdiaphragmatic nodal involvement (e.g., para-aortic, iliac, etc.) |
| IIIE | Tumor with nodal involvement on both sides of the diaphragm |
| IVE | Tumor with extranodal disseminated involvement (e.g., bone marrow, lungs, liver, etc.) |

(PGL) accounts for 5% of all gastric tumors. These are lymphomas of the non-Hodgkin's type and are usually B-cell in origin. They are either high-grade (especially diffuse large cell) or low-grade MALT (mucosa-associated lymphoid tissue) lymphomas. Low-grade MALT lymphomas may contain foci of high-grade lymphoma (52). The gross appearance of PGL is usually that of an exophytic tumor projecting into the lumen, but more diffuse infiltration causing a linitis plastica morphology may occur. The main diagnostic considerations in the differential are gastric adenocarcinoma and the various benign causes of thickened folds previously mentioned.

Gastrointestinal lymphomas are staged differently than carcinomas (Table 8-3). Tumors confined to the GI tract are stage IE. Higher stages are assigned to tumors based on the presence and site of nodal involvement (Table 8-3). Patients with stage IE and with low-grade MALT lymphoma have better survival statistics (53,54). Although the depth of penetration into the wall and lateral extent of the tumor do not alter the stage, they may have clinical and treatment implications. The use of EUS in the evaluation and treatment of high-grade lymphomas differs from the techniques used for MALT lymphomas and will be considered separately.

When left untreated, high-grade PGL follows a clinical course similar to that seen with gastric adenocarcinoma. Unlike adenocarcinoma, however, high-grade

PGL does respond well to treatment with radiation and chemotherapy, and these nonsurgical approaches may be used in addition to or instead of surgical resection. Selection of patients for a particular treatment protocol remains difficult. Ideal candidates for primary resection are patients with smaller tumors that can be removed with a subtotal gastrectomy and who do not have nodal involvement. Adjuvant therapy following resection should be given when the tumor invades the muscularis propria or there is nodal involvement. Radiation and chemotherapy remain the primary treatment modalities when there is unresectable disease (Stages IIE2, IIIE, IVE). It is not yet known whether patients with resectable disease (Stages IE and IIE1) can be treated successfully with radiation and chemotherapy alone and thus avoid the risk and complications of surgery. For patients with a large tumor burden that would require total gastrectomy, primary radiation and chemotherapy may be the best option, to avoid the high risk for complications from surgical gastrectomy and because recurrence is common (52). A potential drawback to primary radiation and chemotherapy in these patients is the risk that transmural disease will perforate during therapy, although this may be more a theoretical than an actual risk.

In patients with high-grade PGL, EUS is particularly helpful in providing detailed information as to the extent of disease so that a rational and effective therapeutic protocol can be tailored to the individual patient. Determining local extent of disease, the depth of involvement through the gastric wall and the longitudinal tumor extent from antrum to fundus, are the most important considerations (Figures 8-12 and 8-13). EUS is approximately 90% accurate in determining depth of penetration (55–59). It can also determine longitudinal extent of tumor involvement, although there is a tendency toward underestimating the longitudinal extent of disease (56,57). In one small series, preoperative EUS mapping reduced the need for total gastrectomy (compared to historical controls) while achieving a 100% complete resection rate (56). EUS has also been used to document response to chemotherapy (58).

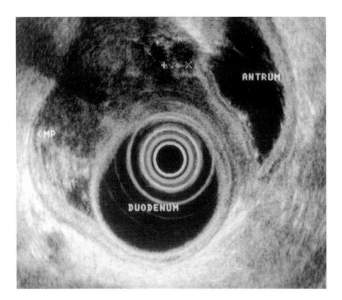

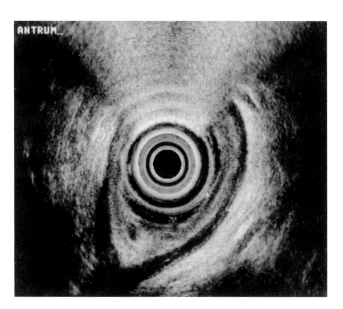

**Figure 8-12.** Lymphoma. This high-grade lymphoma was located in the pylorus and extended into the duodenal bulb. This image is taken from the duodenal bulb, and the water-filled antrum is also seen. The tumor is markedly heterogeneous, containing two 5-mm hypoechoic cystic spaces, and involves all layers of the wall. (12 MHz)

**Figure 8-14.** Gastric lymphoma. This patient with abdominal pain, satiety, and weight loss had a thickened antrum noted on CT. This EUS demonstrates antral thickening to 6 mm with a prominent muscularis propria (fourth) layer. The entire antrum was involved. Large-capacity forceps biopsies using the bite-on-bite technique were nondiagnostic. The diagnosis of lymphoma was made by EUS-guided fine-needle aspiration of an involved celiac lymph node. (12 MHz)

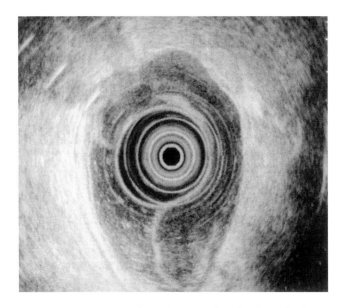

**Figure 8-13.** Gastric lymphoma. This high-grade lymphoma has a very homogeneous and hypoechoic appearance involving all layers of the stomach. This appearance is quite similar to an infiltrating carcinoma and requires biopsy for differentiation (see Figure 8-9). (7.5 MHz)

EUS is also useful in detecting metastatic lymph node involvement in patients with high-grade PGL. Due to the limited depth of penetration of the high-frequency ultrasound used in EUS, only regional (IIE1 and some IIE2) lymph nodes will be seen. Even with this limitation, EUS has been up to 100% sensitive with an average 80% to 90% accuracy for detecting lymph node disease (55–59). Accurate detection of

metastatic lymph nodes is important because nodal tumor may contraindicate the use of surgery as primary therapy. To increase diagnostic accuracy, EUS-guided FNA with flow cytometry of the aspirated specimen has been used to confirm nodal metastasis (60). In one case, I have used EUS-guided FNA of a celiac lymph node to establish the diagnosis of lymphoma in a patient with gastric wall thickening, a prominent muscularis propria on EUS, and negative large-capacity forceps biopsies (unpublished case) (Figure 8-14).

MALT tumors are a unique subset of primary B-cell lymphomas of the stomach with a better prognosis than high-grade PGL (53,54) (Figure 8-15). The pathogenesis of MALT lymphomas is strongly associated with *H. pylori* infection, and successful eradication of the infection has led to complete regression of the lymphoma in some cases (61). However, many patients do not respond to antibiotic treatment and some lymphomas classified as being of the MALT type have foci of both high- and low-grade histology. For these reasons, and because of the questionable ability of standard endoscopy with biopsy to assess persistent submucosal disease, EUS is being actively studied as an adjunct for both diagnosis and monitoring response to therapy (53,61,62). It has already been shown that EUS prior to treatment may predict response to antimicrobial therapy. In a study by Sackmann et al., complete regression occurred in 12 of 14 patients with tumor limited to the mucosa and submucosa on EUS, but none of the 10 patients with either

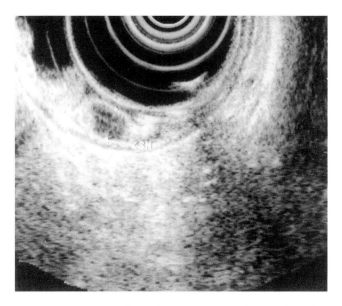

**Figure 8-15.** MALT lymphoma. A 4-mm hypoechoic lesion is seen in the deep mucosa. Note the intact submucosa deep to the lesion (<SM). (12 MHz)

deeper invasion or suspicious lymph nodes present (p < 0.01) responded to antibiotics (61). Similarly, Nobre-Leitao et al. found a high rate of response to antimicrobial therapy in patients staged E1 by EUS (61a). In a study from Memorial Sloan-Kettering Cancer Center, EUS was found to be of help in identifying patients with residual lymphoma following treatment (62). Additionally, they reported four patients with presumptive MALT lymphoma but unremarkable EUS examinations, who were found on subsequent biopsy with immunohistochemical staining and pathologic review to have benign lymphoid aggregates and not lymphoma (62). Therefore, EUS may be useful in the initial evaluation of gastric MALT lymphoma by identifying patients likely to respond to antimicrobial therapy, discriminate between patients with bona fide lymphoma and benign lymphoid hyperplasia, and in follow-up after therapy.

## Summary

EUS is useful in a variety of benign and malignant conditions of the stomach and duodenum. Optimal imaging requires the use of the water-fill technique and scanning at 12 MHz for wall lesions and 7.5 MHz to assess surrounding organs and lymphadenopathy. In the evaluation of thickened gastric folds, EUS can rule out the presence of varices and identify which layers of the stomach are involved. Thickened mucosal layers are seen in benign conditions and indicate that endoscopic large-capacity forceps biopsies will be sufficient to provide a tissue diagnosis and exclude malignancy. The presence of prominently thickened submucosa and

muscularis propria layers should raise the question of an infiltrating malignancy (adenocarcinoma or lymphoma) and requires deep or full-thickness biopsy.

In patients with gastric cancer, EUS provides an accurate assessment of depth of invasion and nodal metastasis, predicting resectability and the likelihood of postoperative recurrence. Following resection, EUS detects anastamotic recurrence at an earlier stage, which may allow for better patient outcome. EUS using higher-frequency ultrasound, perhaps with 20-MHz miniprobes, may allow selection of patients with early gastric cancer for minimally invasive endoscopic resection. In patients with gastric lymphoma, EUS determination of depth, longitudinal spread, and lymph node involvement allows for rational planning among the three treatment modalities: surgery, radiation, and chemotherapy. For low-grade MALT lymphomas, EUS predicts which patients are likely to respond to anti-*Helicobacter* therapy, and is useful in identifying residual and recurrent disease following treatment.

### References

1. Tio TL, Kimmings N, Rauws E, et al. Endosonography of gastroesophageal varices: evaluation and follow-up of 76 cases. Gastrointest Endosc 1995;42:145–150.
2. Kochman ML, Hawes RH. Endoscopic evaluation of submucosal lesions of the gastrointestinal tract. In: Barkin JS, O'Phelan CA, eds. Advanced therapeutic endoscopy. 2nd ed. New York: Raven Press, 1994: 133–145.
3. Faigel DO, Rosen HR, Sasaki AW, Flora K, Benner K. Endoscopic ultrasound in cirrhotics with and without prior variceal hemorrage in comparison to non-cirrhotic controls. Gastrointest Endosc, 2000, in press.
4. Leung VK, Sung JJ, Ahuja AT, et al. Large para-esophageal varices on endosonography predict recurrence of esophageal varices and rebleeding. Gastroenterology 1997;112:1811–1816.
5. Whitaker JA, Deffenbaugh LD, Cooke AR. Esophageal duplication cyst. Am J Gastroeneterol 1980;73: 329–332.
6. Taft DA, Hairston JT. Duplication of the alimentary tract. Am Surg 1976;42: 455–462.
7. Simstein NL. Congenital gastric anomalies. Am Surg 1986;52:264–268.
8. Bhargava BN. Duplication of the stomach. J R Coll Surg 1978;23:34–36.
9. Lavine JE, Harrison M, Heyman MB. Gastrointestinal duplications causing relapsing pancreatitis in children. Gastroenterology 1989;97:1556–1558.
10. Faigel DO, Burke A, Ginsberg GG, et al. The role of endoscopic ultrasound in the evaluation and management of foregut duplications. Gastrointest Endosc 1997;45:99–103.
11. Stelling T, v.Rooj WJJ, Tio TL, et al. Pancreatitis associated with congenital duodenal duplication cyst in an adult. Endoscopy 1987;19:171–173.
12. Geller GA, Wank KK, DiMagno EP. Diagnosis of foregut duplication cysts by endoscopic ultrasonography. Gastroenterol 1995;109:838–842.

13. Al Traif I, Khan MH. Endoscopic drainage of a duodenal duplication cyst. Gastrointest Endosc 1992; 38:64–65.

14. Mendis RE, Gerdes H, Lightdale CJ, Botet JF. Large gastric folds: a diagnostic approach using endoscopic ultrasonography. Gastrointest Endosc 1994;40:437–441.

15. Songur Y, Okai T, Watanabe H, Motoo Y, Sawabu N. Endosonographic evaluation of giant gastric folds. Gastrointest Endosc 1995;41:468–474.

16. Avunduk C, Navab F, Hampf F, Coughlin B. Prevalence of Helicobacter pylori infection in patients with large gastric folds: evaluation and follow-up with endoscopic ultrasound before and after antimicrobial therapy. Am J Gastroenterol 1995;90:1969–1973.

17. Weinstein WM. Gastritis and gastropathies. In: Sleisinger MH, Fordtran JS, eds. Gastrointestinal disease. 5th ed. Philadelphia: WB Saunders. 1993: 545–571.

18. Antonioli D. Gastric carcinoma and its precursors. In: Goldman H, Appelman H, Kaufman N, eds. Gastrointestinal pathology. Baltimore: Williams and Wilkens. 1990:144–180.

19. Parsonnet J, Friedman GD, Vandersteen DP, et al. *Helicobacter pylori* infection and the risk of gastric carcinoma. N Engl J Med 1991;325:1127–1131.

20. Parsonnet J, Hansen S, Rodriguez L, et al. *Helicobacter* infection and gastric lymphoma. N Engl J Med 1994;330:1267–1271.

21. Lightdale CJ. Enlarged gastric folds. Proceedings of the 10th International Symposium on Endoscopic Ultrasonography. 1995:127–134.

21a. Hunerbein M, Ghadimi BM, Haersch W, Schlag PM. Transendoscopic ultrasound of esophageal and gastric cancer using miniaturized ultrasound catheter probes. *Gastrointest Endosc* 1998;48:371–375.

22. Murata Y, Suzuku S, Hashimoto H. Endoscopic ultrasonography of the upper gastrointestinal tract. Surg Endosc 1988;2:180–183.

23. Colin-Jones DG, Rosch T, Dittler HJ. Staging of gastric cancer by endoscopy. Endoscopy 1993;25:34–38.

24. Dittler HJ, Siewart JR. Role of endoscopic ultrasonography in gastric carcinoma. Endoscopy 1993;25: 162–166.

25. Akahoshi K, Misawa T, Fujishima H, et al. Preoperative evaluation of gastric cancer by endoscopic ultrasound. Gut 1991;32:479–482.

26. Tio TL, Schouwink MH, Cikot RJLM. Preoperative TNM classification of gastric cancer invasion by endoscopic ultrasonography: a prospective study of 72 cases. Hepatogastroenterol 1989;36:51–56.

27. Botet JF, Lightdale CJ, Zauber AG, et al. Preoperative staging of gastric cancer: comparison of endoscopic ultrasound and dynamic CT. Radiology 1991;181: 426–432.

28. Rosch T, Lorenz R, Zenker K, et al. Local staging and assessment of resectability in carcinoma of the esophagus, stomach and duodenum by endoscopic ultrasound. Gastrointest Endosc 1992;38:460–467.

29. Grimm H, Binmoeller KF, Hamper K, et al. Endosonography for preoperative locoregional staging of esophageal and gastric cancer. Endoscopy 1993;25: 224–230.

30. Smith JW, Brennan MF, Botet JF, et al. Preoperative endoscopic ultrasound can predict the risk of recurrence after operation for gastric carcinoma. J Clin Oncol 1993;11:2380–2385.

31. Tio TL. The TNM staging system. Gastrointest Endosc 1996;43:S19–S24.

32. Chang KJ, Albers CG, Nguyen P. Endoscopic ultrasound-guided fine needle aspiration of pleural and ascitic fluid. Am J Gastroenterol 1995;90:148–150.

33. Grimm H, Hamper K, Binmoeller KF, Soehendra N. Enlarged lymph nodes: malignant or not? Endoscopy 1992;24 (suppl. 1):320–323.

34. Heintz A, Mildenberger P, Georg M, et al. Endoscopic ultrasonography in the diagnosis of regional lymph nodes in esophageal and gastric cancer—results of studies in vitro. Endoscopy 1993;25:231–235.

35. Bhutani MS, Hawes RH, Hoffman BJ. A comparison of the accuracy of echo features during endoscopic ultrasound (EUS) and EUS-guided fine-needle aspiration for diagnosis of malignant lymph node invasion. Gastrointest Endosc 1997;45:474–479.

36. Nickl NJ, Bhutani MS, Catalano M, et al. Clinical implications of endoscopic ultrasound: the American Endosonography Club Study. Gastrointest Endosc 1996;44:371–377.

36a. Fujino Y, Nagata Y, Oginok, Watahik, H. Evaluation of endoscopic ultrasonography as an indicator for surgical treatment of gastric cancer. 1999;14:540–546.

37. Woodward TA, Levin B. Cancer of the stomach: chemotherapy and radiotherapy. In: Rustgi AK, ed. Gastrointestinal cancers: biology, diagnosis and therapy. Philadelphia: Lippincott-Raven. 1995:261–276.

38. Lightdale CJ, Botet JF, Kelsen DP, et al. Diagnosis of recurrent upper gastrointestinal cancer at the surgical anastamosis by endoscopic ultrasound. Gastrointest Endosc 1989;35:407–412.

38a. Muller C, Kahler G, Scheele J. Endosonographic examination of gastrointestinal anastomoses with suspected locoregional tumor recurrence. Surg Endosc 2000;14:45–50.

39. Lewandrowski KB, Compton CC. The pathology of gastric cancer and conditions predisposing to gastric cancer. In: Rustgi AK, ed. Gastrointestinal cancers: biology, diagnosis and therapy. Philadelphia: Lippincott-Raven. 1995:217–242.

40. Ishi H, Tatsuta M, Okuda S. Endoscopic diagnosis of minute gastric cancer of less than 5 mm in diameter. Cancer 1985;56:655–659.

41. Kodama Y, Inokuchi K, Soejima K, et al. Growth patterns and prognosis in early gastric carcinoma. Superficial spreading and penetrating growth types. Cancer 1985;51:320–326.

42. Yasuda K. Endoscopic ultrasonic probes and mucosectomy for early gastric cancer. Gastrointest Endosc 1996;43:S29–S31.

43. Yanai H, Fujimura H, Suzumi M, et al. Delineation of the gastric muscularis mucosae and assessment of depth of invasion of early gastric cancer using a 20-megahertz endoscopic ultrasound probe. Gastrointest Endosc 1993;39:505–512.

44. Yanai H, Tada M, Karita M, Okita K. Diagnostic utility of 20-megahertz linear endoscopic ultrasonography in

early gastric cancer. Gastrointest Endosc 1996;44: 29–33.

45. Yanai H, Matsumoto Y, Harada T, et al. Endoscopic ultrasonography and endoscopy for staging depth of invasion in early gastric cancer: a pilot study. Gastrointest Endosc 1997;46:212–216.

45a. Akahoshi K, Chijwa Y, Hamada S, et al. Pretreatment staging of endoscopically early gastric cancer with a 15 MHz ultrasound catheter probe. Gastrointest Endosc 1998;48:470–476.

46. Winawer SJ, Posner G, Lightdale CJ, et al. Endoscopic diagnosis of advanced gastric cancer. Gastroenterol 1975;69:1183–1187.

47. Andriulli A, Recchia S, De Angelis C, et al. Endoscopic ultrasonographic evaluation of patients with biopsy negative gastric linitis plastica. Gastrointest Endosc 1990;36:611–615.

48. Bjork JT, Geenen JE, Soergel KH, et al. Endoscopic evaluation of large gastric folds: a comparison of biopsy techniques. Gastrointest Endosc 1997;24: 22–23.

49. Martin TR, Onstad GR, Silvis SE, Vennes JA. Lift and cut biopsy technique for submucosal sampling. Gastrointest Endosc 1976;23:29.

50. Komorowski RA, Caya JG, Geenen JE. The morphological spectrum of large gastric folds: utility of the snare biopsy. Gastrointest Endosc 1986;32:190–192.

51. Miller LS, Liu JB, Barbarevech CA, et al. High-resolution endoluminal sonography in achalasia. Gastrointest Endosc 1995;42:545–549.

52. Thomas CR, Wood B. Gastrointestinal lymphoma and AIDS-related cancer. In: Rustgi AK, ed. Gastrointestinal cancers: biology, diagnosis and therapy. Philadelphia: Lippincott-Raven. 1995:551–574.

53. Cogliatti SB, Schmid U, Schumacher U, et al. Primary B-cell gastric lymphoma: a clinicopathological study of 145 patients. Gastroenterol 1991;101:1159–1170.

54. Muller MF, Maloney A, Jenkins D, et al. Primary gastric lymphoma in clinical practice 1973–1992. Gut 1995;36:679–683.

55. Caletti G, Ferrari A, Brocchi E, Barbara L. Accuracy of endoscopic ultrasonography in the diagnosis and staging of gastric cancer and lymphoma. Surgery 1993;113:14–27.

56. Schuder G, Hildebrandt U, Kreissler-Haag D, et al. Role of endosonography in the surgical management of non-Hodgkin's lymphoma of the stomach. Endoscopy 1993;25:509–512.

57. Palazzo L, Roseau G, Ruskone-Fourmestraux A, et al. Endoscopic ultrasonography in the local staging of primary gastric lymphoma. Endoscopy 1993;25: 502–508.

58. Fujishima H, Misawa T, Maruoka A, et al. Staging and follow-up of primary gastric lymphoma by endoscopic ultrasonography. Am J Gastroeneterol 1991; 86:719–724.

59. Tio TL, den Hartog Jager FCA, Tytgat GNJ. Endoscopic ultrasonography of non-Hodgkin lymphoma of the stomach. Gastroenterol 1986;91:401–408.

60. Wiersema MJ, Gatzimos K, Nisi R, Wiersema LM. Staging of non-Hodgkin's gastric lymphoma with endosonography-guided fine-needle aspiration biopsy and flow cytometry. Gastrointest Endosc 1996;44: 734–736.

61. Sackmann M, Morgner A, Rudolph B, et al. Regression of gastric MALT lymphoma after eradication of *Helicobacter pylori* is predicted by endosonographic staging. Gastroenterol 1997;113:1087–1090.

61a. Nobre-Leitao C, Lage P, Cravo M, et al. Treatment of gastric MALT lymphoma by *Helicobacter pylori* eradication: a study controlled by endoscopic endosonography. Am J Gastroenterol 1998;93:732–736.

62. Pavlick AC, Gerdes H, Portlock CS. Endoscopic ultrasound in the evaluation of gastric small lymphocytic mucosa-associated lymphoid tumors. J Clin Onc 1997;15:1761 1766.

# 9

# Gastrointestinal Submucosal Masses

## Thomas J. Savides

The term *submucosal mass* describes any gastrointestinal tract mass with normal overlying mucosa. Usually these lesions are detected incidentally as smooth masses on endoscopy or barium studies. Because these lesions are located below the mucosal layer, endoscopic biopsies reveal only normal mucosa.

Before the development of endoscopic ultrasound, submucosal masses were generally assumed to be benign, and often were assumed to be either lipomas or leiomyomas. The accuracy of these assumptions can now be tested with EUS because the actual wall layer from which these lesions originate can now be defined. Submucosal masses can be located in the histologic submucosa, muscularis propria, or as extrinsic compression by a structure adjacent to the GI tract (Table 9-1). Because EUS allows much more accurate diagnosis, the technique can help to decide which lesions require additional tissue sampling, endoscopic follow-up, or surgical resection (1–3).

## Endoscopic Findings

Standard video endoscopy is usually performed prior to EUS visualization of submucosal masses because direct visual imaging is still far superior to the fiber-optic or video imaging of echoendoscopes. In the future, the use of two scopes may not be necessary.

Endoscopy is important in identifying the actual location of the mass in relation to other structures (i.e., the GE junction or the ampulla), noting overlying mucosal ulceration, and identifying other lesions. Duodenal submucosal masses should also be examined with a side viewing ERCP scope to accurately characterize the lesion and the relationship to the ampulla.

Careful endoscopic evaluation of submucosal masses may help suggest the etiology of the mass, although superficial biopsy of these masses usually reveals normal mucosa. The characteristic endoscopic findings of lipomas include the *cushion sign*, in which the biopsy forceps indent the lesion as if it were a pillow, and the ability to separate or "tent" the normal overlying mucosa easily from the underlying lipoma with a biopsy forceps. Stromal cell tumors may appear as bilobar or dumbbell-shaped masses. Varices appear tubular and blue. Some submucosal masses disappear with insufflation, such as varices, cysts, and thick folds.

## EUS Imaging Techniques

Endoscopic ultrasound is very useful in identifying the exact histologic layer from which submucosal masses arise. Imaging can be performed with dedicated echoendoscopes (radial scanning or linear array) and with catheter-based ultrasound probes. For small lesions and esophageal lesions, catheter probes may be especially useful because the probe can be placed against the lesion under direct visualization.

Submucosal masses are best imaged with the lesion submerged in water and by using very little water in the balloon around the transducer. The water bath provides the acoustical imaging medium to allow the transducer to be placed 1 to 2 cm away from the lesion, which is the focal length of most transducers. A liquid interface allows the most accurate ultrasound images of the normal five-layer wall pattern, and also prevents physical distortion of the lesion by the probe. In order to prevent air bubbles, which can produce ultrasound artifact, simethicone is usually added to the water, and the water is slowly infused into the lumen (4). Great care must always be taken when infusing large amounts of water into the upper GI tract for imaging to

**Table 9-1.** Differential Diagnosis of Submucosal Masses.

| **Submucosal** |
| --- |
| Lipoma |
| Carcinoid |
| Pancreatic Rest |
| Varices |
| Duplication Cyst |
| Granular Cell Tumor |

| **Muscularis Propria** |
| --- |
| Stromal Cell Tumor |

| **Extrinsic Compression** |
| --- |
| Adjacent Normal Organs (i.e., liver or spleen) |
| Lymph Nodes |
| Malignancy |
| Pseudocyst |

avoid the possibility of regurgitation and aspiration. When using the water-filled stomach technique, the head of the patient's bed should be elevated at least 45 degrees, the least amount of water possible should be instilled, all air should be removed with suction, and the nurse should watch for signs of regurgitation.

The larger the submucosal mass, the easier it is to image with a dedicated echoendoscope. Large masses require an echoendoscope that can penetrate several centimeters of thickness. Very small lesions (less than 1 cm in diameter) can be extremely difficult to image with echoendoscopes, and often are better seen using catheter-based ultrasound probes passed through a standard endoscope.

## Esophagus

Imaging in the esophagus can be challenging because of the inability to create a pool of water in the esophagus. It is generally not practical to infuse much water into the esophagus, because the water may either flow proximally and place the patient at risk for aspiration, or the water will rapidly flow into the stomach. Esophageal masses are often very small, and the ultrasound transducer should be placed against the lesion under direct visualization, if possible. All air should be removed with suction. Very little balloon inflation is needed, and may be detrimental if it distorts or collapses the lesion. Small lesions in the esophagus are often better imaged with a catheter probe.

## Stomach

Imaging in these areas should be done with the lesion submerged under water. As much as 500 ml of water may be needed to obtain an adequate water bath. The head of the patient should be elevated in order to mini-

mize the risk of aspirating the water. Lesions along the greater curve of the stomach can be imaged with the patient in the standard left lateral decubitus position. Lesions along the lesser curve, antrum, and pylorus are more difficult to image when the patient is in the left lateral decubitus position because the water pools in the dependent portion of the fundus. Sometimes these lesions can be imaged by a combination of a large amount of water in the stomach, removing all air from the stomach, and using the water-filled balloon. The patient can also be positioned on the back, stomach, or right side to get the lesion under water, again using great care to avoid aspiration.

## Duodenum

Using a video duodenoscope first to image duodenal submucosal lesions will often result in a better view of the lesion than with a standard forward viewing endoscope, and will also allow for visualization in relationship to the ampulla. For EUS, a large amount of water should be instilled into the duodenum to help create an acoustic window. Duodenal motility can interfere with imaging, and administration of intravenous glucagon (0.5–1.0 mg intravenously) will help relax the duodenum. Ultrasound imaging using a standard radial echoendoscope can often be difficult, especially with small lesions or lesions located on an angulated portion or just inside the pyloric channel. These lesions may be better imaged using a catheter probe passed through a standard endoscope or a duodenoscope, or possibly with a linear array scope. EUS should evaluate not only the submucosal lesion, but also examine the ampulla, common bile duct, and pancreatic head for abnormalities.

## Rectum and Colon

Prior to imaging rectal lesions, a bowel prep with two enemas should be given. Flexible sigmoidoscopy should first be performed to identify the lesion, characterize the overlying mucosa, and to remove any remaining fecal material. Water should be instilled into the rectum and the patient positioned such that the lesion is covered with water. Rectal EUS examinations are usually performed without the use of intravenous sedation or glucagon.

EUS is performed after filling the rectum with water and aspirating any residual air. A small amount of water in the balloon may be needed. Ultrasound imaging should document not only the location of the lesion, but also the relationship to the adjacent organs, including the prostate, seminal vesicles, bladder, and uterus.

Colonic submucosal lesions located proximal to the low sigmoid colon usually require a catheter-probe

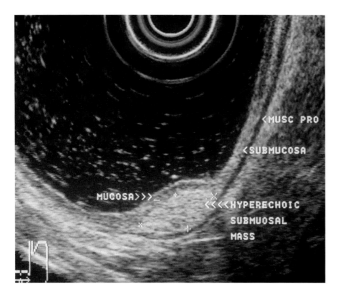

**Figure 9-1.** Gastric lipoma. Note the characteristic hyperechoic mass in the submucosal layer. *Musc prop* = muscularis propria.

ultrasound or dedicated colonic echoendoscope in order to reach the area of interest. Occasionally, sigmoid lesions may be within reach of a standard upper echoendoscope.

## Lesions Located in the Submucosa

### Lipomas

Lipomas represent benign hyperplasia of mature lipocytes and are usually found in the submucosal layer (5). They can involve any part of the intestinal tract, and are usually asymptomatic. Gastric lipomas account for about 5% of all gastrointestinal lipomas, and 75% are located in the antrum (6). Usually they are discovered incidentally during endoscopy, but occasionally they cause symptoms such as pain, bleeding, or obstruction.

Characteristic endoscopic findings include a yellow color. Pressing against the surface of a submucosal lipoma with a closed biopsy forceps leaves an indentation, as if it were a pillow (cushion sign). Grasping the normal overlying mucosa with biopsy forceps can easily pull the mucosa away from the underlying mass (tent sign). Routine biopsies yield normal mucosa, as the lesion is in the submucosa. Deep-well biopsy or fine-needle aspiration may reveal lipocytes. Endoscopic ultrasound shows a characteristic hyperechoic mass located in the submucosa (Figure 9-1). This finding is virtually diagnostic of a lipoma. Because of the high accuracy of EUS in diagnosing lipomas, biopsies or fine-needle aspiration are not needed.

Though lipomas are by definition benign, transformation to malignant liposarcoma has been reported.

Surgical removal of these lesions should be performed for symptomatic or enlarging lesions. Additionally, lesions that seem to be infiltrating multiple wall layers or do not have an echo pattern entirely consistent with a lipoma should be considered for resection. Small, asymptomatic lesions that appear to be lipomas on EUS may not need any further follow-up, or at most perhaps periodic re-evaluation to confirm no increase in size.

There have been reports of snare resection of gastrointestinal lipomas (7). However, the risk of perforation seems to greatly increase if the lipoma is greater than 2 cm in diameter (8). Given that lipomas are almost universally benign, it does not seem that routine removal of lipomas is worth the potential risk of perforation (9).

### Carcinoid Tumors

Carcinoid tumors are neuroendocrine tumors, sometimes also referred to as amine precursor uptake and decarboxylation (APUD) tumors. The term *carcinoid* was originally used to describe tumors of a characteristic pathologic appearance arising in the epithelial layer but with a less aggressive clinical course than that of typical adenocarcinoma. They are thought to originate from the peripheral neuroendocrine system in the mucosa, and then penetrate the muscularis mucosa to form a submucosal lesion (10,11). Histologically they appear as small, round, or polygonal uniform cells arranged in nests and often stain argentaffin positive.

Carcinoid tumors can produce a variety of functionally active substances, including serotonin, histamine, gastrin, somatostatin, pituitary hormones, catecholamines, kinins, and prostaglandins. Most of these tumors produce very small amounts of these substances, and therefore are clinically silent.

Carcinoid tumors are divided into foregut, midgut, and hindgut neoplasms based on their anatomic location and functional characteristics. Foregut carcinoids include the bronchi, stomach, duodenum, and pancreas. Foregut carcinoids may cause flushing. Patients with pernicious anemia are at increased risk of gastric carcinoid tumors because the enterochromaffin-like cells (ECL) are stimulated by the elevated levels of gastrin, resulting in hyperplasia and, in some cases, carcinoid tumors. Midgut carcinoids involve the small bowel, appendix, and right colon. Midgut carcinoids are associated with the carcinoid syndrome (flushing, diarrhea, and asthma) once they have metastasized to the liver. One-third of all carcinoid tumors in the United States are appendiceal in origin. Hindgut carcinoids involve the transverse colon, sigmoid colon, and rectum. These patients rarely present with systemic symptoms, but rather with local complications. In the United States, most cases are located in the appendix, rectum, and ileum, and in Japan they are located in the stomach, rectum, and duodenum (11,12).

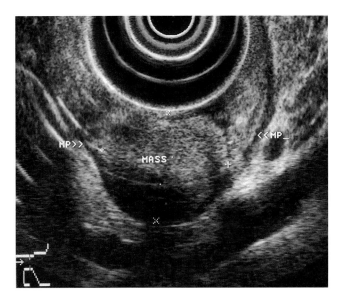

**Figure 9-2.** Duodenal carcinoid tumor. The submucosal mass has mixed hypo- and hyperechoic areas and is clearly different from the typical hyperechoic lipoma or hypoechoic stromal tumor.

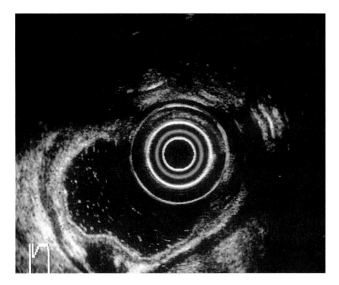

**Figure 9-3.** Granular cell tumor of the stomach. Note the slightly irregular hypoechoic mass in the submucosa with internal echoes. This is different from a typical lipoma or stromal cell tumor.

Features associated with increased metastatic risk of duodenal or rectal carcinoid tumors include size greater than 2 cm and involvement of the muscularis propria (13–15). Endoscopically, carcinoids usually appear as smooth, round, yellowish masses, which can have a central erythematous depression or ulceration (16). Unlike other submucosal tumors, the diagnosis of carcinoids can often be made with standard biopsy forceps (16,17).

The EUS appearance of carcinoid tumors is a hypoechoic, homogenous lesion with distinct smooth margins, located in the submucosal layer (Figure 9-2) (17). The lesions are less hypoechoic than the second or fourth layers. EUS has an accuracy rate of 90% for diagnosing the exact wall layer involved (17). Lymph node metastases tend to occur in lesions greater than 15 mm in diameter by EUS, and there can be malignant lymph node invasion in tumors limited to the submucosa (17).

Treatment of carcinoids depends on their location. Gastric carcinoids may be multicentric and, at least in Japan, have a high risk of metastases (17). Small lesions (< 1 cm) located in the mucosa can be endoscopically resected, but larger lesions (> 2 cm) located in the submucosa or muscularis propria should be considered for surgical resection. Duodenal carcinoids do not seem to metastasize until they have penetrated the muscularis propria, which allows endoscopic resection of small lesions in the mucosa (14,17). Rectal carcinoid tumors should be surgically resected if the diameter is greater than 15 mm. Small rectal carcinoids (less than 10 mm) limited to the mucosa or submucosa, and without adjacent lymphadenopathy can be considered for endoscopic resection (17).

Any patient with a carcinoid tumor that is endoscopically resected should have follow-up endoscopy with biopsies and endoscopic ultrasound to ensure there is no recurrence over time. With the increasing use of EUS in identifying and staging carcinoid tumors, long-term follow-up after endoscopic resection using EUS is needed to help determine the value of nonsurgical management in preventing metastatic disease.

### Granular Cell Tumors

Granular cell tumors originate from either Schwann cells or smooth muscle (5). They are usually found in the tongue, oropharynx, skin, subcutaneous tissue, and breast, but can be found anywhere in the body (18). In the gastrointestinal tract, the most common site is the tongue, followed by the esophagus, stomach, and colon. These lesions are usually found in the mucosa or submucosal layers (19). Histologically they consist of large polygonal cells containing numerous eosinophilic granules. Up to 15% of patients with granular cell tumors will have multiple tumors.

Granular cell tumors are detected incidentally during endoscopy. Endoscopically, they appear as polypoid masses that may have a yellowish color. Esophageal granular cell tumors are usually found in the distal esophagus. Deep mucosal biopsies will often yield the diagnosis. A recent EUS study found that among 21 granular cell tumors, 95% were less than 2 cm in diameter, 95% were located in the mid or distal esophagus, 100% had a hypoechoic appearance, 95% had smooth margins, and 71% seemed to originate from the second hypoechoic layer and 24% from the third hyperechoic layer (Figure 9-3) (20).

The natural history of these lesions seems to be benign, based on long-term follow-up of lesions diagnosed by biopsy and not removed, as well as by lesions that were removed endoscopically (21). The rare malignant granular cell tumors of the esophagus have ranged in size from 4 to 10 cm in diameter (21). This preliminary data suggests that perhaps surgical resection could be reserved for lesions causing symptoms, measuring greater than 2 cm diameter, with EUS findings suggesting infiltration through the intestinal wall, or increasing in size on serial endoscopy or EUS. Tumors that are not removed should be followed with EUS every one to two years to monitor growth.

Endoscopic removal of small granular cell tumors can be performed with multiple biopsies using pinch forceps (22). Snare polypectomy has also been used in order to obliterate the lesion (23,24). There have also been case reports of tumor ablation using alcohol, polidocanol, and laser (25–27). Longer-term follow-up to determine the natural history of these lesions, based on their EUS characteristics, will help decide optimal patient management.

## Duplication Cysts

Duplication cysts arise during embryonic development, and can be located anywhere within or adjacent to the luminal gastrointestinal tract (28). They are spherical or tubular, contain mucin, possess a smooth muscle layer, and are lined by the same mucosa as the adjacent bowel. They occasionally communicate with the adjacent intestinal lumen. Approximately 50% of duplication cysts are found in the small intestine, with the remainder in the esophagus, stomach, and colon.

Duplication cysts are usually asymptomatic, but can result in symptoms due to mass effect, bleeding, or perforation (29). Cysts located near the ampulla of Vater may cause pancreatitis (30). Most cysts are diagnosed in infants or children, and there is a female preponderance. When located in the mediastinum, these cysts can be confused with bronchogenic cysts and therefore may also be referred to as foregut cysts. Duplication cysts rarely have been reported to undergo malignant transformation (31,32).

EUS of duplication cysts usually reveals a round, anechoic lesion in the third hypoechoic layer (Figure 9-4) (33,34). They may have endosonographic findings of distinct wall layers. EUS may also show the cysts to be located adjacent to the tubular GI tract (35). They have been reported to have echogenic material due to thick mucinous material or debris (36). There can be a fluid interface seen between the debris in the cyst and the rest of the fluid (37). The diagnosis can be confirmed with fine-needle aspiration of the fluid, although this is not generally necessary (34,38).

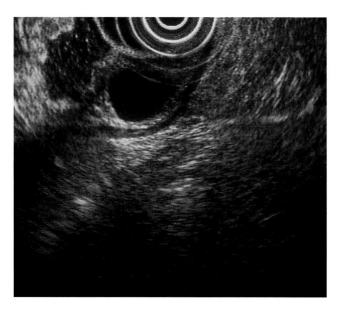

**Figure 9-4.** Duplication cyst in the gastric antrum. Note the round, anechoic structure in the third (submucosal) layer.

Treatment of symptomatic or enlarging lesions has traditionally been surgical resection or marsupialization. Endoscopic treatment has been successfully achieved by needle aspiration and needle-knife cystostomy (30,35,39,40). The optimal management of asymptomatic cysts is not yet defined, and could include surgical resection, endoscopic treatment, or simply periodic EUS surveillance to observe for enlargement.

## Heterotopic Pancreas (Pancreatic Rest)

Heterotopic pancreas, also known as pancreatic rest or ectopic pancreas, is usually found within a few centimeters of the gastroduodenal junction. Seventy-five percent are found in the stomach, duodenum, or jejunum. They are incidental findings in 1% to 14% of autopsies (41). The lesions are thought to form during rotation of the foregut when portions of the pancreas become separated. Histologically, they contain a mixture of pancreatic tissue, including ducts and parenchyma.

Endoscopically, they appear as submucosal masses that may have a central umbilication through which secretions drain. With EUS, the pancreatic rest appears hypoechoic or has intermediate echogenicity and may be found in any layer of the intestinal wall (33). Usually a tissue diagnosis can be made with deep mucosal biopsies.

Heterotopic pancreas is usually asymptomatic and found incidentally during endoscopy. Any pathology that can affect the pancreas can also occur in the pancreatic rest, such as malignancy, cysts, and islet cell tumors. Incidentally found asymptomatic pancreatic rests require no further evaluation or treatment (41).

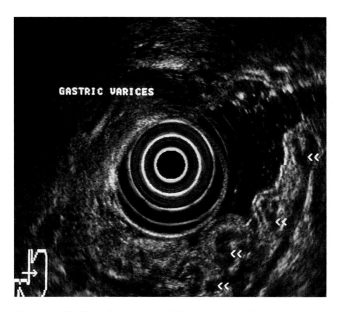

**Figure 9-5.** Gastric varices. The *arrows* point to hypoechoic, tubular structures in the submucosal layer, which correspond to intramural varices.

## Varices

Endoscopic ultrasound can visualize many aspects of the normal portal venous system, such as the portal vein, splenic vein, superior mesenteric vein, and azygous vein. In the setting of portal hypertension, esophageal and gastric submucosal veins, periesophageal and perigastric collateral veins, and perforating veins connecting the adventitial and submucosal veins can be easily seen (Figure 9-5) (42). Compared to standard video endoscopy, EUS using a dedicated echoendoscope does not help in the detection of esophageal varices but does improve diagnosis of gastric varices (42–44). EUS appears accurate for diagnosing moderate or large esophageal varices, but not small varices (44).

## Lesions Located in the Muscularis Propria

### Gastrointestinal Stromal Cell Tumors (GISTs)

These lesions, formerly known as leiomyomas and leiomyosarcomas, are mesenchymal tumors, which are usually composed of spindle cells, and were originally considered to be of smooth muscle origin. However, recent studies suggest that many of these lesions have little evidence of smooth muscle or neural differentiation (5). In fact, the only consistent immune marker has been for vimentin, a primitive cell filament that does not occur in mature smooth muscle cells of the gut muscularis, but does occur in endothelium and in fibroblasts (5). Recent work suggests that

some GIST lesions may originate from the Interstitial Cells of Cajal, the so-called "pacemaker cells" for the gastrointestinal tract.

Histologically, stromal tumors can appear as spindle cell or epitheliod tumors (5). Some pathologists divide GISTs into four major categories, based on their phenotypic features: 1) tumors showing differentiation toward smooth muscle cells, 2) tumors showing differentiation toward neural elements, 3) tumors showing dual differentiation with both smooth muscle and neural elements, 4) tumors lacking differentiation toward either smooth muscle or neural cells (45). None of the phenotypic features or immune markers seem to have any certain prognostic significance for stromal tumors, and generally are not clinically useful.

Approximately two-thirds of all gastrointestinal stromal tumors occur in the stomach. The reported incidence of gastric stromal tumors is quite variable, ranging from 0.18% to 46% based on autopsy or surgical resection specimens (46). Using a whole organ stepwise cutting method, Yamada showed that in 286 resected stomachs the rate of leiomyomas was 16%, with most being less than 5 mm in diameter and located in the upper half of the stomach (46). GIST lesions are often detected as incidental findings during other imaging studies, but may present with bleeding, pain, or obstructive symptoms.

Malignant stromal tumors can metastasize to the liver, peritoneum, and lungs (47). The malignant potential of these tumors is classified into three categories: no malignant potential, low (or uncertain) malignant potential, or high malignant potential (5). High-risk factors for malignancy include size greater than 5 cm, greater than 5 mitoses per 50 high-power fields, tumor necrosis, nuclear pleomorphism, dense cellularity, microscopic invasion of the lamina propria or blood vessels, and an alveolar pattern in the epithelioid variant (5). Stromal tumors thought to have high malignant potential have one unequivocal or two high-risk factors. Stromal tumors of uncertain malignant potential have only one high-risk factor and benign stromal tumors have no high-risk factors. Nevertheless, any prognostic pathologic staging for GISTs should be considered with caution because there are reports of metastatic disease occurring years after removal of small, benign-appearing stromal cell tumors (48).

Carney's triad is the rare association of gastric leiomyosarcomas with pulmonary chondroma and functioning extra-adrenal paragangliomas (49,50). Carney's triad is usually found in women less than 40 years of age, and is diagnosed in patients with two triad components. In young or middle-aged women with stromal cell tumors of indeterminate or high malignant potential, consideration should be give to obtaining a chest x-ray and urine catecholamines (50). GISTs have also been associated with von Recklinghausen's disease (51,52).

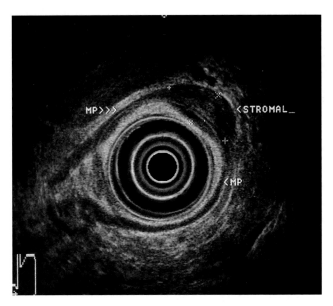

**Figure 9-6.** Stromal cell tumor of stomach. Note that this lesion is located within the muscularis propria (*MP*), which is typical for stromal cell tumors.

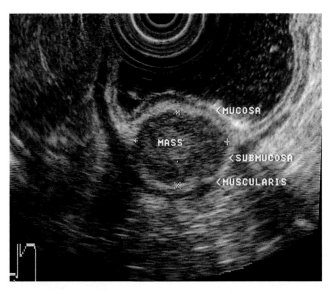

**Figure 9-7.** Stromal cell tumor of the stomach. Note that this lesion is diffusely hypoechoic and located in the submucosa. This tumor probably developed as a bud from either the muscularis propria or muscularis mucosa, and grew within the submucosa.

Endoscopy of stromal tumors reveals a submucosal mass that is often dumbbell shaped and may have a central umbilication or ulceration. Endoscopic biopsies usually reveal only overlying normal mucosa. The EUS appearance of stromal cell tumors is usually a hypoechoic mass originating from the muscularis propria (fourth hypoechoic layer) (Figure 9-6) (53). Occasionally, the hypoechoic lesion may be seen in the submucosa (third hyperechoic layer), and have a suggestion of origination from either the muscularis mucosa or muscularis propria (Figure 9-7).

The EUS features associated with malignant stromal tumors include tumor size greater than 4 cm, irregular extraluminal border, echogenic foci (greater than 3 mm), and cystic spaces (greater than 4 mm) (54). The cystic spaces seen in stromal cell tumors of high malignant potential may correspond to cystic degeneration and liquefaction necrosis (55,56). If two or more of these criteria are present, the lesion is likely of high malignant potential, and if none of the criteria are present, then it is probably benign (54). However, expert endosonographers using the above criteria had only fair agreement using kappa statistics (54). At present, EUS cannot accurately differentiate benign from malignant GIST, and EUS criteria should not be the only basis for classification of malignant potential.

Deep mucosal biopsies and fine-needle aspiration do not yield enough tissue for accurate pathologic assessment of the malignant potential of these lesions. Biopsy and FNA of suspected stromal tumors should be performed only if there is doubt regarding the diagnosis of the submucosal mass, and if the tissue diagnosis will change clinical management.

The optimal management of submucosal masses that are suspected to be stromal cell tumors by EUS is unknown. Surgical resection should be performed for all lesions causing symptoms (i.e., bleeding, obstruction, pain), lesions greater than 3 cm in diameter, lesions with suspicious EUS findings as above, and lesions that increase in size on serial EUS exams. Small (less than 3 cm diameter), asymptomatic, incidentally discovered lesions that are suspected to be benign stromal cell tumors may be observed with repeat EUS every 6 to 12 months. These small lesions might never become clinically significant, especially given their high incidence in resection studies, and therefore serial EUS might be a reasonable alternative to surgery. If the lesions increase in size, develop suspicious-appearing EUS features, or become symptomatic, they should be resected.

Endoscopic resection of stromal tumors has been reported (57–61). This should be considered only in cases where the lesion is less than 2 cm and seems to originate from the muscularis mucosa and not the muscularis propria. Follow-up endoscopy and EUS may be helpful to make sure there is no residual stromal tumor.

## Extrinsic Compression Lesions

Normal abdominal organs can cause indentations in the gastrointestinal tract, which may mimic a submucosal

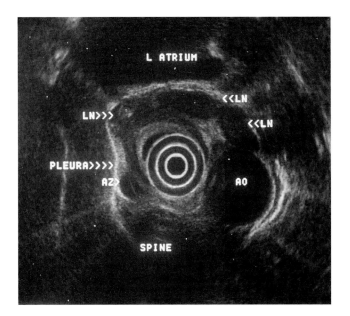

**Figure 9-8.** Posterior mediastinal lymph nodes (*LN*). These are suspected to be due to histoplasmosis infection. *AO* = aorta, *AZ* = azygous vein, *L* = left.

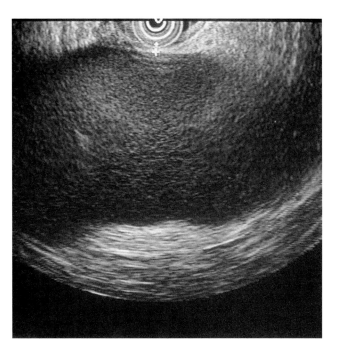

**Figure 9-9.** Pancreatic pseudocyst pressing against the stomach.

tumor. In the esophagus, compressions can be seen by the aortic arch and left atrium. Pathologic compression in the esophagus may occur from malignant lymph nodes or masses, especially from lung cancer. Benign lymph nodes, such as due to histoplasmosis, can sometimes present as a submucosal esophageal mass (Figure 9-8) (62). In the stomach, the left lobe of the liver and the spleen can cause compression. Pancreatic pseudocysts or extrinsic tumors can cause extrinsic compression (Figure 9-9). In the rectum, the prostate or cervix can cause an extrinsic compression, which may mimic a submucosal mass. Accurate diagnosis of these extrinsic compressions can prevent further expensive testing.

## Comparison of Imaging Studies for Submucosal Masses

Rosch compared EUS versus barium upper GI series versus CT scan and found that EUS detected 37 of 37 lesions, barium study detected 11 of 13 lesions, and CT detected 16 of 24 lesions (63). These tumors ranged in size from 0.5 cm to 10.0 cm, with a mean of 2.8 cm.

## Endoscopic Tissue Sampling
### Which Lesions Need Sampling?

EUS results can help determine when it is safe and useful to obtain tissue sampling by fine-needle aspiration or

large particle biopsy. Although various techniques can obtain tissue for cytologic or histopathologic diagnosis, they should be used selectively in only those cases in which the information will change management. For example, a hyperechoic structure in the submucosa is almost certainly a lipoma, and needs no confirmation with FNA. A hypoechoic lesion in the muscularis propria is almost certainly a stromal cell tumor, and FNA cytology or even large-particle biopsies will not yield enough tissue for the pathologist to determine the malignant potential of the lesion. FNA and snare resection are potentially very useful when the diagnosis is in doubt, such as a heterogeneous lesion in the submucosal layer, which could be a carcinoid, granular cell tumor, pancreatic rest, or other lesion. Contraindications to FNA or snare resection are EUS findings of a vascular lesion such as varices, or an extrinsic mass causing the observed "mucosal" abnormality such as compression by the liver or spleen. Submucosal masses that are not typical lipomas or stromal cell tumors should have tissue sampling performed. Extrinsic masses that are suspicious for malignancy should be considered for transintestinal FNA.

### Biopsy Forceps

Jumbo biopsy forceps (3.2 mm diameter) should be used to maximize the chances of obtaining deep tissue. Biopsies should be obtained from any areas of mucosal ulceration. The "deep-well" or "tunneling" biopsy technique can also be tried, in which successive biopsies are taken from the same spot, with the idea of removing the mucosa with the first biopsy and then obtaining deeper tissue—from the underlying lesion—with the next biopsy.

### Fine-Needle Aspiration

Fine-needle aspiration can be performed either through a standard endoscope or through a dedicated FNA echoendoscope (64). Various FNA needles exist, ranging from sclerotherapy type needles, which are 15 mm long and 23 Fr, to dedicated EUS FNA needles, which are 22 Fr and up to 8 cm long. Generally, the needle is passed into the lesion, the stylet is removed, and suction is appled while the needle is moved in and out of the lesion. Suction on the syringe is then released, the needle is retracted, the catheter is removed, and the contents are then placed onto a glass slide. Several passes are often needed to obtain adequate tissue. Caletti has devised a needle for sampling submucosal lesions in which there is a guillotine device that obtains samples 8 mm in length and 1 to 2 mm in diameter (65).

### Mucosectomy Followed by Deep Biopsy

Another means of obtaining tissue from beneath the mucosal layer is by first removing the overlying mucosa, and then biopsying the underlying lesion. The process of endoscopic mucosectomy is performed with snare resection of a portion of the overlying mucosa. This may be preceded by either submucosal saline or epinephrine injection to raise the mucosa off the underlying mass, or by rubber band ligation of mucosa overlying the lesion, followed by snare resection. Mucosectomy usually provides access to the underlying lesion, which can then be directly biopsied. Occasionally the entire lesion may actually extrude through the unroofed mucosa following mucosectomy.

## Endoscopic and Larascopic Resection of Submucosal Masses

If EUS shows the mass to be located in the submucosal layer and to be less than 2 cm in diameter, endoscopic removal may be the method of choice for obtaining a definitive diagnosis (23,61). In general, a submucosal lesion with the classic characteristics of a lipoma does not need resection and stromal cell tumors should not be removed endoscopically if they communicate with the muscularis propria.

Pre-injection with saline or epinephrine beneath the lesion may potentially decrease the risk of perfora-

tion or bleeding during attempted resection. Very small lesions can also be managed with rubber band ligation to form a more protruding polypoid shape that can then be removed with snare cautery (60).

Gastric submucosal masses that require surgical removal can sometimes be resected using a laparoscopic approach. Intraoperative endoscopy during laparoscopy is very useful not only to identify the lesion but also to push it into a favorable position for laparoscopic transection with a stapling device. There has also been a case reported of performing endoscopic resection of a 2-cm stromal cell tumor during simultaneous laparoscopy to confirm lack of perforation at the time of resection (59).

Regardless of the technique used to remove a submucosal tumor, attention should be given to complete removal of the tissue. If residual tumor tissue is suspected, periodic endoscopic ultrasound surveillance should be performed.

## Utility of EUS for Management of Submucosal Masses

### Interobserver Agreement of EUS for Evaluating Submucosal Masses

Interobserver agreement regarding the finding of submucosal masses during EUS is generally good. In one study, six experienced endosonographers reviewed videotapes of EUS examinations. There was excellent agreement for cystic lesions and extrinsic compression, good agreement for lipomas, and fair agreement for stromal tumors and vascular lesions (66).

### Outcome Studies

Preliminary reports of outcome studies suggest that EUS is useful for evaluating and managing submucosal masses. In one large multicenter trial, endosonographers were asked to determine whether EUS findings changed patient management plans. They reported that EUS resulted in major changes in diagnostic and/or therapeutic strategies in two-thirds of patients with submucosal tumors (67). Additional outcome studies are in progress to further define and quantify the benefits of endoscopic ultrasound in evaluating patients with submucosal lesions in the upper gastrointestinal tract.

## Conclusion

EUS is the most accurate imaging modality for lesions located within, or compressing, the gastrointestinal wall. EUS findings can be diagnostic based on ultrasound characteristics alone and can identify lesions that require tissue sampling. With the ability of EUS to diagnose submucosal lesions of the upper gastrointestinal tract with a high degree of accuracy, the natural history of these lesions can be better understood with more rational selection of candidates for surgical resection.

## References

1. Boyce GA, Sivak-MV J, Rosch T, et al. Evaluation of submucosal upper gastrointestinal tract lesions by endoscopic ultrasound. Gastrointest Endosc 1991;37:449–454.
2. Caletti G, Zani L, Bolondi L, et al. Endoscopic ultrasonography in the diagnosis of gastric submucosal tumor. Gastrointest Endosc 1989;35:413–418.
3. Inai M, Sakai M, Kajiyama T, et al. Endosonographic characterization of duodenal elevated lesions. Gastrointest Endosc 1996;44:714–719.
4. Yiengpruksawan A, Lightdale CJ, Gerdes H, Botet JF. Mucolytic-antifoam solution for reduction of artifacts during endoscopic ultrasonography: a randomized controlled trial. Gastrointest Endosc 1991;37:543–546.
5. Lewin KJ, Riddell RH, Weinstein WM. Mesenchymal tumors. In: Lewin KJ, Riddell RH, Weinstein WM, eds. Gastrointestinal pathology and its clinical implications. New York: Igaku-Shoin, 1992:284–341.
6. Maderal F, Hunter F, Fuselier G, et al. Gastric lipomas—an update of clinical presentation, diagnosis, and treatment. Am J Gastroenterol 1994;79:964–967.
7. Nakamura S, Iida M, Suekane H, et al. Endoscopic removal of gastric lipoma: diagnostic value of endoscopic ultrasonography. Am J Gastroenterol 1991;86:619–621.
8. Pfeil SA, Weaver MG, Abdul KF, Yang P. Colonic lipomas: outcome of endoscopic removal. Gastrointest Endosc 1990;36:435–438.
9. Christie JP. The removal of lipomas. Gastrointest Endosc 1990;36:532–533.
10. Matsuyama M, Suzuki H. Differentiation of immature mucous cells into parietal, argyrophil, and chief cells in stomach grafts. Science 1970;169:385–387.
11. Soga J. Histogenesis of carcinoids in relation to ordinary carcinomas. Acta Med Biol 1982;30:17–33.
12. Godwin JD. Carcinoid tumors, an analysis of 2837 cases. Cancer 1974;36:560–569.
13. Morgan JC, Mark C, Hearn D. Carcinoid tumors of gastrointestinal tract. Ann Surg 1974;180:720–727.
14. Burke AP, Sobin LH, Federspiel BH, et al. Carcinoid tumors of the duodenum: a clinicopathologic study of 99 cases. Arch Pathol Lab Med 1990;114:700–704.
15. Federspiel BH, Burke AP, Sobin LH, Shekitka KM. Rectal and colonic carcinoids: a clinicopathologic study of 84 cases. Cancer 1990;65:135–140.
16. Nakamura S, Iida M, Yao T, Fujishima M. Endoscopic features of gastric carcinoids. Gastrointest Endosc 1991;37:535–538.
17. Yoshikane H, Tsukamoto Y, Niwa Y, et al. Carcinoid tumors of the gastrointestinal tract: evaluation with endoscopic ultrasonography. Gastrointest Endosc 1993;39:375–383.
18. Lack EE, Worsham GF, Callihan MD, et al. Granular cell tumor: a clinicopathologic study of 110 patients. J Surg Oncol 1980;13:301–316.
19. Brady PG, Nord HJ, Connar RG. Granular cell tumor of the esophagus: natural history, diagnosis, and therapy. Dig Dis Sci 1988;33:1329–1333.
20. Palazzo L, Landi B, Cellier C, et al. Endosonographic features of esophageal granular cell tumors. Endoscopy 1997;29:850–853.
21. Orlowska J, Pachlewski J, Gugulski A, Butruk E. A conservative approach to granular cell tumors of the esophagus: four case reports and literature review. Am J Gastroenterol 1993;88:311–315.
22. Giacobbe A, Facciorusso D, Conoscitore P, et al. Granular cell tumor of the esophagus. Am J Gastroenterol 1988;83:1398–1400.
23. Yasuda I, Tomita E, Nagura K, et al. Endoscopic removal of granular cell tumors. Gastrointest Endosc 1995;41:163–167.
24. Tada S, Iida M, Yao T, et al. Granular cell tumor of the esophagus: endoscopic ultrasonographic demonstration and endoscopic removal. Am J Gastroenterol 1990;85:1507–1511.
25. Maccarini MR, Michieletti G, Tampieri I, et al. Simple endoscopic treatment of a granular-cell tumor of the esophagus. Endoscopy 1996;28:730–731.
26. Choi PM, Schneider L. Endoscopic Nd:YAG laser treatment of granular cell tumor of the esophagus. Gastrointest Endosc 1990;36:144–146.
27. Moreira LS, Dani R. Treatment of granular cell tumor of the esophagus by endoscopic injection of dehydrated alcohol. Am J Gastroenterol 1992;87:659–661.
28. Lewin KJ, Riddell RH, Weinstein WM. Small and large bowel structure, developmental and mechanical disorders. In: Lewin KJ, Riddell RH, Weinstein WM, eds. Gastrointestinal pathology and its clinical implications. New York: Igaku-Shoin. 1992:734–736.
29. Wieczorek RL, Seidman I, Ranson JHC, Ruoff M. Congenital duplication of the stomach: case report and review of the English literature. Am J Gastroenterol 1984;79:597–602.
30. Al Traif I, Khan MH. Endoscopic drainage of a duodenal duplication cyst. Gastrointest Endosc 1992;38:64–65.
31. Olsen JB, Clemmensen O, Andersen K. Adenocarcinoma arising in a foregut cyst of the mediastinum. Ann Thorac Surg 1991;51:497–499.
32. Coit DG, Mies C. Adenocarcinoma arising within a gastric duplication cyst. J Surg Oncol 1992;50:274–277.
33. Yasuda K, Cho E, Nakajima M, Kawai K. Diagnosis of submucosal lesions of the upper gastrointestinal tract by endoscopic ultrasonography. Gastrointest Endosc 1990;36:S17–S20.
34. Van Dam J, Rice TW, Sivak MV J. Endoscopic ultrasonography and endoscopically guided needle aspiration for the diagnosis of upper gastrointestinal tract foregut cysts. Am J Gastroenterol 1992;87:762–765.
35. Faigel DO, Burke A, Ginsberg GG, et al. The role of endoscopic ultrasound in the evaluation and management

of foregut duplications. Gastrointest Endosc 1997;45: 99–103.

36. Bhutani MS, Hoffman BJ, Reed C. Endosonographic diagnosis of an esophageal duplication cyst. Endoscopy 1996;28:396–397.

37. Geller A, Wang KK, DiMagno EP. Diagnosis of foregut duplication cysts by endoscopic ultrasonography. Gastroenterology 1995;109:838–842.

38. Ferrari AP, Van Dam J, Carr LD. Endoscopic needle aspiration of a gastric duplication cyst. Endoscopy 1995;27:270–272.

39. Woolfolk GM, McClave SA, Jones WF, et al. Use of endoscopic ultrasound to guide the diagnosis and endoscopic management of a large gastric duplication cyst. Gastrointest Endosc 1998;47:76–79.

40. Johanson JF, Geenen JE, Hogan WJ, Huibregtse K. Endoscopic therapy of a duodenal duplication cyst. Gastrointest Endosc 1992;38:60–64.

41. Dolan RV, ReMine WH, Dockerty MB. The fate of heterotopic pancreatic tissue. Arch Surg 1974;109:762.

42. Caletti G, Brocchi E, Baraldini M, et al. Assessment of portal hypertension by endoscopic ultrasonography. Gastrointest Endosc 1990;36:S21–S27.

43. Burtin P, Cales P, Oberti F, et al. Endoscopic ultrasonographic signs of portal hypertension in cirrhosis. Gastrointest Endosc 1996;44:257–261.

44. Choudhuri G, Dhiman RK, Agarwal DK. Endosonographic evaluation of the venous anatomy around the gastro-esophageal junction in patients with portal hypertension. Hepatogastroenterology 1996;43:1250–1255.

45. Rosai J. Stromal cell tumors and lymphomas. In: Rosai J, ed. Ackerman's surgical pathology. 8th ed. St. Louis: Mosby, 1996:645–647.

46. Yamada Y, Kato Y, Yanagisawa A, et al. Microleiomyomas of human stomach. Hum Pathol 1988;19:569–572.

47. Ng EH, Pollock RE, Romsdahl MM. Prognostic implications of patterns of failure for gastrointestinal leiomyosarcomas. Cancer 1992;69:1334–1341.

48. Suster S. Gastrointestinal stromal tumors. Semin Diagnostic Path 1996;13:297–313.

49. Carney JA. The triad of gastric epitheliod leiomyosarcoma, pulmonary chondroma, and functioning extraadrenal paraganglioma: a five-year review. Medicine 1983;62:159–169.

50. Margulies KB, Sheps SG. Carney's triad: guidelines for management. Mayo Clin Proc 1988;63:496–502.

51. Fuller CE, Williams GT. Gastrointestinal manifestations of type 1 neurofibromatosis (von Recklinghausen's disease). Histopathology 1991;19:1–11.

52. Schaldenbrand JD, Appelman HD. Solitary solid stromal gastrointestinal tumors in von Recklinghausen's disease with minimal smooth muscle differentiation. Hum Pathol 1984;15:229–232.

53. Tio TL, Tytgat GNJ, den Hartog Jager FCA. Endoscopic ultrasonography for the evaluation of smooth muscle tumors in the upper gastrointestinal tract: an experience with 42 cases. Gastrointest Endosc 1990;36:342–350.

54. Chak A, Canto MI, Rosch T, et al. Endosonographic differentiation of benign and malignant stromal cell tumors. Gastrointest Endosc 1997;45:468–473.

55. Yamada Y, Kida M, Sakaguchi T. A study on myogenic tumors of the upper gastrointestinal tract by endoscopic ultrasonography—with special reference to the differential diagnosis of benign and malignant lesions. Dig Endosc 1992;4:396–408.

56. Nakazawa S, Yoshino J, Yamanaka T, et al. Endoscopic ultrasonography of gastric myogenic tumor: a comparative study between histology and ultrasonography. J Ultrasound Med 1989;8:353–359.

57. Yu JP, Luo HS, Wang XZ. Endoscopic treatment of submucosal lesions of the gastrointestinal tract. Endoscopy 1992;24:190–193.

58. Binmoeller KF, Grimm H, Sohendra N. Endoscopic closure of a perforation using metallic clips after snare excision of a gastric leiomyoma. Endoscopy 1993;39:172–174.

59. Wolfsohn DM, Savides TJ, Easter DW, Lyche KD. Laparoscopy-assisted endoscopic removal of a stromal-cell tumor of the stomach. Endoscopy 1997;29:679–682.

60. Chang KJ, Yoshinaka R, Nguyen P. Endoscopic ultrasound-assisted band ligation: a new technique for resection of submucosal tumors. Gastrointest Endosc 1996;44:720–722.

61. Kajiyama T, Sakai M, Torii A, et al. Endoscopic aspiration lumpectomy of esophageal leiomyomas derived from the muscularis mucosae. Am J Gastroenterol 1995;90:417–422.

62. Savides TJ, Gress FG, Wheat LJ, et al. Dysphagia due to mediastinal granulomas: diagnosis with endoscopic ultrasonography. Gastroenterology 1995;109:366–373.

63. Rosch T, Lorenz R, Dancygier H, et al. Endosonographic diagnosis of submucosal upper gastrointestinal tract tumors. Scand J Gastroenterol 1992;27:1–8.

64. Wiersema MJ, Hawes RH, Tao LC, et al. Endoscopic ultrasonography as an adjunct to fine needle aspiration cytology of the upper and lower gastrointestinal tract. Gastrointest Endosc 1992;38:35–39.

65. Caletti GC, Brocchi E, Ferrari A, et al. Guillotine needle biopsy as a supplement to endosonography in the diagnosis of gastric submucosal tumors. Endoscopy 1991;23:251–254.

66. Gress F, Schmitt C, Savides T, et al. Interobserver agreement among endosonographers for endoscopic ultrasound (EUS) evaluation of submucosal masses. Gastrointest Endosc 1998;45:AB173. Abstract.

67. Nickl NJ, Bhutani MS, Catalano M, et al. Clinical implications of endoscopic ultrasound: the American Endosonography Club study. Gastrointest Endosc 1996;44:371–377.

# 10

# Endoscopic Ultrasound of the Biliary Tract

## Peter D. Stevens
## Charles J. Lightdale

The gastrointestinal endoscopist continues to play a central role in the evaluation and management of biliary diseases, despite the advancements in noninvasive imaging and minimally invasive surgery. While ERCP has been the principal modality used by endoscopists for evaluating the biliary tree, there is an increasing understanding of the role of endosonography as a complementary imaging method available to endoscopists. Extrahepatic biliary imaging with EUS has been possible because of the close apposition of the gastric antrum and duodenum with the porta-hepatis and the extrahepatic biliary tree. This juxtaposition creates an acoustical window through which a high-frequency ultrasound transducer, incorporated into an echoendoscope, can be manouvered into position within the antrum and duodenum to produce clear images. Recently, ultrasound probes have been developed that can be placed into the bile ducts or gallbladder via either the transpapillary or percutaneous routes, and these may expand the usefulness of EUS for biliary diseases. This chapter will describe the technique of biliary EUS imaging and review the recent literature regarding the role of EUS in specific benign and malignant biliary conditions.

## Instruments

### Endoscope-Based Probes

Both mechanically rotating radial scanning and electronic curvilinear array echoendoscopes can be used to image the biliary tree. Although the radial scanning instruments make orientation easier, the curvilinear array systems are necessary if EUS-guided puncture will be performed. Also, when imaging in the region of the hepatic hilum or the pancreatic head with the curvilinear array instruments, the availability of Doppler is useful in helping to determine whether an anechoic tubular structure is a vessel or a duct (Figures 10-1 and 10-2).

### Catheter-Based Probes

The availability of high-frequency catheter-based ultrasound probes has made it possible to obtain ultrasound images from within the biliary tree. These mechanically rotating high-frequency ultrasound probes, now equipped with transducer frequencies between 7.5 and 30 MHz, vary in width between 1.4 and 3.2 mm and were first developed for percutaneous use (1,2). Recently, they have been increasingly used by endoscopists via the transpapillary route (3–7). For the endoscopic approach, a sphincterotomy is sometimes necessary to facilitate the insertion of standard catheter-based instruments across the papilla without damaging the ultrasound transducer. However, wire-guided instruments are now available that allow efficient passage of these probes across native papilla, through strictures, and into the intrahepatic biliary tree (8). In addition, these probes can be placed via the transpapillary route through the cystic duct into the gallbladder (9) for high-frequency imaging of small mural lesions. Recently, a specially designed catheter-based system has been developed to produce three-dimensional images of the bile duct (10), although clinical experience with this system is limited at present.

## Technique

When compared to other endoscopic procedures, and even to EUS of the gastrointestinal tract wall, EUS of the biliary tree is difficult. The endoscopist must obtain the images by maneuvering the tip of the scope

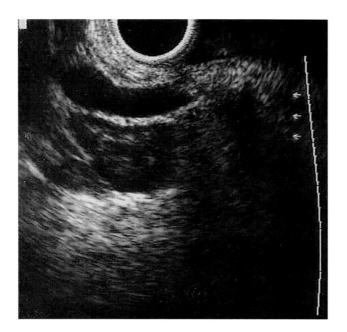

**Figure 10-1.** This image was obtained using the Olympus UC30P curvilinear echoendoscope and shows a periduodenal lymph node just beyond a hypoechoic tubular structure that might represent the bile duct or a blood vessel.

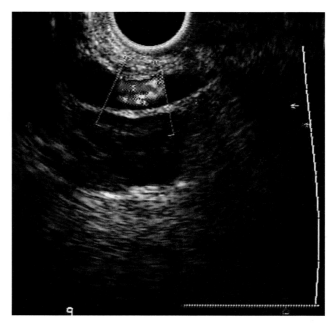

**Figure 10-2.** This image was taken moments after the image shown in Fig. 10-1 using color Doppler. The vascular nature of the tubular structure is clearly demonstrated.

between the duodenal bulb and the second portion of the duodenum "blindly." The real-time EUS image is used as a guide to supplement the endoscopist's "muscle memory" of how to maneuver the sometimes cumbersome echoendoscope upstream and downstream in this region. It is important to avoid compressing important structures or trapping multiple duodenal folds and/or air between the transducer and areas of interest. As a result, one needs both considerable endoscopic skill and a detailed understanding of the regional cross-sectional anatomy in order to obtain and interpret images of the biliary tree. The basic technical aspects of our approach to bile duct imaging with the radial scanning instrument are described in the following paragraphs.

There are two general methods of examining the bile duct, depending on whether the imaging begins in the duodenal bulb or at the level of the papilla. To begin imaging from the bulb, advance the echoendoscope tip across the pylorus and bulb until it lodges in the superior duodenal angle. Achieving this position will be facilitated by tipping gently downward once the transducer is at the superior duodenal angle. Aspirate any air and partially fill the water balloon to improve acoustical contact. Over-filling the balloon will decrease the mobility of the tip of the endoscope. At this position the portal vein is usually easily identified running 1 or 2 centimeters deep to the transducer along the left side of the screen from the liver on the top left of the screen to the portal venous confluence and pancreas at the bottom of the screen. The common bile

duct and common hepatic duct are seen in their long axis alongside the portal vein and superficial to it. If the duct is dilated, recognition of this prominent structure is usually immediate. However, if it is not dilated, identification may be more difficult. Once identified, the bile duct can be traced from the confluence of the right and left hepatic ducts, past the confluence of the common hepatic duct and cystic duct, down to the papilla, or confluence of the pancreatic duct and bile duct. The endoscopist should keep these conjunctions in mind while imaging the duct, and attempt to identify all three. Usually, the tubular image of the common bile duct obtained from the bulb transmutes into an oval and then a circle as the echoendoscope is passed deeper into the duodenum toward the papilla. In contrast to the sometimes evasive bile duct, the gallbladder is usually easily identified from the bulb and may also be imaged from the antrum or occasionally from deeper in the duodenum.

When the bile ducts are not dilated, it may be best to begin imaging at the level of the papilla. In this position, the endoscopist can confirm visually that the EUS images represent the peripapillary pancreas and ducts, which may appear as small slits, ovals, or circles in this region. Once the bile duct has been identified in the peripapillary pancreas, it can be traced upstream to the level of the liver hilum and gallbladder. As mentioned, in practice both of these methods are used in tandem as the bile duct is imaged repeatedly in the upstream and downstream directions in order to collect adequate information.

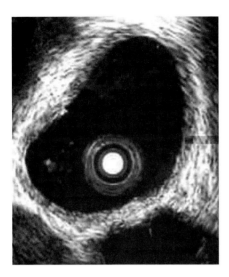

**Figure 10-3.** This figure shows an intraductal ultrasound (IDUS) image obtained with a 20-MHz catheter probe (Olympus UM 3R, Olympus America, Melville, NY) that has been placed within the bile duct under endoscopic and fluoroscopic guidance. The normal three-layer wall of this dilated bile duct is demonstrated.

## Normal Anatomy

### Bile Duct

The normal bile duct can be imaged as a three-layer structure: the inner hyperechoic layer represents the mucosa with a border echo, the middle hypoechoic layer represents the smooth muscle fibers and fibroelastic tissue, and the outer hyperechoic layer represents the thin and loose connective tissue with a border echo (11). However, when imaging with an echoendoscope through the duodenum, the bile duct may appear as a single-layer structure because of a thin second (muscular) layer. Occasionally, only two layers are imaged. In this situation, the inner hypoechoic layer represents both the mucosa and the muscular layer. When imaging with higher-frequency intraductal probes (Figure 10-3), the three-layer pattern is more consistent and has the same anatomic correlates as detailed above (3,12).

### Gallbladder

The gallbladder wall typically appears as a three-layer structure both by echoendoscopic imaging and by intraluminal probe imaging (9,13). The first layer is hyperechoic and represents the mucosa; the second layer is hypoechoic and represents the muscular layer; the third layer represents the subserosal and serosal layers. Unfortunately, in some cases the gallbladder may be positioned such that part of the wall is too far from the transducer for adequate imaging and thus may limit the usefulness of EUS.

## Applications

### Bile Duct

#### Cancer Detection

Although there has been less information published concerning the role of endosonography for the detection and staging of bile duct cancers than there has been for esophageal, gastric, or pancreatic cancer, it does appear to have a role in identifying and characterizing biliary cancers, especially for smaller tumors. Primary bile duct cancers usually present with painless obstruction of the biliary tree and jaundice. Ultrasound and CT reliably show that the ductal system is obstructed and at what level, but they usually cannot precisely localize tumors, especially if the lesions are less than 2 cm in diameter.

The typical endosonography image of a bile duct tumor cancer shows a round or fusiform hypoechoic area arising from or surrounding the bile duct wall. Although distal common bile duct tumors are usually easily imaged in a dilated duct, more proximal tumors may be difficult to detect due to limited penetration of the echoendoscope transducers. For the detection of small bile duct tumors, endosonography is as sensitive as ERCP and superior to US, CT, and angiography (14,15).

EUS is highly sensitive for the detection of abnormalities of the bile duct, but it has not yet been shown to be able to reliably distinguish benign from malignant thickening of the bile duct wall (5). For excluding malignant disease, however, the finding of a normal bile duct wall on EUS has a very high negative predictive value (16).

#### Staging

Endosonographic staging of bile duct tumors is based on the TNM system (17). The primary tumor is staged as follows: T1 tumors involve only the mucosa and/or muscle layer; T2 tumors involve the perimuscular connective tissue, and T3 tumors involve adjacent structures including the liver, pancreas, duodenum, gallbladder, colon, stomach, and/or major blood vessels. Invasion is diagnosed when there is continuation of the hypoechoic tumor mass into adjacent structures. Regional lymph nodes are staged as either N0—no regional lymph nodes—or N1 when regional lymph nodes including celiac lymph nodes are present. In general, size criteria have not been used in EUS studies of bile duct cancer staging; rather, lymph nodes with a hypoechoic texture and sharp boundaries, or those penetrated by the hypoechoic tumor mass are considered malignant. Lymph nodes with a hyperechoic pattern and indistinct boundaries are considered benign (18,19).

Qilian et al. (20) evaluated the use of EUS for the preoperative assessment of 18 patients with extrahepatic bile duct tumors. The overall accuracy for T stage was 72% and for N stage 61%. In an earlier study,

Mukai et al. (11) reported the accuracy of EUS for determining the T and N stage of CBD tumors in 16 patients. All 16 patients underwent resection. The extent of malignant invasion (T stage) was accurately diagnosed by EUS in 81% of patients. Overstaging occurred in one patient due to inflammation around the CBD and understaging occurred in two patients because of microscopic tumor invasion. The accuracy for lymph node staging was also 81%.

Tio et al., who reported their updated series on so-called Klatskin tumors in 1993, have conducted the largest volume of work on EUS for staging of proximal bile duct cancers. They found that the overall accuracy of EUS for T stage was 86% and for N stage was 64% (18). Although the accuracy of T staging is excellent, the accuracy for lymph nodes is less impressive. The problems with lymph node diagnosis should be largely addressed by EUS-guided fine-needle aspiration biopsy, which has an overall accuracy of about 91% (20).

For determining resectability of bile duct cancer, portal venous invasion remains a key factor. This particular aspect of staging was the subject of a recent comparative trial reported by Sugiyama et al. (15). In their trial, EUS was prospectively compared to ultrasound, computed tomography, and angiography for the detection of portal venous system invasion in 19 bile duct cancers. All of the 19 lesions were resected, with or without portal venous resection, and underwent careful histopathologic staging. The authors of this study separated the degree of apparent involvement of the portal vein by tumor, as imaged by EUS, into four grades. In Grade 1, the tumor was not near the portal vein. In Grade 2, the tumor was in contact with the portal vein, but the echogenic interface was intact. In Grade 3, the tumor was contiguous with the portal vein and the echogenic interface was lost. In Grade 4, the tumor was seen in the vein or was occluding the vein. The authors defined EUS Grades 1 and 2 as negative for invasion, and EUS Grades 3 and 4 as positive for invasion. Using this system, they found that the accuracy for determining portal venous invasion was 93% for EUS, compared to 74% for US, 84% for CT, and 89% for angiography.

### Catheter-Probe Based Intraductal Ultrasound (IDUS)

The normal bile duct wall appears as a two- or three-layered structure on intraductal ultrasound and is similar to that seen with standard EUS (21–24). In contrast to EUS, IDUS is able to evaluate the proximal bile duct and surrounding structures at the hilum of the liver, including the portal vein, right hepatic artery, and contents of the hepatoduodenal ligament.

***Cancer Detection and Staging with IDUS***   The usefulness of IDUS for diagnostic imaging (Figures 10-3

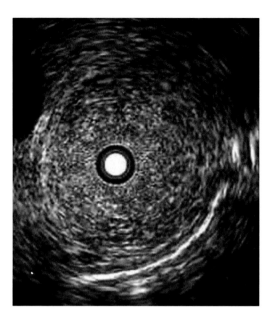

**Figure 10-4.** This figure shows an IDUS image of the distal portion of the bile duct shown in Figure 10-3. At this level, corresponding to a stricture on fluoroscopy, there is effacement of the wall layers and expansion of the wall by a hypoechoic process that extends into the surrounding pancreatic parenchyma.

through 10-5) is based on its ability to detect early lesions, to determine the maximal longitudinal extent of the bile duct cancer, and to determine the presence of extension into other organs or major blood vessels when the tumor is not well-defined by other imaging methods (Figure 10-4). Intraductal ultrasound has been shown to be useful in determining invasion into the portal vein, right hepatic artery, and pancreatic parenchyma (23–26), with a diagnostic accuracy approaching 100%.

While IDUS alone cannot determine with a high degree of certainty whether any stricture is benign or malignant (5), Tamada et al. suggest that the IDUS findings can help direct management. If the IDUS of a stricture shows that a wall-layer structure is interrupted by a protruding tumor, prompt surgical exploration is appropriate, even without tissue confirmation of malignancy. If the IDUS shows a normal wall, further invasive testing is unnecessary. On the other hand, when the IDUS shows a lesion that leaves the wall layers undisturbed, direct biopsies should be obtained if possible, because only some of these will prove to be malignant (12).

There are several important limitations of IDUS technology. First, there is limited penetration depth with these high-frequency probes, and certain structures are not well seen as a result, such as the main hepatic artery and the left hepatic artery. Also, because these probes cannot resolve the fibromuscular layer from the perimuscular connective tissue (both may appear as a single hypoechoic layer), differentiation between T1 and T2 cancers is not reliable (27). Another potential problem for IDUS is the influence of biliary drainage catheters on bile duct thickness. In one study (12), it was demonstrated that bile duct wall thickness as measured by IDUS appears to be increased after placement of a biliary drainage catheter. This could lead to an overestimation of the longitudinal (upstream or downstream) spread of disease. Further work is needed in this important area to try to distinguish patterns of malignant and benign thickening of the bile duct wall.

## Gallbladder

### Evaluation of Polypoid Lesions of the Gallbladder
Sugiyama et al. (28) evaluated the accuracy of EUS in diagnosing small (<20 mm) polypoid lesions of the gallbladder. They retrospectively reviewed the preoperative EUS and transabdominal ultrasound in 65 patients who had undergone gallbladder resection for small polypoid lesions. The lesions resected were cholesterol polyp, n = 40; adenomyomatosis, n = 9; adenoma, n = 4; and adenocarcinoma, n = 12. They found that EUS showed a tiny echogenic spot or an aggregation of echogenic spots with or without echopenic areas in 95% of patients with cholesterol polyps, and multiple microcysts or comet-tail artifacts in all patients with adenomyomatosis. Adenomas and adenocarcinomas were not associated with finding echogenic spots, microcysts, or artifacts. The authors concluded that a polypoid lesion (sessile or on a pedicle) without those features should be considered a neoplasm. Overall, EUS was superior to transabdominal ultrasound in differentiating the nature of these gallbladder lesions (97% compared with 71%).

Uchida et al. reported the use of intraductal probes for evaluating polypoid gallbladder lesions in four patients, and was able to image the lesion of interest in three of the four patients studied (9). Although this technique might improve image quality slightly over that obtained with endoscope-based EUS, it is quite difficult to insert the probe into the gallbladder and requires the use of a guide wire. The utility of this approach has not been proved, and further studies are awaited.

### Gallbladder Cancer Staging
Mitake et al. (29) performed EUS in 39 patients before surgical resection for gallbladder carcinoma. They found that EUS accurately evaluated the depth of tumor infiltration with an overall T stage accuracy of 79.5%. The N stage accuracy was 89.7%. Although there was some difficulty in distinguishing between T1 and T2 cancers and in evaluating gallbladders with multiple gallstones, the authors concluded that en-

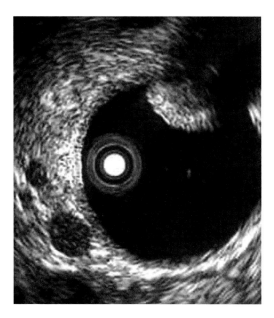

**Figure 10-5.** This figure shows an IDUS image of a common bile duct stone, which is seen in the upper right corner of the intraductal image as a curvilinear hyperechoic structure with a strong acoustic shadow.

dosonography is useful in the clinical staging of gallbladder carcinoma.

### Gallbladder and Bile Duct Stones
When performing EUS, common bile duct stones are easily identified as curvilinear hyperechoic foci with strong acoustic shadowing using either standard or catheter-based EUS (Figure 10-5). A number of studies have demonstrated the exceptional accuracy of EUS for common bile duct stones, even in small bile ducts harboring small distal stones (30–38). In studies with more than 50 patients, the sensitivity ranges from 84% to 100%, and the specificity ranges from 95% to 100%. EUS may also be useful for detecting small gallbladder stones missed on transabdominal imaging, especially those located in the neck of the gallbladder, where duodenal gas can obscure the image generated by conventional ultrasound.

Among the studies comparing EUS to ERCP for the detection of bile duct stones, most have used ERCP as the gold standard. However, when Prat et al. compared the two procedures, they used endoscopic exploration of the bile duct with a balloon and basket as the gold standard. The procedures were similar in sensitivity (EUS 93%, ERCP 89%), specificity (EUS 97%, ERCP 100%), positive predictive value (EUS 98%, ERCP 100%), and negative predictive value (EUS 88%, ERCP 83%) (33).

Although EUS involves conscious sedation and requires the peroral introduction of an endoscope, the entire procedure can be performed efficiently in less than 15 minutes, and can be followed immediately by ERCP and stone extraction if needed (37,39).

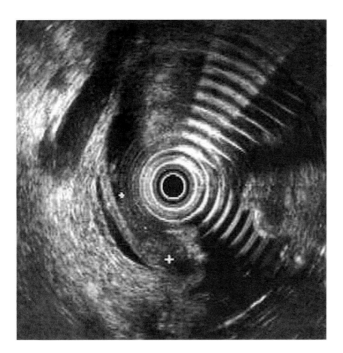

**Figure 10-6.** This figure shows an EUS image obtained with the mechanical radial scanning echoendoscope (Olympus GF-UM130) in a patient with idiopathic pancreatitis after standard imaging procedures. The cursor marks (+) are placed to show the layering biliary sludge partially occluding the bile duct just upstream of the papilla. The pancreatic duct is seen deep to the bile duct in the seven- to nine-o'clock position and the portal vein is seen deep to the bile duct in the nine- to eleven-o'clock position.

EUS may prove most useful for evaluating patients who are at moderate risk of harboring bile duct stones in whom a diagnostic ERCP might carry too great a risk of pancreatitis. EUS can be followed immediately by therapeutic ERCP during the same endoscopic session, if needed. Patients who might benefit from combined EUS/ERCP are those scheduled for laparoscopic cholecystectomy who are suspected of having common bile duct stones. In a recent preliminary report of a randomized clinical trial, we found that combined preoperative EUS/ERCP was equivalent to laparoscopic cholangiogram and transcystic common bile duct exploration for patients at a moderate risk for common bile duct stones in terms of overall success rate, length of hospital stay, and total hospital charges, but was associated with significantly shorter operating room times and fewer failed procedures (40).

### Biliary Sludge

Biliary sludge, or microlithiasis, may be associated with biliary colic and acute cholecystitis and it may be responsible for up to 60% of cases of "idiopathic" pancreatitis (41,42). There are reports that EUS can identify very small amounts of sludge in vitro (43) and that EUS is more sensitive than US in patients with idiopathic pancreatitis for detecting biliary microlithiasis (44) (Figure 10-6). Dill et al. (45) reported that the detection of biliary sludge within the gallbladder by EUS predicted the response to cholecystectomy in patients with biliary-type pain from unsuspected cholecystitis. If these studies are confirmed, EUS will come to occupy a pivotal role in the evaluation of patients with unexplained right upper quadrant pain or idiopathic pancreatitis.

## Summary

Endoscopic ultrasound is a minimally invasive imaging modality that provides high-resolution images of the extrahepatic biliary tree and the surrounding structures. It has been shown to be accurate for the detection and staging of bile duct and gallbladder cancers, and is especially useful for small tumors. Intraductal techniques, which are still in evolution, may provide even more information about the etiology and extent of biliary strictures and mural tumors. EUS has also been shown to be useful for the detection of biliary stones and sludge when transabdominal ultrasound is not diagnostic. In many cases, diagnostic EUS can be followed immediately by therapeutic ERCP if needed. The instruments and techniques for endosonography continue to improve, and at present EUS can be considered a promising minimally invasive tool for evaluating the biliary tree.

### References

1. Engstrom CF, Wiechel KL. Endoluminal ultrasound of the bile ducts. Surg Endosc 1990;4:187–190.
2. Gerdes H, Botet J, Lightdale CJ. Percutaneous biliary endosonography in the evaluation of patients with recurrent obstructive jaundice. Gastrointest Endosc 1991;37:245.
3. Cushing GL, Fitzgerald PJ, Bommer WJ, et al. Intraluminal ultrasonography during ERCP with high-frequency ultrasound catheters. Gastrointest Endosc 1993;39:432–435.
4. Yasuda K, Mukai H, Nakajima M, Kawai K. Clinical application of ultrasonic probes in the biliary and pancreatic duct. Endoscopy 1992;24(suppl 1):370–375.
5. Gress F, Chen YK, Sherman S, et al. Experience with a catheter-based ultrasound probe in the bile duct and pancreas. Endoscopy 1995;27:178–184.
6. Waxman I. Characterization of a malignant bile duct obstruction by intraductal ultrasonography [see comments]. Am J Gastroenterol 1995;90:1073–1075.
7. Chak A, Canto M, Stevens PD, et al. Clinical applications of a new through-the-scope ultrasound probe: prospective comparison with an ultrasound endoscope. Gastrointest Endosc 1997;45:291–295.
8. Chak A, Isenberg G, Kobayashi G, et al. Prospective evaluation of over-the-wire catheter ultrasound probe. Gastrointest Endosc 1999;49:AB154.

9. Uchida N, Ezaki T, Hirabayashi S, et al. Scanning of polypoid gallbladder lesions by ultrasonic micro-probes using transpapillary catheterization. Endoscopy 1996;28:302–305.

10. Kanemaki N, Nakazawa S, Inui K, et al. Three-dimensional intraductal ultrasonography: preliminary results of a new technique for the diagnosis of diseases of the pancreatobiliary system. Endoscopy 1997; 29:726–731.

11. Mukai H, Nakajima M, Yasuda K, et al. Evaluation of endoscopic ultrasonography in the pre-operative staging of carcinoma of the ampulla of Vater and common bile duct. Gastrointest Endosc 1992;38:676–683.

12. Tamada K, Tomiyama T, Ichiyama M, et al. Influence of biliary drainage catheter on bile duct wall thickness as measured by intraductal ultrasonography. Gastrointest Endosc 1998;47:28–32.

13. Morita K, Nakazawa S, Kimoto E. Gallbladder diseases. In: Kawai K, ed. Endoscopic ultrasonography in gastroenterology. 1st ed. Tokyo: Igaku-Shoin, 1988: 87–95.

14. Yasuda K, Nakajima M, Kawai K. Diseases of the biliary tract and papilla of Vater. In: Kawai K, ed. Endoscopic ultrasonography in gastroenterology. 1st ed. Tokyo: Igaku-Shoin, 1988:96–105.

15. Sugiyama M, Hagi H, Atomi Y, Saito M. Diagnosis of portal venous invasion by pancreatobiliary carcinoma: value of endoscopic ultrasonography. Abdom Imaging 1997;22:434–438.

16. Tamada K, Ueno N, Tomiyama T, et al. Characterization of biliary strictures using intraductal ultrasonography: comparison with percutaneous cholangioscopic biopsy. Gastrointest Endosc 1998; 47:341–349.

17. Anonymous. American Joint Committee on Cancer. Ann Surg 1999.

18. Tio TL, Reeders JW, Sie LH, et al. Endosonography in the clinical staging of Klatskin tumor. Endoscopy 1993;25:81–85.

19. Qilian Z, Weidong N, Lando Z, Jinyu L. Endoscopic ultrasonography assessment in preoperative staging for carcinoma of ampulla of Vater and extrahepatic bile duct. Chinese Med J 1996;109:622–625.

20. Hoffman BJ, Hawes RH. Endoscopic ultrasonography-guided puncture of the lymph nodes: first experience and clinical consequences. Gastrointest Endosc Clin North Am 1995;5:587–594.

21. Tamada K, Ido K, Ueno N, et al. Preoperative staging of extrahepatic bile duct cancer with intraductal ultrasonography (IDUS). Am J Gastroenterol 1994;89: 239–246.

22. Furukawa T, Naito Y, Tsukamoto Y, et al. New technique using intraductal ultrasonography for the diagnosis of diseases of the pancreatobiliary system. Ultrasound Med 1992;11:607–612.

23. Kuroiwa M, Tsukamoto Y, Naitoh Y, et al. New technique using intraductal ultrasonography for the diagnosis of bile duct cancer. Ultrasound Med 1994; 13:189–195.

24. Tamada K, Ido K, Ueno N, et al. Assessment of portal vein invasion by bile duct cancer using intraductal ultrasonography. Endoscopy 1995;27:573–578.

25. Tamada K, Ido K, Ueno N, et al. Assessment of the course and variations of the hepatic artery in bile duct cancer by intraductal ultrasonograhy. Gastrointest Endosc 1996;44:249–256.

26. Tamada K, Ueno N, Ichiyama M, et al. Assessment of pancreatic parenchymal invasion by bile duct cancer using intraductal ultrasonography. Endoscopy 1996; 28:492–496.

27. Tamada K, Kanai N, Ueno N, et al. Limitations of intraductal ultrasonography in differentiating between bile duct cancer in stage T1 and stage T2: in-vitro and in-vivo studies. Endoscopy 1997;29:721–725.

28. Sugiyama H, Xie XY, Atomi Y, Saito M. Differential diagnosis of small polypoid lesions of the gallbladder: the value of endoscopic ultrasonography. Ann Surg 1999;229:498–504.

29. Mitake M, Nakazawa S, Naitoh Y, et al. Endoscopic ultrasonography in diagnosis of the extent of gallbladder carcinoma. Gastrointest Endosc 1990;36:562–566.

30. Norton SA, Alderson D. Prospective comparison of endoscopic ultrasonography and endoscopic retrograde cholangiopancreatography in the detection of bile duct stones. Brit J Surg 1997;84:1366–1369.

31. Sugiyama M, Atomi Y. Endoscopic ultrasonography for diagnosing choledocholithiasis: a prospective comparative study with ultrasonography and computed tomography. Gastrointest Endosc 1997;45: 143–146.

32. Palazzo L, Levy P, Bernades P. Usefulness of endoscopic ultrasonography in the diagnosis of choledocholithiasis. [Review] [51 refs]. Abdom Imaging 1996; 21:93–97.

33. Prat F, Amouyal G, Amouyal P, et al. Prospective controlled study of endoscopic ultrasonography and endoscopic retrograde cholangiography in patients with suspected common-bileduct lithiasis [see comments]. Lancet 1996;347:75–79.

34. Shim CS, Joo JH, Park CW, et al. Effectiveness of endoscopic ultrasonography in the diagnosis of choledocholithiasis prior to laparoscopic cholecystectomy [see comments]. Endoscopy 1995;27:428–432.

35. Palazzo L, Girollet PP, Salmeron M, et al. Value of endoscopic ultrasonography in the diagnosis of common bile duct stones: comparison with surgical exploration and ERCP. Gastrointest Endosc 1995;42: 225–231.

36. Amouyal P, Amouyal G, Levy P, et al. Diagnosis of choledocholithiasis by endoscopic ultrasonography [see comments]. Gastroenterology 1994;106:1062–1067.

37. Edmundowicz SA, Aliperti G, Middleton WD. Preliminary experience using endoscopic ultrasonography in the diagnosis of choledocholithiasis. Endoscopy 1992;24:774–778.

38. Strohm WD, Kurtz W, Classen M. Detection of biliary stones by means of endosonography. Scand J Gastroenterol Suppl 1984;94:60–64.

39. Canto M. Endoscopic ultrasonography and gallstone disease. [Review] [43 refs]. Gastrointest Endosc 1996; 43:S37–43.

40. Shah VH, Stevens PD, Memmo P, et al. Preoperative EUS/ERCP vs. intraoperative cholangiography in

patients with suspected CBD stones: a prospective randomized trial. Gastrointest Endosc 1999;49:AB227.

41. Ros E, Navarro S, Bru C, et al. Occult microlithiasis in "idiopathic" acute pancreatitis: prevention by cholecystectomy of ursodeoxycholic acid therapy. Gastroenterology 1991;101:1701–1709.

42. Lee SP, Nicholls JF, Park HZ. Biliary sludge as a cause of acute pancreatitis. New Eng J Med 1992;326: 589–593.

43. Stevens PD, Lightdale CJ, Saha SA, Abedi M. In-vitro comparison of endoscope-based vs. catheter-based endoscopic ultrasound for the detection of biliary sludge. Gastrointest Endosc 1996;43:S57.

44. Amouyal G, Amouyal P, Levy P. Value of endoscopic ultrasonography in the diagnosis of ideopathic acute pancreatitis. Gastroenterology 1994; 106:A283.

45. Dill JE, Hill S, Callis J, et al. Combined endoscopic ultrasound and stimulated biliary drainage in cholecystitis and microlithiasis—diagnoses and outcomes. Endoscopy 1995;27:424–427.

# 11

# Endoscopic Ultrasonography of the Pancreas

## Peter D. Stevens
## Sandeep Bhargava

Although pancreatic imaging, using the gut wall as an acoustical window, has been a primary focus of endosonographers since the earliest papers began to appear (1,2), pancreatic endosonography (EUS) remains a difficult technique to master. In the view of most experts, obtaining and interpreting endosonographic images of the pancreas represents one of the greatest challenges for both students and skilled endosonographers alike. Once mastered, however, EUS can provide an exceptional degree of anatomical detail allowing accurate identification and precise staging of a variety of conditions and lesions. This chapter describes the methods for EUS imaging of the pancreas and reviews the role of EUS in pancreatic diseases.

## Instruments

### Echoendoscopes

In Chapter 3, two types of echoendoscopes were described in detail, those with mechanically rotating transducers (e.g., radial scanning instruments, GF-UM 130, Olympus America, Melville, NY), and those with electronic, curvilinear array transducers (e.g., CLA instruments: GF-UC30P, Olympus America, Melville, NY and FG36UX, Pentax Precision Instruments Co., Orangeburg, NY). For pancreatic imaging, both types of instruments are useful and have their own advantages and disadvantages.

The radial instruments provide a 360-degree tomographic image of the anatomical structures adjacent to the echoendoscope. The complete scanning arc and radial orientation simplify the identification of anatomic structures. This is especially useful when imaging the pancreas and major retroperitoneal vessels. Unfortunately, this instrument does not provide Doppler imaging and the radial orientation of the ultrasound plane does not facilitate EUS-guided fine-needle biopsy or puncture.

The CLA instrument is equipped with a multi-element electronic transducer that produces an image oriented in the plane of the endoscope's accessory channel and allows for real-time guidance of accessories, such as fine-needle biopsy devices, into areas of interest for tissue acquisition and therapeutic injection. These instruments are also able to produce both color flow mapping and duplex Doppler. Many of the specific uses for this instrument have been aimed at pancreatic conditions. These "interventional" applications, which are discussed in detail in Chapter 12, include fine-needle aspiration (FNA) biopsy for the diagnosis of primary pancreatic lesions, metastatic lymph nodes, and fluid collections; fine-needle injection (FNI) therapy, such as celiac plexus block (3,4) and pancreatic pseudocyst drainage.

For imaging alone, both radial scanning and linear array instruments produce excellent results. In the single study that compared the two types of instruments for accuracy in pancreatic cancer staging, they were found to be equivalent (5). From a more qualitative standpoint, the radial instruments produce a 360-degree view that makes orientation easier for novice endosonographers and completes survey examinations faster for experienced endosonographers. However, the availability of FNA puncture and the convenience of Doppler to help distinguish ducts and cysts from vessels make the CLA instrument irreplaceable for the advanced pancreaticobiliary endosonographer.

### Catheter-Based Probes

Small mechanically rotating transducers have been incorporated into catheter sized probes (7.5–30 MHz).

These probes, designed initially for intravascular imaging, have been placed into the bile ducts via both percutaneous and transpapillary approaches, and into the pancreas duct via the endoscopic retrograde method (6–8). Recently, wire-guided probes have been introduced (UM-4R, Olympus America, Melville, NY) that have eliminated the need for sphincterotomy. These probes should be easier to introduce in the bile and pancreatic ducts and may prove more durable than standard probes. Results of catheter-based intraductal ultrasound (IDUS) for pancreatic imaging will be discussed below.

## Endoscopic Ultrasound of the Pancreas: Method of Examination

### Body and Tail Imaging

Although obtaining the skills to efficiently perform and accurately interpret an EUS examination of the pancreas takes a great deal of experience, the novice should begin to explore the pancreas whenever the echoendoscope is passed into the stomach. In our unit, each upper examination, regardless of clinical indication, affords the opportunity to learn a bit more about imaging the pancreas. From the stomach, the pancreas body and tail can be easily identified. In most patients, with the scope reasonably straight and inserted to about 50 cm from the incisors, the splenic vein can be identified several centimeters deep to the gastric wall and running parallel to it. The pancreas lies between the splenic vein and the wall of the stomach.

Once the splenic vein is identified, it is often helpful to electronically rotate the image so that the splenic vein is running left to right across the 6-o'clock position on the screen. It may also be helpful and sometimes necessary to instill up to about 300 ml of deaerated water into the stomach. With slow and deliberate combinations of movements including tip deflection, torque, and insertion/withdrawal, the vein can be followed to the portal confluence on the anatomic right (screen left) and to the splenic hilum on the anatomic left (screen right).

During this portion of the exam, the echoendoscope tip is moving like a pendulum along the path of the splenic vein. In most cases, slight withdrawal of the scope is required to fully examine the tail of the pancreas. In addition, within 5 cm of insertion or withdrawal from the position where the splenic vein is seen adjacent to the body of the pancreas, one should be able to identify the splenic artery, the portal confluence, the superior mesenteric artery near the neck of the pancreas, the left kidney, the left adrenal gland, and the spleen near the tail of the pancreas.

### Pancreatic Head Imaging

The head of the pancreas and uncinate process can be difficult to examine. While there is a technical limitation to ultrasound in those rare lesions that may be "isoechoic," and can be overlooked, most missed lesions are simply missed. In order to avoid missing lesions, it is important to image the pancreas head region multiple times using more than one technique. Our method is to image this area dynamically, during pullback and insertion, from 3 separate starting positions, identifying the pancreas primarily by its relation to major vessels.

The first starting position is in the horizontal duodenum or as close to that position as possible. There, the aorta and inferior vena cava (IVC) can be imaged in the long view. The echoendoscope is locked with rightward tip deflection and the image electronically rotated so that the aorta and IVC are running top-to-bottom on the left side of the screen. During a pullback from this position, the endosonographer keeps the tip of the scope adjacent to the pancreas with upward tip deflection while maintaining acoustical contact using a small amount of water in the lumen and in the balloon. The scope is continuously withdrawn slowly, while maintaining pancreas imaging, until the scope falls upstream out of the pylorus.

Imaging at the start of the pullback, from the third portion of the duodenum, reveals the uncinate process, identified by the "salt and pepper" parenchyma adjacent to the duodenum and surrounded by the SMA, SMV, and aorta. From the second portion of the duodenum, in the region of the papilla, the pancreatic duct and bile duct can be seen approaching the duodenal wall and sometimes can be seen crossing the muscularis propria and entering the papilla. Care should be taken to avoid confusing the superior duodenal artery (SDA) from the common bile duct. The SDA appears closest to the duodenal wall. From the bulb, the bile duct can be seen running into the parenchyma of the pancreas (Figure 11-1). Often, with the scope positioned between the second portion of the duodenum and the bulb, the pancreatic duct can be seen running adjacent to the common bile duct in the head of the pancreas producing an endosonographic "stack sign" (9) (Figure 11-2).

After the pullback is repeated several times, the pancreas can be imaged starting in the bulb and moving downstream toward the papilla in a manner physically identical to that described for the bile duct (Chapter 10). Finally, we begin imaging from directly opposite the papilla, with water in the lumen and while turning the patient to a more supine position, thereby focusing on the periampullary region. The ampullary area is often compressed and obscured by gathered folds, making this last position crucial to an adequate ampullary exam.

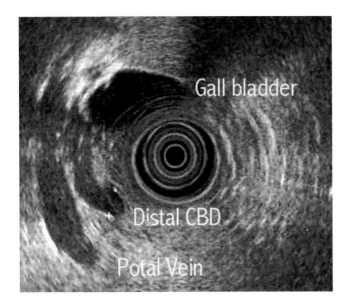

**Figure 11-1.** Radial EUS image showing normal pancreatic parenchyma in the region of the head. The CBD is running parallel to the portal vein.

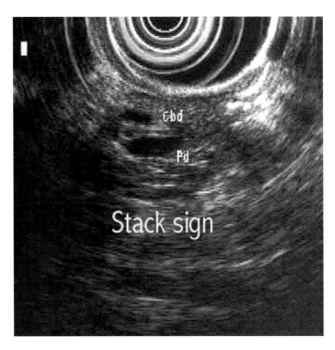

**Figure 11-2.** Radial EUS image of the endosonographic "stack sign."

**Table 11-1.** EUS for detection of pancreatic tumors

|                | Sensitivity | Specificity | PPV | NPV | Accuracy |
|----------------|-------------|-------------|-----|-----|----------|
| Snady, 1992    | 85          | 80          | 89  | 73  | 83       |
| Rosch, 1991    | 99          | 100         | 100 | 97  | 76       |
| Akahoshi, 1998 | 89          | 97          | 94  | 93  | 94       |
| Baron, 1997    | 95          | 88          | 95  | 88  |          |
| Legmann, 1998  | 100         | 93          |     |     |          |
| Muller, 1994   | 94          | 100         |     |     | 96       |
| Yasuda, 1993   |             |             |     |     | 100      |

NPV = negative predictive value
PPV = positive predictive value

## EUS of the Normal Pancreas

The pancreas is easily recognized not only by its position with respect to major blood vessels and organs but also by its characteristic ultrasound appearance. The gland is generally a homogeneous echogenic structure with a granular salt-and-pepper echo texture. From the stomach, the anechoic pancreatic duct is identified as a longitudinal structure running parallel to the splenic vein, and often can be traced to the tail of the pancreas in the spleno-renal angle. From the duodenum, the echotexture is similar. A particularly confusing EUS characteristic of the pancreas is that the primitively ventral pancreas appears as a hypoechoic structure within the pancreas and could be misconstrued as focal pancreatitis or tumor. In a well-illustrated report of their prospective experience in 100 patients undergoing EUS for a variety of indications, Savides and colleagues (10) described this finding in 75% of normal individuals and 40% of patients with suspected pancreatic disease. The differential appearance is due to the higher fat content of the primitively dorsal pancreas compared to the primitively ventral pancreas.

## Pancreatic Cancer

### Diagnosis

**Pancreatic Tumor Detection**

There is an abundance of data indicating that EUS is the most sensitive method for detection of pancreatic tumors with the larger series demonstrating sensitivities in the range of 90% or better (Table 11-1) (11–21).

EUS is especially helpful for smaller lesions (17, 19,20). In most studies, EUS is superior to transabdominal ultrasound (US) and computed tomography (CT) and equivalent to ERCP for lesions 3 cm or less. Two other studies have demonstrated that EUS was superior to the *combination* of CT and ERCP for lesions less than 3 cm (21). In one study comparing EUS, dynamic CT, and MRI for the evaluation of patients with possible pancreatic tumors, endosonography had a sensitivity, specificity, and overall accuracy superior to these other modalities. For tumors less than 3 cm, the sensitivities were 93% (EUS), 67% (MRI), and 53% (CT) (19).

More recently, EUS has compared favorably with spiral CT for the detection of pancreatic tumors. Legmann and colleagues (16) compared dual-phase spiral CT with endosonography in patients with suspected pancreatic tumors and showed that the two modalities were statistically equivalent in yield. The diagnostic sensitivity was 100% for EUS and 92% for spiral CT.

There is also developing evidence that EUS may be able to identify subtle abnormalities in the pancreas that correspond to histologic dysplasia before tumors develop. In a study of early diagnosis and treatment of pancreatic dysplasia in patients with a family history of pancreatic cancer, EUS was able to detect every patient who had pancreatic dysplasia at surgery (22).

### Differential Diagnosis of Pancreatic Tumors

Most tumors are relatively hypoechoic compared to the normal pancreatic parenchyma, although the echo pattern becomes mixed and more variable the larger the size. Pancreatic adenocarcinomas tend to have an irregular margin, sometimes with extending pseudopodia, but malignant lesions smaller than 3.0 cm may have a smooth margin. Unfortunately, it has become clear that areas of focal inflammation can have a similar hypoechoic pattern, sometimes with an equally irregular margin of demarcation (12,20).

The specificity of EUS for differentiating pancreatic cancer from focal pancreatitis is disappointingly low at about 70% (12,20). The inability to differentiate benign from malignant pancreatic lesions must be kept in mind as a current limitation of EUS, although EUS-FNA may help to resolve this issue.

### *Staging*

At present, the only curative treatment available for pancreatic adenocarcinoma is surgery. Unfortunately, only a small proportion of patients with pancreatic cancer will be resectable for cure. Therefore, accurate staging for determination of resectability is crucial in order to prevent unnecessary exploratory surgery. Using the TNM staging system (Table 11-2) promoted by the International Union Against Cancer and the American Joint

**Table 11-2.** AJCC staging of pancreatic carcinoma

**Primary Tumor (T)**

| | |
|---|---|
| T1 | Limited to pancreas, <2cm |
| T2 | Limited to pancreas, >2cm |
| T3 | Extension into duodenum, CBD |
| T4 | Extension into vessels (not splenic), stomach, spleen and colon |

**Regional Lymph Nodes (N)**

| | |
|---|---|
| N0 | No nodal metastases |
| N1 | Regional nodal metastases |

**Distant Metastases (M)**

| | |
|---|---|
| M0 | No distant metastases |
| M1 | Distant metastases |

**Stage Grouping**

| Stage | T | N | M |
|---|---|---|---|
| I | 1 | 0 | 0 |
| | 2 | 0 | 0 |
| II | 3 | 0 | 0 |
| III | 1 | 1 | 0 |
| | 2 | 1 | 0 |
| | 3 | 1 | 0 |
| IV A | 4 | Any | 0 |
| IV B | Any | Any | 1 |

CBD = Common bile duct

Committee on Cancer, EUS has been shown to be particularly accurate at staging the primary tumor (T stage) (5,11,14,16–19,21,23–29). In this system, T1 and T2 tumors are limited to the pancreas and are differentiated by their size, either smaller than 2 cm (T1) or larger (T2). T3 tumors infiltrate the duodenal wall, common bile duct. T4 tumors infiltrate the stomach, spleen, colon, or adjacent blood vessels (Figure 11-3). Please note that this is a new change in the AJCC TNM classification for Pancreatic Cancer Staging. Regional lymph nodes are either present (N0) or not present (N1). Lymph nodes can be identified with good sensitivity, but specificity is lower (18,19,22–26) due to the problem of differentiating metastatic from reactive nodes. Nevertheless, EUS has been found to be more accurate for N stage than dynamic CT (19).

In the evaluation of resectability, EUS appears to be the most accurate method to detect invasion of branches of the portal venous system, which usually correlates with a tumor that cannot be completely resected (30). EUS criteria for invasion vary somewhat from study to study but typically include direct tumor extension into the vessel lumen, irregular venous wall, loss of the bright parenchymal-vascular interface, proximity of the mass to the vessel, and the presence of regional collateral vessels (23,27,28,31). Portal venous involvement

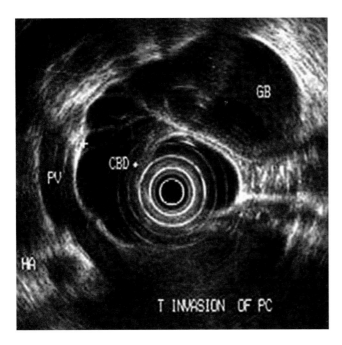

**Figure 11-3.** Radial scanning image from the duodenum showing invasion of the portal vein by a pancreatic head carcinoma.

correlates highly with arterial involvement, which is not well seen on EUS. Distant metastases must be demonstrated by other means (e.g., by CT or laparoscopy), but local resectability has been predicted by EUS with an accuracy of 80% (26). A summary of the results of staging studies is presented in Table 11-3.

Using prospectively collected data on 45 patients with pancreatic cancer who ultimately underwent resection, Brugge and colleagues calculated that the clean (R0) resection rate would be increased from 60% if angiographic staging had been used alone to 78% if EUS were used alone. Using both modalities, the rate for clean resection would be highest at 86%. The improvement in the clean resection rate with the addition of angiography results from the ability of angiography to detect superior mesenteric vein involvement more accurately than EUS (28).

In another study investigating the role of multiple-modality staging, Awad and colleagues (25) evaluated the use of EUS, contrast-enhanced CT, visceral angiography, and laparoscopy for determining resectability. They computed the predictive value of resectability (PVR), and predictive value of unresectability (PVUR) in 30 patients with pancreatic cancer. They found that the PVR and PVUR were between 50% and 60% for each modality alone; however, when EUS, CT, angiography, and laparoscopy were combined, the PVR and PVUR were 100% and 71%, respectively.

Apart from predicting resectablity, EUS staging has been shown in a preliminary report to accurately pre-

dict clinical outcome in both operated and nonoperated patients (32). Patients with T1 tumors survived longer (mean = 52.8 months) than patients with T2 and T3 tumors (mean = 11.9 and 8.8 months, respectively). In this prospective series, while T1 patients appeared to benefit from surgery, there was no difference in survival between the operated and non-operated patients whose tumors were staged T3 and/or N1.

There is increasing interest in demonstrating that the improved staging of pancreatic cancer provided by EUS can be translated into improvements in clinical and economic outcomes. Although there is little data from prospective trials, decision analytic models were recently applied to this question (33). The authors compared four strategies for evaluating patients with pancreatic cancer for resectability. They found that EUS followed by laparoscopy (for patients without local invasion by EUS) resulted in the lowest cost per patient and reduced the number of open explorations by 71%. When angiography was used to confirm local invasion determined by EUS, the rate of curative resections was increased by 2.4 per 100 patients staged, albeit at a cost of $111,000 per curative resection.

### EUS-Guided Fine-Needle Aspiration for Diagnosing Pancreatic Cancer

As mentioned, EUS is limited in its ability to differentiate benign from malignant lesions of the pancreas. However, the recent development of EUS-FNA has allowed endoscopists to obtain tissue from lesions outside the gastrointestinal wall (Figure 11-4). This has particular importance for pancreatic cancer, where both the lesion and regional lymph nodes may be sampled by this technique for accurate diagnosis and staging.

Two case reports appeared in 1992 describing the use of EUS-guided fine needle puncture of the pancreas to sample a tumor (34) and for treatment of a pseudocyst (35). Subsequently, multiple case reports (36) and clinical series (37) have suggested that EUS-FNA has a sensitivity of 73 to 90% and a specificity of 94 to 100% for pancreatic cancer diagnosis (Table 11-3).

Although percutaneous fine-needle aspiration is possible under sonographic or CT guidance, these imaging methods are limited by their inability to define small lesions. In addition, there is some concern about seeding of tumor along the line of puncture when the percutaneous approach is used (38). EUS-FNA may at least partially overcome the limitations of percutaneous puncture. EUS is able to detect small lesions, and given the short distance traveled by the needle during EUS-FNA, the likelihood of tumor seeding should be small. In addition, for patients who undergo resection, the needle tract will be excised at the time of operation.

Recently, an international multicenter group detailed their experience with EUS-FNA (39). In the four

**Table 11-3.** EUS staging for pancreatic carcinoma

|  | Sensitivity | Specificity | PPV | NPV | Accuracy |
|---|---|---|---|---|---|
| Yasuda 1988 |  |  |  |  |  |
| Venous invasion | 79 | 87 |  |  | 81 |
| Snady 1992 |  |  |  |  |  |
| Assessment of resectability | 91 | 62 | 67 | 89 | 75 |
| Yasuda 1993 |  |  |  |  |  |
| Stage I |  |  |  |  | 100 |
| Stage II |  |  |  |  | 71 |
| Stage III |  |  |  |  | 64 |
| Stage IV |  |  |  |  | 100 |
| Ant invasion |  |  |  |  | 79 |
| Duo invasion |  |  |  |  | 83 |
| Retro invasion |  |  |  |  | 79 |
| Nodal invasion |  |  |  |  | 66 |
| Palazzo 1993 |  |  |  |  |  |
| Nodal staging | 62 | 100 | 100 | 55 | 74 |
| Vascular invasion | 100 | 79 | 89 | 100 | 92 |
| Muller 1994 |  |  |  |  |  |
| T staging |  |  |  |  | 82 |
| N staging accuracy |  |  |  |  | 64 |
| N1 |  |  |  |  | 40 |
| N0 |  |  |  |  | 83 |
| Brugge 1996 |  |  |  |  |  |
| Mass localization |  |  |  |  | 80 |
| Vascular invasion |  |  |  |  |  |
| Irregular wall | 47 | 100 |  |  | 87 |
| Loss of interface | 59 | 84 |  |  | 78 |
| Proximity | 89 | 69 |  |  | 73 |
| Size > 2.5 cm | 67 | 33 |  |  | 39 |
| Tio 1996 |  |  |  |  |  |
| T1 |  |  |  |  | 100 |
| T2 |  |  |  |  | 78.3 |
| T3 |  |  |  |  | 84.8 |
| Lymph node staging | 92 | 26 | 70 | 62 | 69 |
| Awad 1997 |  |  |  |  |  |
| Staging and resection | 50 | 63 |  |  |  |
| Gress 1997 |  |  |  |  |  |
| Staging accuracy with linear scope |  |  |  |  |  |
| T |  |  |  |  | 94 |
| N |  |  |  |  | 71 |
| Staging accuracy with radial scope |  |  |  |  |  |
| T |  |  |  |  | 88 |
| N |  |  |  |  | 75 |
| Akahoshi 1998 |  |  |  |  |  |
| T1 |  |  |  |  | 100 |
| T2 |  |  |  |  | 33 |
| T3 |  |  |  |  | 73 |
| N |  |  |  |  | 50 |
| Legmann 1998 |  |  |  |  |  |
| Staging |  |  |  |  | 93 |
| Resectability |  |  |  |  | 90 |
| Unresectability |  |  |  |  | 86 |
| Palazzo 1998 |  |  |  |  |  |
| Staging |  |  |  |  |  |
| T |  |  |  |  | 82 |
| N |  |  |  |  | 68 |
| Venous involvement |  |  |  |  | 85 |
| Buscail 1999 |  |  |  |  |  |
| Vascular involvement | 67 | 100 | 100 | 83 | 87 |
| Midwinter 1999 |  |  |  |  |  |
| PV and SMV involvement | 81 | 86 | 87 | 80 |  |
| SMA involvement | 17 | 67 | 17 | 67 |  |
| Nodal status | 44 | 93 | 80 | 72 |  |

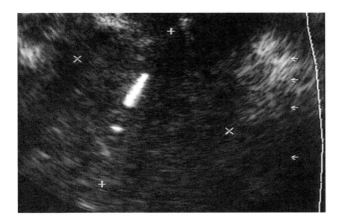

**Figure 11-4.** Curvilinear image showing EUS-guided FNA of a pancreatic head mass.

centers, a total of 124 patients underwent EUS-FNA of pancreatic lesions, with or without associated lymph nodes. In the hands of these experienced endosonographers, the operating characteristics were: sensitivity, 86%; specificity, 94%; positive predictive value, 100%; negative predictive value, 86%; and accuracy 88%. In the same report, the authors detailed the complications related to 554 EUS-FNA procedures directed at gastrointestinal wall lesions, extra-luminal masses, lymph nodes, or cystic lesions. There were 5 complications overall (1.1%), and the rate was higher for cystic lesions (14%) than for solid lesions (0.5%). The complications were: fever after EUS-FNA of cystic lesions, 2 patients; pancreatic pseudocyst hemorrhage, 1 patient; duodenal perforation, 1 patient; and esophageal perforation during dilation of a stricture, 1 patient. No complications were fatal and none occurred in the last 12 months of the study.

### Clinical Application of EUS for Pancreatic Mass Lesions

Based on current data and our own experience, we currently use EUS as part of a strategic assessment of suspected pancreatic mass lesions. For patients who have a suspected pancreatic lesion after either CT or US, we perform EUS of the pancreas. EUS-FNA of suspicious lesions or nodes is conducted during the same examination. In this situation, we reserve ERCP for cases in which the EUS is inconclusive.

For patients with a potentially resectable pancreatic mass identified on CT or US for whom biliary drainage is not required, we stage the tumor with EUS and perform EUS-FNA of imaged lesions, including celiac axis lymph nodes. If biliary drainage is required, we initially perform ERCP with biliary and pancreatic stricture tissue sampling followed by biliary duct stenting. This procedure is followed, usually on a separate day in our institution, by EUS staging (including peri-

pancreatic and celiac lymph node FNA). EUS-guided FNA of the primary tumor is done only if ERCP tissue sampling was nondiagnostic.

Subsequent therapy is largely determined by the staging information provided by endosonography. Patients with T1, T2, or T3 lesions undergo laparoscopy and if no metastatic disease is identified, have subsequent surgical resection. Patients with T4 lesions are candidates for palliative chemotherapy or neoadjuvant chemoradiation protocols but do not undergo resection as primary treatment. Patients with small peripancreatic nodes are managed according to the T stage of the lesion at our institution, while patients with metastatic celiac lymph nodes are offered palliative chemotherapy.

## Neuroendocrine Tumors

With the recognized ability of EUS to image small pancreatic lesions, there has been a keen interest in using this modality to localize gastrointestinal neuroendocrine tumors, especially gastrinomas and insulinomas (40–49). As discussed, many patients are referred for pancreatic EUS after a conventional imaging test such as a sonogram or CT suggests or documents a lesion. In contrast, patients with suspected neuroendocrine tumors are referred when there is documentation of unregulated hormone production and yet conventional imaging tests are normal.

From a practical point of view, the EUS technique for localizing a neuroendocrine tumor varies little from the standard pancreaticobiliary exam described above. However, this is absolutely not a screening test: the patient must have an endocrinologic diagnosis of a hypersecreting tumor. In addition, a generous amount of time should be set aside to perform the procedure. The tumors are usually small, hypoechoic and discrete and may be located within the pancreas or adjacent to the gland attached by a pedicle. Some tumors may arise outside the pancreas and attention must be paid to any structure that is not explained, such as a single periportal or peripancreatic "lymph node" (Figure 11-5). In addition, since recent literature suggests that more gastrinomas may be found in the duodenal wall than in the pancreas (50), a careful videoendoscopic examination of the duodenum, perhaps with a side viewing instrument, is essential when that type of tumor is suspected.

A number of recent studies have reported that EUS is a highly accurate modality for the localization of pancreatic endocrine tumors (PET) (40–43,45–47,51) with a sensitivity between 82 and 89%. EUS compares favorably with somatostatin receptor scintigraphy (SRS) for pancreatic gastrinoma localization, and both tests are clearly superior to CT. However, both EUS and SRS may miss a significant proportion of duodenal

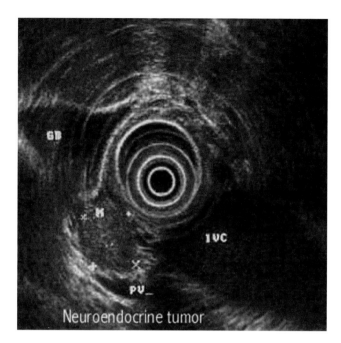

**Figure 11-5.** Radial scanning EUS image demonstrating a small neuroendocrine tumor adjacent to the portal vein.

gastrinomas (50). For the localization of insulinomas, which have a low density of high affinity octreotide receptors and are often missed by SRS, EUS is clearly the imaging method of choice with a reported sensitivity of between 82 and 89%.

Bansal and colleagues (49), recently reported a cost-effectiveness analysis on the use of EUS for the preoperative localization of PETs. In their case-control study, 36 patients who underwent EUS localization were compared to a matched group of 36 patients treated before the introduction of EUS to their institution, who underwent standard localization procedures (diagnostic angiography and selective venous sampling) and/or operative exploration. The EUS group had significantly reduced charges for preoperative localization studies ($2620 vs. $4846), largely due to a decrease in the number of diagnostic angiograms and venous sampling procedures, and also had reduced surgical and anesthesia times. The cost-effectiveness ratio for the EUS group was $3144 per tumor localized compared with $5628 per tumor localized for the group treated before EUS became available.

In one prospective study of insulinoma localization (48), the sensitivity of EUS was noticeably lower (57%) than in previous studies. The authors reported both false negative and false positive examinations, with lesions in the tail being most difficult to detect. In an accompanying editorial (4), the possible role for EUS-guided FNA to exclude false positive findings in this situation was raised. Recently, a preliminary report found that FNA could significantly increase the accuracy rate of EUS for the detection of PETs (51a).

In summary, EUS in experienced hands has been shown to be a highly accurate method for the localization of neuroendocrine tumors. Additional information is now needed to assess the potential usefulness of EUS-FNA for these tumors and to assess the overall impact of EUS on patient outcome.

## Cystic Masses

With the wide availability of abdominal imaging studies including transabdominal ultrasound, CT, and MRI, cystic pancreatic masses (CPMs) of the pancreas are being identified with increased frequency. The majority of these lesions are incidental findings, and there is considerable controversy over their management. Conventional imaging alone may not be sufficient for the complete evaluation of these lesions, especially when they are less than 2 to 3 cm in diameter. There is increasing evidence that EUS imaging, with or without fine needle aspiration of cyst contents, may provide critical information concerning the management of CPMs.

The differential diagnosis of cystic pancreatic masses is presented in Table 11-4. From a practical point of view, there are two typical clinical situations in which determining the nature of the CPM will change management. First, in patients with a large, symptomatic CPM, pseudocysts can be drained by a variety of methods, while other cystic lesions, regardless of whether they are benign or malignant or even their specific etiology, will need to be removed. Second, in the case of incidentally discovered lesions less than 3 cm in size, some lesions may need to be removed (e.g., mucinous cystadenomas and cystadenocarcinomas) while others may be safely followed with serial studies (e.g., serous cystadenoma).

Koito and colleagues (52) correlated pathologic and EUS data from 52 pancreatic solitary cystic tumors in order to assess the ability of EUS to determine the nature of CPMs. The lesions included mucinous cystadenoma (10), mucinous cystadenocarcinoma (7), serous cystadenoma (5), ductectatic mucinous tumor (10), solid and papillary epithelial neoplasm (5) and nonneoplastic cysts (15). EUS was performed with the radial instrument and interpreted by two endosonographers who were not aware of the pathologic findings. The resected specimens were meticulously sectioned and the gross appearances of the longitudinally cut lesions were classified into six different patterns. These patterns, shown in Figure 11-6, are the thick wall type, tumor protruding type, thick septal type, microcystic type, thin septal type, and simple type. The thick wall type showed a thick wall and, in some cases, the presence of multiple cysts in the tumor. The tumor protruding type showed mural nodules

**Table 11-4.** Classification of cystic or cystic-appearing lesions of the pancreas

Congenital true cysts
   Polycystic disease
   Von Hippel-Lindau disease
   Cystic fibrosis
   Dermoid cysts
Angiomatous cysts
Cystic neoplasms
   Mucinous tumors
      Mucinous cystadenoma (macrocystic adenoma) and
         cystadenocarcinoma
      Intraductal mucin hypersecreting neoplasm; "Mucinous ductal ectasia"
   Nonmucinous tumors
      Serous cystadenoma (microcystic adenoma)
      Papillary cystic tumor
      Cystic cavitation of pancreatic adenocarcinoma or
         lymphoma
   Acquired cysts
      Central cavitary aneurysm
      Pseudocyst
      Parasitic cyst
   Misdiagnosed nonpancreatic lesions
      Splenic artery aneurysm
      Choledochal cyst
      Mesenteric cyst
      Duodenal duplication cyst

### EUS Classification of Cysts

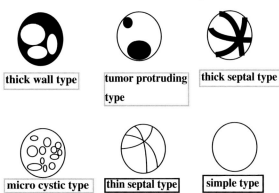

**Figure 11-6.** This illustration shows the six types of cystic lesions of the pancreas (provided by Koito and colleagues).

with or without papillary projections. The thin and thick septal types were differentiated by the breadth of the septae, thin being characterized as less than 3 mm. The microcystic type consisted of at least six small cysts less than 2 cm in diameter within the mass lesion. The simple type had a thin rim and no internal components. In their 52 cases, all the neoplastic tumors were classified as thick wall, thick septal, tumor protruding, or microcystic types. Interestingly, all serous cystadenomas were microcystic and no other cysts fit that classification. EUS imaging was able to accurately classify 94% of the lesions.

In another study of cystic pancreatic lesions, Sugiyama and colleagues focused on the role of endosonography to diagnose and classify a particular cystic lesion: intraductal papillary tumor, or IPT (53). This interesting lesion is characterized by dilation of a portion of the pancreatic duct (main duct, branch ducts, or both) with copious secretion of mucin. The tumor, which is often resectable and has a favorable prognosis even when malignant, is also known as mucin-hypersecreting carcinoma, intraductal mucin-hypersecreting neoplasm, mucin-producing tumor, intraductal carcinoma, intraductal mucin-producing tumor, ductectatic mucinous cystadenoma and cystadenocarcinoma, and mucinous duct ectasia. In Sugiyama's report, they compared EUS, ERCP, and conventional (US) images to surgical findings in 28 patients with IPT and in 38 patients with other pancreatic cystic lesions and found

that EUS was helpful in identifying these lesions, in defining their extent within and outside of the pancreas, and in predicting malignancy based on the presence of mural nodules.

There is continued interest in using information from cyst contents, aspirated under EUS guidance, to determine the nature of cystic pancreatic lesions. In one preliminary report (54), cyst contents were examined for cytology, mucin staining, and a variety of tumor markers (CEA, CA-125, CA 19-9, CA 72-4, TPA, and CA 15-3). They found that the specificity of cytology was 100% for malignant lesions, but that the sensitivity of cytology was low (0.57). In their experience, the addition of tumor marker analysis seemed to increase the overall accuracy of the examination in terms of both detection of mucinous lesions and detection of malignant lesions.

## Pancreatic Ductal Imaging

Using catheter-like probes, it is possible to image from within the pancreatic duct, but the clinical utility of this approach for pancreatic tumor assessment or cancer diagnosis has not yet been established. Furakowa and colleagues (55) have used very high frequency (30 MHz) catheter probes introduced into the pancreatic duct at ERCP in 40 patients with pancreatic diseases, including 11 adenocarcinomas and 15 with chronic pancreatitis. They also examined surgical and autopsy specimens from these and other patients, and were convinced that echo patterns obtained in this way can distinguish benign from malignant disease in most cases. This method may have special utility in detecting early adenocarcinomas in high-risk patients. Papillary neoplastic lesions confined to the wall of the pancreatic duct were described in 4 cases (1 cancer, 3 adenomas). Overall, complications of the procedure were infrequent; mild pancreatitis occurred in only 1 of the 40 cases. Prospective studies of high frequency pancreatic duct imaging will be required to confirm these observations.

## Chronic Pancreatitis

With the high-resolution images of the pancreas provided by EUS, it is reasonable to assume that this modality would be useful for the evaluation of the structural changes of chronic pancreatitis. ERCP has traditionally been considered the gold standard for structural changes in the pancreatic ducts consistent with the diagnosis of chronic pancreatitis. EUS has emerged as a very sensitive modality for the evaluation of chronic pancreatitis (56–60). It has the advantage over other imaging studies in that it can detect abnormalities of both ductular and parenchymal abnormalities. Morphology provides detailed images of both the pancreatic duct and the surrounding parenchyma. EUS is more sensitive than ERCP for the parenchymal changes of chronic pancreatitis (Figure 11-7).

Wiersema and colleagues (61) studied 69 patients with chronic abdominal pain with EUS followed by ERCP and/or PPJ: 11 ductular and parenchymal features were assessed with EUS. The EUS findings were considered consistent with chronic pancreatitis if any three features were abnormal. Among the 69 patients with pain, 30 were shown to have chronic pancreatitis based on clinical, ERCP and/or PPJ data. EUS was abnormal in 24 of these 30, while ERCP was abnormal in only 19. All 19 patients with abnormal ERCPs also had abnormal EUS examinations. There were eight features found to be indicative of chronic pancreatitis using the logistic regression analysis:

1. Echogenic foci within the gland
2. Focal areas of reduced echogenicity within the gland
3. Increased echogenicity/thickness of the main pancreatic duct wall
4. Accentuation of the glands lobular pattern
5. Cysts
6. Irregular contour of the main pancreatic duct
7. Dilation of the main pancreatic duct
8. Side branch dilation

When generation of a receiver operating characteristic curve was performed, it revealed that when three or more of the criteria were present, the sensitivity, specificity and accuracy were 80%, 86%, and 86%, respectively.

In another study, Nattermann and colleagues (58) performed a prospective study of EUS and ERCP in 114 patients, 94 of whom had acute or chronic pancreatitis.

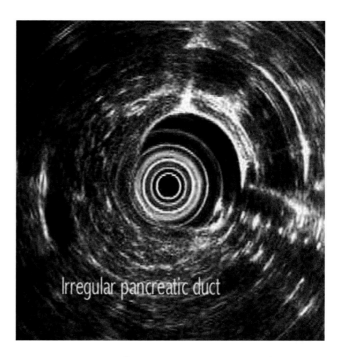

**Figure 11-7.** Radial EUS image showing changes of chronic pancreatitis including echogenic foci within the gland and a hyperechoic border of the main pancreatic duct.

They used a set of ductular and parenchymal EUS features similar to that used by Weirsema and colleagues to determine the presence or absence of chronic pancreatitis. Abnormal EUS features were found in all patients with grades 2 and 3 chronic pancreatitis by Cambridge classification on ERCP. They found that 88 percent of patients with grade 1 pancreatitis on ERCP had an abnormal EUS. In addition, 63% of patients with chronic pancreatitis and a normal ERCP also had an abnormal EUS. The parenchymal and ductal changes were not seen in the 20 control subjects.

The EUS findings of parenchymal heterogeneity and lobulations were similar to those described by Nakazawa and Lees. The generally accepted concept that these findings correspond to progressive fibrosis and scar formation (echogenic) alternating with sites of inflammation (hypoechoic) was reinforced by these authors.

Catalano and colleagues (57) reported on the utility of EUS for the diagnosis of chronic pancreatitis in a group of patients with idiopathic recurrent pancreatitis. In their study, 80 consecutive subjects underwent EUS, ERCP, and a secretin test. To avoid confounding factors, patients were excluded if they were over 60 years of age or had acute pancreatitis within 6 weeks of examination. When clinical history was combined with ERCP and functional testing, 38 of the 80 patients were found to have chronic pancreatitis. When at least three EUS features were used to diagnose chronic pancreatitis, the sensitivity and specificity were 86% and 98%, respectively.

In a population with a high prevalence of disease, Sahai and colleagues (62) reported on the accuracy of EUS to diagnose, rule out, and establish the severity of chronic pancreatitis found by ERCP. Their large number of patients, 126 in all, allowed a more sophisticated analysis of the EUS features of chronic pancreatitis that have been used for over a decade. On univariate analysis, the following were found to predict the Cambridge class and/or chronic pancreatitis: all EUS criteria except hyperechoic duct margin and cyst, the total number of positive EUS criteria (the greater the number, the more significant) and a positive history of alcohol abuse. Multivariate analysis showed that the independent predictors were calcifications, a positive history of alcohol abuse, and total number of EUS criteria on examination. The PPV was greater than 85% when more than 2 criteria were present. When more than 6 criteria were present, the PPV for moderate to severe pancreatitis was above 85%. Moreover, moderate to severe chronic pancreatitis was unlikely (NPV >85%) when fewer than 3 criteria were present.

In each of the studies discussed above, there were patients who had EUS criteria for chronic pancreatitis but had normal ERCPs. However, without histology or long-term clinical follow-up it is not possible to confirm if these patients truly have chronic pancreatitis. A recent study by Hastier and colleagues (63) assessed the significance of these isolated EUS parenchymal changes by documenting their natural history during a follow-up period. In their study, 72 patients with alcoholic cirrhosis were examined with EUS and ERCP. Chronic pancreatitis was diagnosed in 14 patients by both methods. Isolated EUS parenchymal findings consistent with chronic pancreatitis were observed in 18 patients. After a mean follow-up of 22 months, during which the subjects continued to consume alcohol, there was no progression of the earlier EUS appearance.

In summary, the ability of EUS to identify subtle pancreatic parenchymal abnormalities has made it a valuable tool for evaluating patients with symptoms compatible with chronic pancreatitis. For patients with moderate to severe pancreatitis by Cambridge classification, EUS is effective at making the diagnosis and may avoid unnecessary pancreatography. In patients with suspected mild disease, a normal EUS is able to exclude chronic pancreatitis as a diagnostic possibility. However, in patients who are found to have minimal changes on EUS, additional work is needed to determine the significance, if any, of the EUS findings.

## Acute Pancreatitis

EUS has a more limited role in the evaluation of patients with acute pancreatitis. It is clear that EUS is at least as accurate as ERCP for the detection of CBD

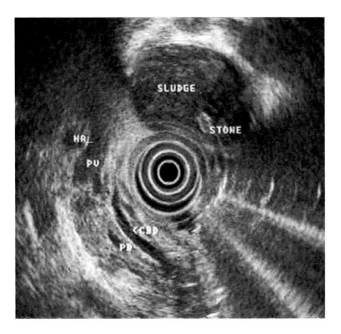

**Figure 11-8.** Radial EUS image in a patient with recurrent pancreatitis demonstrating biliary sludge and stones in the gallbladder. Also seen in this image are the hepatic artery, portal vein, CBD, and PD.

stones. This has been shown in a variety of patient populations including patients with acute pancreatitis (64–67). As such, it is reasonable to assume that performing EUS rather than ERCP in patients with severe acute pancreatitis may prevent unnecessary negative ERCPs. At present however, there is no prospective data to support or refute this assumption. The use of EUS to determine the severity of acute pancreatitis as suggested by some authors needs further investigation (64,65).

In patients with recurrent idiopathic pancreatitis EUS may be useful to identify patients with biliary sludge who may benefit from cholecystectomy, ursodeoxycholic acid therapy or sphincterotomy (Figure 11-8). Liu and colleagues (68) recently reported a prospective study on the use of EUS in patients with idiopathic pancreatitis with gallbladder in situ. Of 89 consecutive patients with acute pancreatitis, 18 were classified as idiopathic after reviewing the clinical history and conventional imaging, that is, US or CT scanning. Of these 18, 14 had small gallbladder stones and 3 of these had concomitant CBD stones. This proportion of patients (78%) who were found to have unsuspected calculous disease is similar to the proportion of patients found to have microlithiasis or sludge on microscopic examination of bile in two previous studies of idiopathic pancreatitis (42,68). The higher sensitivity of EUS versus conventional ultrasound for biliary sludge is supported by both a clinical study in patients with biliary colic (69) and a preliminary report using an in vitro gallbladder model (70).

## Pancreatic Pseudocysts

EUS has been used to assist or direct endoscopic puncture and drainage of pancreatic pseudocysts by a number of investigators (4,71–73). Fockens and colleagues (73) focused on demonstrating the utility of EUS in this situation. They used EUS in 32 patients to determine the distance between the pseudocyst and the gut wall, identify interposed vascular structures, and to determine the optimal site for drainage. EUS determined that in 37.5% of cases endoscopic drainage was either not appropriate or feasible due to a variety of reasons. In the future, it is likely that EUS will play a pivotal role in the evaluation and management of pancreatic pseudocysts.

## Pancreas Divisum and Other Anomalies

EUS has been used in the evaluation of a variety of congenital pancreatic anomalies and variants (9,74,75). Bhutani and colleagues (6) evaluated the utility of the "stack sign" for excluding the diagnosis of pancreas divisum. They identified the "stack sign" in 25 of 30 patients without pancreas divisum and in only 2 of 6 patients with the abnormality (p = 0.04).

Sugiyama and Atomi (74) demonstrated that EUS is capable of diagnosing an anomalous pancreaticobiliary junction. In their hands, EUS was able to detect a long common channel (12 mm or more) in 9 of 10 patients. Gress and colleagues (75) described a band-like stricture in continuity with and without the same echogenicity as the head of the pancreas in 2 patients with annular pancreas. Endosonographers need to be aware of these unusual diagnoses that may be encountered in patients referred for EUS.

### Celiac Plexus Neurolysis

Endosonography may also be useful for the treatment of intractable pain in patients with pancreatic cancer. Recently, Wiersema and colleagues (4) described EUS-guided celiac plexus neurolysis for the palliation of pain in 30 patients with intra-abdominal malignancy, the majority of which were pancreatic cancers. Bupivacaine (25%) and absolute ETOH was injected on both sides of the aorta under real-time endosonographic guidance using the Pentax convex linear array echoendoscope and a 23-gauge needle. The procedure, which was performed at the same time as the initial EUS staging and/or FNA exam, resulted in a significant reduction in pain score for 91% of surviving patients at follow-up evaluations conducted up to 12 weeks after EUS CPN. Gress and colleagues (3) performed a similar study, but as a randomized trial, comparing EUS and CT-guided celiac plexus blocks for managing the abdominal pain associated with chronic pancreatitis. In

this study, they used a combination of triamcinolone and bupivacaine, instead of ethanol, and reported a significant reduction in the pain scores for the EUS-guided celiac block group when compared to the CT group. Further studies with larger sample populations are now needed.

## Conclusion

Endosonography produces detailed images of the pancreas and surrounding blood vessels and provides both accurate detection and staging of malignant lesions and the means for making a tissue diagnosis. The staging information obtained from EUS is useful in directing the subsequent management of these patients, and will be increasingly important as additional stage-dependent treatment options become available. Also, the ability to obtain tissue efficiently during the staging examination facilitates the administration of appropriate palliative therapy if initial resection is not advisable. For the diagnosis of chronic pancreatitis, EUS appears to be a valuable tool and is probably more sensitive than other current imaging methods. Potential therapeutic applications of EUS for pancreatic diseases include EUS-guided celiac plexus block for pain control and the EUS-guided delivery of tumoricidal agents. Although long-term prospective evaluation is needed to determine to what degree this new endoscopic modality impacts on the clinical and economic outcomes of patients with pancreatic diseases, it seems likely to occupy a central role in the management of these patients for the foreseeable future.

### References
1. DiMagno EP, Buxton JL, Regan PT, et al. Ultrasonic endoscope. Lancet 1980;1:629–631.
2. Strohm WD, Kurtz W, Hagenmuller F, Classen M. Diagnostic efficacy of endoscopic ultrasound tomography in pancreatic cancer and cholestasis. Scand J Gastroenterol Suppl 1984;102:18–23.
3. Gress F, Schmitt C, Sherman S, Ikenberry S, Lehman G. A prospective randomized comparison of endoscopic ultrasound and CT guided celiac plexus block for managing chronic pancreatitis pain [see comments]. Am J Gastroenterol 1994;44:900–905.
4. Wiersema MJ, Wiersema LM. Endosonography guided celiac plexus neurolysis. Gastrointest Endosc 1996;44:656–662.
5. Gress F, Savides T, Cummings O. Radial scanning and linear array endosonography for staging pancreatic cancer: a prospective randomized comparison. Gastrointest Endosc 1997;45:138–142.
6. Furukawa T, Tsukamoto Y, Naitoh Y, Mitake M, Hirooka Y, Hayakawa T. Differential diagnosis of pancreatic diseases with an intraductal ultrasound system. Gastrointest Endosc 1994;40:213–219.

7. Mukai H, Nakajima M, Yasuda K, Mizuno S, Kawai K. Evaluation of endoscopic ultrasonography in the pre-operative staging of carcinoma of the ampulla of Vater and common bile duct. Gastrointest Endosc 1992;38:676–683.

8. Chak A, Canto M, Stevens PD, et al. Clinical applications of a new through-the-scope ultrasound probe: a prospective comparison with an ultrasound endoscope. Gastrointest Endosc 1997;45:291–295.

9. Bhutani MS, Hoffman BJ, Hawes RH. Diagnosis of pancreas divisum by endoscopic ultrasonography. Endoscopy 1999;31:167–169.

10. Savides TJ, Gress FG, Zaidi SA, Ikenberry SO, Hawes RH. Detection of embryologic ventral pancreatic parenchyma with endoscopic ultrasound. Gastrointest Endosc 1996;43:14–19.

11. Yasuda K, Mukai H, Fujimoto S, Nakajima M, Kawai K. The diagnosis of pancreatic cancer by endoscopic ultrasonography. Gastrointest Endosc 1988;34:1–8.

12. Kaufman AR, Sivak MV Jr. Endoscopic ultrasonography in the differential diagnosis of pancreatic disease. Gastrointest Endosc 1989;35:214–219.

13. Tio TL, Sie LH, Kallimanis G, et al. Staging of ampullary and pancreatic carcinoma: comparison between endosonography and surgery. Gastrointest Endosc 1996;44:706–713.

14. Palazzo L, Roseau G, Gayet B. Endoscopic ultrasonography in the diagnosis and staging of pancreatic adenocarcinoma. Results of a prospective study with comparison to ultrasonography and CT scan [see comments]. Endoscopy 1993;25:143–150.

15. Baron PL, Aabakken LE, Cole DJ. Differentiation of benign from malignant pancreatic masses by endoscopic ultrasound. Ann Surg Oncol 1997;4:639–643.

16. Legmann P, Vignaux O, Dousset B. Pancreatic tumors: comparison of dual-phase helical CT and endoscopic sonography. AJR Am J Roentgenol 1998; 170.1315–1322.

17. Akahoshi K, Chijiiwa Y, Nakano I. Diagnosis and staging of pancreatic cancer by endoscopic ultrasound. Br J Radiol 1998;71:492–496.

18. Yasuda K, Mukai H, Nakajima M, Kawai K. Staging of pancreatic carcinoma by endoscopic ultrasonography [see comments]. Endoscopy 1993;25:151–155.

19. Muller MF, Meyenberger C, Bertschinger P, Schaer R, Marincek B. Pancreatic tumors: evaluation with endoscopic US, CT, and MR imaging. Radiology 1994; 190:745–751.

20. Rosch T, Lorenz R, Braig C. Endoscopic ultrasound in pancreatic tumor diagnosis. Gastrointest Endosc 1991;37:347–352.

21. Snady H, Cooperman A, Seigel J. Endoscopic ultrasonography compared with computed tomography with ERCP in patients with obstructive jaundice or small peripancreatic mass. Gastrointest Endosc 1992; 38:27–34.

22. Brentnall TA, Bronner MP, Byrd DR, Haggitt RC, Kimmey MB. Early diagnosis and treatment of pancreatic dysplasia in patients with a family history of pancreatic cancer. Ann Int Med 1999;131:247–255.

23. Midwinter MJ, Beveridge CJ, Wilsdon JB, Bennett MK, Baudouin CJ, Charnley RM. Correlation between spiral computed tomography, endoscopic ultrasonography and findings at operation in pancreatic and ampullary tumors. Br Surg 1999;86:189–193.

24. Buscail L, Pages P, Berthelemy P, Fourtanier G, Frexinos J, Escourrou J. Role of EUS in the management of pancreatic and ampullary carcinoma: a prospective study assessing resectability and prognosis. Gastrointest Endosc 1999;50:34–40.

25. Awad SS, Colletti L, Mulholland M. Multimodality staging optimizes resectability in patients with pancreatic and ampullary cancer. Am Surg 1997; 63:634–638.

26. Tio TL, Tytgat GN. Endoscopic ultrasonography in staging local resectability of pancreatic and peri-ampullary malignancy. Scand J Gastroenterol Suppl 1986;123:135–142.

27. Palazzo L. Staging of pancreatic carcinoma by endoscopic ultrasonography [review with 14 refs]. Endoscopy 1998;30 (suppl 1):A103–A107.

28. Brugge WR, Lee MJ, Kelsey PB, Schapiro RH, Warshaw AL. The use of EUS to diagnose malignant portal venous system invasion by pancreatic cancer [see comments]. Gastrointest Endosc 1996;43:561–567.

29. Rosch T, Braig C. Gain T, et al. Staging of pancreatic and ampullary carcinoma by endoscopic ultrasonography. Comparison with conventional sonography, computed tomography, and angiography. Gastroenterology 1992;102:188–199.

30. Rosch T, Lorenz B, Braig C, Classen M. Endoscopic ultrasonography in diagnosis and staging of pancreatic and biliary tumors [review with 33 refs]. Endoscopy 1992;24: (suppl 1):304–308.

31. Snady H, Bruckner H, Siegel J, Cooperman A, Neff R, Kiefer L. Endoscopic ultrasonographic criteria of vascular invasion by potentially resectable pancreatic tumors. Gastrointest Endosc 1994;40:326–333.

32. Gress F, Savides T, Zaidi S. EUS staging of pancreatic cancer accurately predicts patient outcome and survival. Gastrointest Endosc 1995;43:S50. Abstract.

33. Tierney WM, Fendrick AM, Hirth RA, Scheiman JM. The clinical and economic impact of alternative staging strategies for Ademo carcinoma of the pancreas. American Journal of Gastroentemology Press 2000.

34. Vilmann P, Jacobsen GK, Henriksen FW, Hancke S. Endoscopic ultrasonography with guided fine needle aspiration biopsy in pancreatic disease. Gastrointest Endosco 1992;38:172–173. March–April.

35. Grimm H, Binmoeller KF, Soehendra N. Endosonography guided drainage of a pancreatic pseudocyst. Gastrointest Endosc 1992;38:170.

36. Chang KJ, Albers CG, Erickson RA, Butler JA, Wuerker RB, Lin F. Endoscopic ultrasound-guided fine needle aspiration of pancreatic carcinoma. Am J Gastroenterol 1994;89:263–266.

37. Vilmann P, Hancke S, Henriksen FW, Jacobsen GK. Endosonographically-guided fine needle aspiration biopsy of malignant lesions in the upper gastrointestinal tract. Endoscopy 1993;25:523–527.

38. Ferrucci JT, Wittenberg J, Margolies MN, Carey RW. Malignant seeding of the tract after thin-needle aspiration biopsy. Radiology 1979;130:345–346.

39. Wiersema MJ, Vilmann P, Giovannini M, Chang KJ, Wiersema LM. Endosonography-guided fine-needle

aspiration biopsy: diagnostic accuracy and complication assessment. Gastroenterology 1997;112:1087–1095.

40. Rosch T, Lightdale CJ, Botet JF, et al. Localization of pancreatic endocrine tumors by endoscopic ultrasonography. N Engl J Med 1992;326:1721–1726.

41. Lightdale CJ, Botet JF, Woodruff JM, Brennan MF. Localization of endocrine tumors of the pancreas with endoscopic ultrasonography. Cancer 1991;68:1815–1820.

42. Glover JR, Shorvon PJ, Lees WR. Endoscopic ultrasound for localization of islet cell tumors. Gut 1992;33:108–110.

43. Palazzo L, Roseau G, Salmeron M. Endoscopic ultrasonography in the preoperative localization of pancreatic endocrine tumors. Endoscopy 1992;24 (suppl 1):350–353.

44. Zimmer T, Ziegler K, Bader M. Localization of neuroendocrine tumors of the upper gastrointestinal tract. Gut 1994;35:471–475.

45. Ruszniewski P, Amouyal P, Amouyal G, et al. Localization of gastrinomas by endoscopic ultrasonography in patients with Zollinger-Ellison syndrome. Surgery 1995;117:629–635.

46. Thompson NW, Czako PF, Fritts LL, et al. Role of endoscopic ultrasonography in the localization of insulinomas and gastrinomas. Surgery 1994;116:1131–1138.

47. Zimmer T, Stolzel U, Bader M, et al. Endoscopic ultrasonography and somatostatin receptor scintigraphy in the preoperative localization of insulinomas and gastrinomas. Gut 1996;39:562–568.

48. Schumacher B, Lubke HJ, Frieling T, Strohmeyer G, Starke AA. Prospective study on the detection of insulinomas by endoscopic ultrasonography [see comments]. Endoscopy 1996;28:273–276.

49. Bansal R, Tierney W, Carpenter S, Thompson N, Scheiman JM. Cost effectiveness of EUS for preoperative localization of pancreatic endocrine tumors. Gastrointest Endosc 1999;49:19–25.

50. Gibril F, Jensen R. Comparative analysis of diagnostic techniques for localization of gastrointestinal neuroendocrine tumors. Yale Biol Med 1997;70:509–522.

51. Zimmer T, Ziegler K, Liehr RM, Stolzel U, Riecken EO, Wiedenmann B. Endosonography of neuroendocrine tumors of the stomach, duodenum, and pancreas [review with 29 refs]. Ann NY Acad Sci 1994;733:425–436.

51a. Ciaccia D, Harada N, Wiersema MJ, et al. Preoperative localization and diagnosis of pancreatic and peri pancreatic islet cell tumors using EUS-guided FNA. Gastrointest Endoscopy 1997;45(4)584. Abstract.

52. Koito K, Namieno T, Nagakawa T, Shyonai T, Hirokawa N, Morita K. Solitary cystic tumor of the pancreas: EUS-pathologic correlation. Gastrointest Endosc 1997;45:268–276.

53. Sugiyama M, Atomi Y, Saito M. Intraductal papillary tumors of the pancreas: evaluation with endoscopic ultrasonography. Gastrointest Endosc 1998;48:164–171.

54. Mallery S, Quirk D, Lewandowski K, et al. EUS-guided FNA with cyst fluid analysis in pancreatic cystic lesions. Gastrointest Endosc 1998;47:AB149:504.

55. Furukawa T, Tsukamoto Y, Naitoh Y, Hirooka Y, Katoh T. Evaluation of intraductal ultrasonography in the diagnosis of pancreatic cancer [see comments]. Endoscopy 1993;25:577–581.

56. Sahai AV, Zimmerman M, Aabakken L. Prospective assessment of the ability of endoscopic ultrasound to diagnose, exclude or establish the severity of chronic pancreatitis found by ERCP [see comments]. Gastrointest Endosc 1998;48:18–25.

57. Catalano MF, Geenen JE. Diagnosis of chronic pancreatitis by endoscopic ultrasonography. Endoscopy 1998;30 (suppl 1):A111–A115.

58. Nattermann C, Goldschmidt AJ, Dancygier H. Endosonography in chronic pancreatitis; a comparison between endoscopic retrograde pancreatography and endoscopic ultrasonography [see comments]. Endoscopy 1993;25:565–570.

59. Wiersema MJ, Wiersema LM. Endosonography of the pancreas: normal variation versus changes of early chronic pancreatitis [review with 24 refs]. Gastrointest Endosc Clin N Am 1995; 5:487–496.

60. Zuccaro GJ, Sivak MV, Jr. Endoscopic ultrasonography in the diagnosis of chronic pancreatitis. Endoscopy 1992;24 (suppl 1):347–349.

61. Wiersema MJ, Hawes RH, Lehman GA, Kochman ML, Sherman S, Kopecky KK. Prospective evaluation of endoscopic ultrasonography and endoscopic retrograde cholangiopancreatography in patients with chronic abdominal pain of suspected pancreatic origin [see comments]. Endoscopy 1993;25:555–564.

62. Kulling D, Sahai AV, Knapple WL, Cunningham JT, Hoffman BJ. Diagnostic endoscopic ultrasound of the pancreas may cause acute pancreatitis. Endoscopy 1998;30:S7–S8.

63. Hastier P, Buckley MJ, Francois E. A prospective study of pancreatic disease in patients with alcoholic cirrhosis: comparative diagnostic value of ERCP and EUS and long-term significance of isolated parenchymal abnormalities. Gastrointest Endosc 1999;49:705–709.

64. Chak A, Hawes RH, Cooper GS. Prospective assessment of the utility of EUS in the evaluation of gallstone pancreatitis. Gastrointest Endosc 1999;49:599–604.

65. Sugiyama M, Atomi Y. Acute biliary pancreatitis: the roles of endoscopic ultrasonography and endoscopic retrograde cholangiopancreatography. Surgery 1998;124:14–21.

66. Prat F, Amouyal G, Amouyal P. Prospective controlled study of endoscopic ultrasonography and endoscopic retrograde cholangiography in patients with suspected common bile duct lithiasis [see comments]. Lancet 1996;347:75–79.

67. Palazzo L, Borotto E, Cellier C. Endosonographic features of pancreatic metastases. Gastrointest Endosc 1996;44:433–436.

68. Liu CL, Lo CM, Chan JFK, Poon RTP, Fan ST. EUS for detection of occult cholelithiasis in patients with idiopathic pancreatitis. Gastrointest Endosc 2000;51:28–32.

69. Dill JE. Symptom resolution or relief after cholecystectomy correlates strongly with positive combined endoscopic ultrasound and stimulated biliary drainage. Endoscopy 1997;29:646–648.

70. Stevens PD, Lightdale CJ, Saha SA. In vitro comparison of endoscope based vs. catheter based endoscopic ultrasound for the detection of biliary sludge. Gastrointest Endosc 1996;43:S57. Abstract.

71. Gerolami R, Giovannini M, Laugier R. Endoscopic drainage of pancreatic pseudocysts guided by endosonography. Endoscopy 1997;29:106–108.

72. Fockens P, Johnson TG, van Dullemen HM, Huibregtse K, Tytgat GN. Endosonographic imaging of pancreatic pseudocysts before endoscopic transmural drainage. Gastrointest Endosc 1997;46:412–416.

73. Giovannini M, Bernardini D, Seitz JF. Cystogastrotomy entirely performed under endosonography guidance for pancreatic pseudocyst; results in six patients [see comments]. Gastrointest Endosc 1998;48:200–203.

74. Sugiyama M, Atomi Y. Anomalous pancreaticobiliary junction without congenital choledochal cyst. Br J Surg 1998;85:911–916.

75. Gress F, Yiengpruksawan A, Sherman S. Diagnosis of annular pancreas by endoscopic ultrasound [review with 27 refs]. Gastrointest Endosc 1996;44:485–489.

# 12

# Colorectal Endoscopic Ultrasonography

## Manoop S. Bhutani

## Instruments for Colorectal Endosonography

### Rigid Probes

Rigid probes do not incorporate fiber-optic bundles and thus do not provide simultaneous endoscopic and ultrasound images. The use of rigid probes has been limited to the rectum. The most frequently used rigid probe is an instrument with a single-element 7.5-MHz transducer that provides a 360-degree radial image at right angles to the long axis of the probe (Bruel and Kjaer; Naerum, Denmark/Marlborough, MA). A balloon around the transducer provides acoustic coupling with the gut wall. Rigid probes with linear array imaging are also available (Hitachi, Tarrytown, NY, and Acuson, Mountainview, CA).

### Echoendoscopes

These instruments are endoscopes that have high-frequency ultrasound transducers incorporated in the distal tip, thus providing both an endoscopic and a high-frequency ultrasound image.

1. A dedicated echocolonoscope is available that has front viewing optics with a 7.5-MHz rotating transducer (CFUM20, Olympus, Milville, NY). The front viewing endoscopic image allows the instrument to be advanced under direct vision up to the level of the cecum in a similar fashion to regular colonoscopy.
2. A side viewing upper gastrointestinal echoendoscope (GFUM20 & GFUM30 Olympus, Milville, NY) providing radial images at 7.5 and 12 MHz can be inserted into the rectum, but usually cannot be advanced beyond the distal sigmoid colon due to the side viewing optics.

3. Linear upper echoendoscopes such as the FG32UA (Pentax, Orangeburg, NY) provide a linear image and can also be inserted into the rectum, but usually not beyond the distal sigmoid due to the side viewing optics. Of note, linear echoendoscopy allows real-time EUS-guided FNA of pericolonic lymph nodes and masses.
4. Recently, small, high-frequency miniprobes have become available that can be passed through the biopsy channels of standard endoscopes (see Chapter 15). These miniprobes can then be used to image the gastrointestinal wall and focal lesions by direct application of the miniprobe to the target lesion under endoscopic vision. Such miniprobes are available from a number of manufacturers (Olympus, Fujinon, Microvasive).

## Examination Technique

Preparation for colonic examination by endosonography varies depending on the area to be imaged. Laxative enemas similar to the preparation for flexible sigmoidoscopy are sufficient for anorectal and sigmoid lesions. For colonic endosonography proximal to the sigmoid colon, a per-oral lavage similar to that used for colonoscopy is desirable. A quick, flexible sigmoidoscopy should be routinely performed prior to EUS to assess the quality of the preparation and to ensure that the recto-sigmoid lumen is free of stool (1). An awareness of other potential artifacts during trans-rectal ultrasound is also desirable (2) (Figure 12-1). Endosonographic examination is then conducted with one of the available instruments. If one of the blind rectal probes is being used, it is lubricated and inserted into the anus and advanced into the rectal vault. A balloon

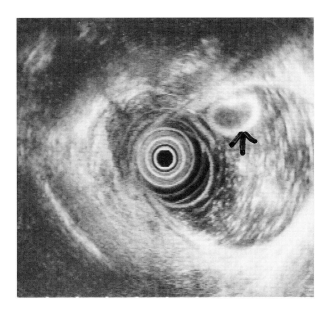

**Figure 12-1.** A mirror image artifact (*arrow*) during radial EUS in the rectum.

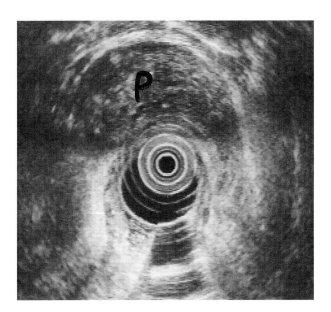

**Figure 12-2.** Prostate gland (*P*) seen anterior to the rectum during endosonography with a radial transducer.

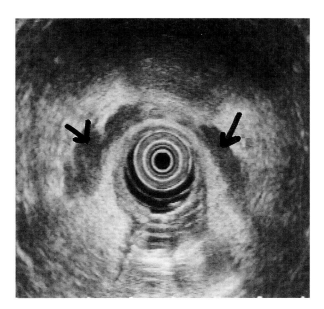

**Figure 12-3.** Hypoechoic, elongated structures (*arrows*) are seminal vesicles seen during rectal EUS. These should not be confused with lymph nodes.

and then under endoscopic visualization advanced to the distal sigmoid colon. We have imaged sigmoid lesions with this technique as far as 45 centimeters from the anal verge ( 3 ). However, caution needs to be exercised because advancing the side viewing echoendoscopes "blindly" proximal to the sigmoid colon may cause colonic perforation. The echocolonoscope has front viewing optics and can be easily advanced under direct vision to the cecum.

## Colorectal Cancer Staging by EUS
### Tumor (T) Stage

Malignant colorectal tumors appear as hypoechoic masses by EUS. A tumor that by EUS appears to be limited to the mucosa or the submucosa (first three echo layers) is classified as a T1 lesion (Figure 12-4). A colorectal carcinoma invading into the muscularis propria (hypoechoic fourth EUS layer) but with an intact outer margin of the muscularis propria and with no penetration completely through the muscularis propria is a T2 lesion (Figure 12-5). A T3 lesion penetrates through the rectal wall and all of the EUS layers, has irregular outer margins, or has tumor pseudopodia extending beyond the five echo layers (Figure 12-6). A T4 lesion is a colorectal cancer that is locally invading into an adjacent organ such as the prostate.

### N Stage

Lymph nodes during EUS may be seen as round, oval, or sometimes triangular structures that have variable

at the tip of the rigid probe creates the acoustic interface between the rectum and the transducer.

Regardless of the type of transducer, familiarity with normal rectal anatomy as seen with that particular transducer is essential (Figures 12-2 and 12-3). If the examination is being performed of the anal sphincter only, the instrument is withdrawn so that the transducer provides images of the internal and external anal sphincter. The side viewing upper endoscopic ultrasound instruments can also be inserted into the rectum

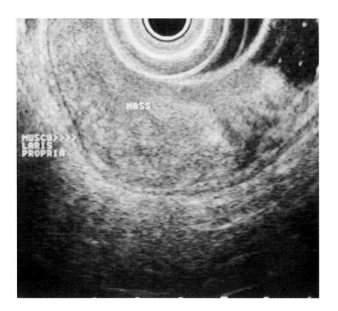

**Figure 12-4.** A T1 rectal adenocarcinoma arising within a large villous adenoma (mass). The muscularis propria under the mass is intact without invasion.

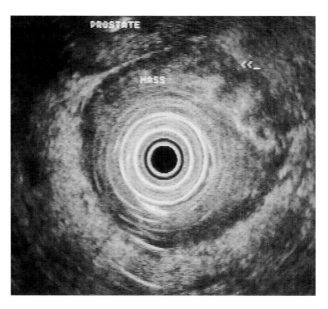

**Figure 12-6.** A hypoechoic rectal carcinoma that has an irregular outer margin (*arrows*) and has penetrated through the muscularis propria (T3).

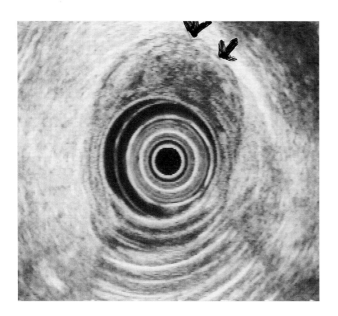

**Figure 12-5.** A rectal carcinoma seen by EUS as invading the muscularis propria (*arrows*) but not penetrating through it (T2).

echogenicity. Moving the ultrasound probe and following these structures ultrasonographically helps to ensure that a round hypoechoic/anechoic area initially suggestive of a lymph node does not elongate into a long, tubular structure that is a blood vessel. If color Doppler is available, it may further help in differentiating a vascular structure from a lymph node. When no lymph nodes are seen during EUS or if the lymph nodes visualized during EUS are considered reactive and not malignant, the N-stage is classified as N0.

When lymph nodes visualized during EUS are believed to be malignant, EUS stage N1 is assigned.

## Accuracy of T- and N-Staging

The accuracy of EUS T-staging for colorectal carcinoma varies between 78% and 92% (3–10) although it has been as low as 60% to 69% in some studies (11,12). Both overstaging and understaging may occur. Overstaging seems to be a greater problem than understaging. Overstaging has been attributed to the occurrence of peritumoral tissue reaction (13). N-staging by EUS has been somewhat less accurate, in the range of 73% to 83% (10). This is due to the fact that all visualized lymph nodes are not necessarily malignant. Multiple echo features of the visualized lymph nodes have been studied, including size, sharpness of margins, echogenicity, presence of an echogenic center, round or oval shape, and so on. Lymph nodes that are greater than 1 cm, round, with distinct margins, and hypoechoic have been considered to have a much greater chance of malignant invasion (14). However, there is no universal agreement among endosonographers about the features most predictive of malignant invasion (15). In addition, there is interobserver variability in both T- and N-stage interpretation. This seems to be a greater problem with lymph node evaluation; in a group of rectal cancer patients there was 88% agreement in T-stage but only 78% agreement in N-stage (16). EUS-guided FNA is an important adjunct to accurate lymph node assessment during EUS (15) and it has been applied in patients with rectal cancer (17).

### Importance of T- and N-Staging in Colorectal Cancer

In rectal cancer, preoperative T- and N-staging is important because sphincter-saving trans-anal excision of an early (T1 N0) lesion can be performed instead of the more radical abdominoperineal resection (10,18).

Although there is as yet no defined role for EUS in studying colon polyps, EUS may be useful in predicting malignant transformation in, for example, a rectal villous adenoma prior to surgical excision. If invasion to the muscularis propria is seen with a villous adenoma, overt malignancy is likely to be present, and a trans-anal excision would not be appropriate. However, determination of malignancy within a large adenoma at the level of the anal sphincters may be technically very difficult due to artifacts (19). T- and N-staging by EUS in rectal cancer is important for T-stage-dependent preoperative chemotherapy and radiation protocols.

The role of EUS staging in colon cancers in the rest of the colon is less clear as these patients usually undergo laparotomy and resection if no distant metastases are present. However, EUS may have an important role as a staging modality. For proximal colon cancers minimally invasive laparoscopic and endoscopic mucosal resection (20–23) techniques are more commonly used.

## EUS for Local Recurrence of Colorectal Carcinoma

Local recurrence of colorectal cancer after attempted curative resection occurs in 2.6% to 32% of patients (24). Endosonography may be useful in the diagnosis of suspected local recurrence when no lesions arising from the mucosa are seen during conventional colonoscopy. In such cases EUS may reveal hypoechoic areas (or areas of mixed echogenicity) outside the colorectal wall. Endosonographic alterations due to the primary surgery need to be kept in mind. Fibrosis at the site of surgery appears hyperechoic and the surgical anastomosis is seen as an interruption of the five-layer echo structure (25). If staples were used during surgery, they create a very bright localized echo (26).

After an area of suspected recurrence is identified by EUS, confirmation of recurrent cancer by pathologic examination is required and can be obtained by EUS-guided FNA, percutaneous transperineal FNA, or a CT-guided biopsy. Alternatively, immunoscintigraphy may be used to confirm suspected recurrence and has a sensitivity of 80% to 91% (25). When EUS and CT were compared for imaging an area of recurrence, CT appeared to be slightly superior to EUS (94.5% versus 89%) (27, 28). A multicenter trial with larger numbers

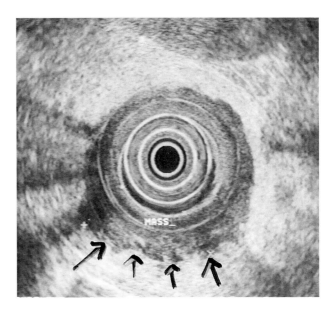

**Figure 12-7.** A T3 rectal carcinoma imaged by radial endosonography after chemotherapy and radiation. The lesion still appears T3 with irregular outer margins (*arrows*) and penetration through the muscularis propria.

of patients comparing all of the different imaging and biopsy modalities is needed.

## Restaging after Chemotherapy and Radiation

Neo-adjuvant chemoradiation is often utilized for "down" staging of a rectal cancer prior to surgical resection. Although EUS is very accurate in T- and N-staging for rectal cancer prior to initiating any treatment, restaging after chemoradiation is problematic. Inflammation and necrosis after chemoradiation appears hypoechoic and indistinguishable from malignant tissue. This results in the obvious problem of overstaging by EUS after radiation and chemotherapy (29,30) (Figure 12-7).

Similarly, lymph nodes visualized prior to treatment may still be present, but commenting on whether they are benign or malignant may not be accurate. In a recent study comparing digital rectal examination, computed tomography, endorectal ultrasound, and magnetic resonance imaging for predicting T1N0 disease after irradiation of rectal cancers, digital exam had the highest negative predictive value, but still detected only 24% of patients to be free of disease. Endoscopic ultrasound failed to detect the absence of disease in 83% of patients (30). Similar problems with overstaging after chemoradiation occurs in esophageal cancer (29). A recent study suggested that the decrease in the maximal thickness of the tumor pre- and post-EUS in esophageal cancer was more predictive of a response to chemoradiation than

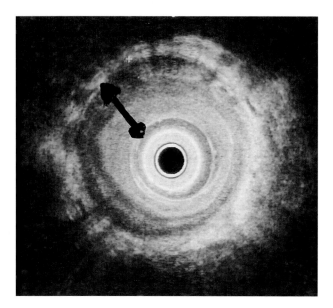

**Figure 12-8.** Rectal linitis plastica image by radial EUS. There is marked thickening of the rectal wall with loss of the five-layer echoarchitecture.

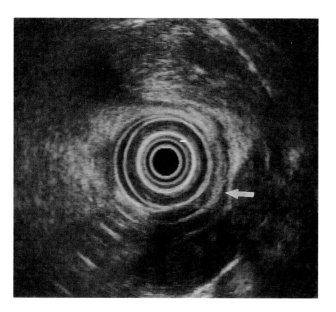

**Figure 12-9.** Endosonographic image of a colonic lipoma (*arrow*). The lesion is echogenic, homogeneous, and contiguous with the muscularis propria.

an effort to try to discern the T-stage post treatment based on the conventional echo layer encroachment approach (31). A similar strategy may be useful in rectal cancer but needs further evaluation.

## Linitis Plastica of the Rectum

Linitis plastica of the rectum (RLP) is a rare phenomenon. It may be a primary rectal carcinoma or metastases from another primary site such as the stomach, breast, or prostate. Endoscopy generally reveals rectal stenosis with induration and thickening of the folds and an endoscopic mucosal biopsy is positive in only a small number of these cases. EUS in RLP classically reveals circumferential thickening of the rectal wall with a mean thickness of 12 mm, with either a thickening of the submucosa/muscularis propria or disruption of the five-layer echo architecture (32–34). Peri-rectal fat infiltration, ascites, or lymph nodes may also be seen. However, EUS cannot differentiate between primary and secondary rectal linitis plastica (Figure 12-8). EUS has been used to monitor treatment response in patients with RLP receiving chemotheapy (32).

## Anal Sphincter Defects

Trans-rectal ultrasound provides a unique method to image the external and internal anal sphincters (35). The internal anal sphincter is seen as a thin hypoe-

choic zone surrounding the anal canal. The external anal sphincter is seen as a heterogeneous echogenic area lateral to the internal anal sphincter. Defects in the continuity of the external and internal anal sphincters can be visualized by trans-rectal sonography. Imaging of these defects is useful in evaluation of patients with fecal incontinence who may have anatomic defects in their anal sphincters (36). In fact, sphincter defects visualized during anal sonography do correlate with physiologic defects by anal needle electromyography (37–39). Patients with anorectal inflammatory conditions such as Crohn's disease, ileoanal pouch with infectious complications, and radiation proctitis have increased thickness of anal wall dimensions when studied by anal sonography (40).

## Submucosal Compression of the Colorectal Wall

It is difficult to predict the cause of an endoscopically visible bulge into the gastrointestinal lumen when the overlying mucosa is normal. Such submucosal compression can be from an intramural lesion arising from the deeper layers of the gastrointestinal wall or from an extramural process. EUS is extremely useful in evaluating lower gastrointestinal submucosal lesions. In the American Endosonography Club Study on the clinical utility of EUS, EUS had the greatest influence on clinical management in patients with submucosal lesions (41). Typically, a lipoma is characterized by a homogeneous, echogenic appearance that is contigu-

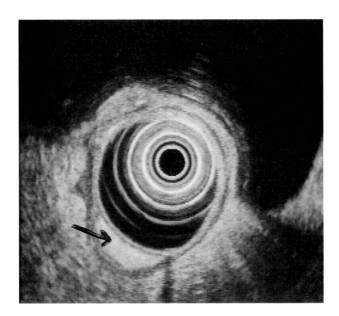

**Figure 12-10.** A rectal myogenic lesion (*M*) appearing as a hypoechoic mass which is contiguous with the muscularis propria (*arrow*), the fourth EUS layer.

ous with the third echo layer (the submucosa) (Figure 12-9). Most lipomas are benign and malignant transformation is a rare phenomenon. Thus, there is controversy about the need for endoscopic removal once a lipoma is diagnosed by EUS (42). However, EUS should be a prerequisite prior to contemplating endoscopic removal of a lipoma. EUS may also help in monitoring such lesions if they are left in situ.

A myogenic tumor appears as a hypoechoic mass that is contiguous with the fourth echo layer (muscularis propria) (Figure 12-10). The differential diagnosis of a myogenic tumor includes a leiomyoma, leiomyosarcoma, or leiomyoblastoma. A myogenic tumor that is greater than 4 cm in diameter, has an irregular margin, with cystic or echogenic foci is more likely to be a malignant lesion (43). However, there is overlap between benign and malignant myogenic lesions, and resection of the entire lesion is optimal to ensure absence of malignancy (44). EUS may be useful if a decision is made to monitor a myogenic lesion that appears benign. Any change in ultrasonographic features such as size, echogenicity, margins, or appearance of new lymphadenopathy warrants surgical resection of the mass.

Myogenic lesions may also arise superficial to the muscularis propria from the muscularis mucosa of the colorectal mucosa. Such lesions, if limited to the mucosa and if small (< 1 cm), may be removed by local excision (42). Enteric endometriosis also appears as a hypoechoic lesion arising from the muscularis propria (the fourth echo layer). However, enteric endometriosis is usually shaped like a spindle or a half-moon while

myogenic tumors are more likely to be lobulated, especially if the lesion is large (44).

Carcinoid tumors of the rectum are not uncommon (45,46). They generally appear as a firm, small, submucosal nodule (47). By endoscopic ultrasound a rectal carcinoid appears as a hypoechoic mass arising from the second echo layer and sometimes compresses the submucosa or expands beyond it. Lesions that are less than 2 cm in size, with no extension beyond the submucosa by EUS may be treated locally by endoscopic or trans-anal surgical excision (48–50). A more aggressive surgical approach is necessary for rectal carcinoids that are larger than 2 cm or reveal invasion into the muscularis propria or regional lymphadenopathy.

Colonic lymphangiomas can also produce submucosal compression. By endosonography they appear as multiple, anechoic (cystic) lesions with echogenic septations located within the third echo layer (the submucosa) (44,51–53). These lesions are generally benign and do not require therapy unless they cause symptoms such as bleeding, intestinal obstruction, or intussusception (53). Colitis cystic profunda has echo features similar to that of colonic lymphangiomas (54,55). There have also been isolated case reports of endosonography in colonic pneumatosis cystoides intestinalis (56) and polypoid prolapsing mucosal folds associated with colonic diverticular disease (57). Recurrence of colorectal carcinoma, malignant lymphoma, and appendical mucocele may also cause submucosal elevation in the colorectum (44). Rectal varices may produce multiple submucosal elevations in the rectum. If there is a question about the diagnosis of rectal varices, EUS can help by showing multiple anechoic tubular and circular structures in the submucosa and just outside the rectal wall—the classical EUS image of varices (58) (Figure 12-11).

## Peri-Anorectal Abscess and Fistula

Endosonography is a useful method to study perianorectal abscesses and fistulae (42,59–60). A fistula during EUS will appear as an anechoic or hypoechoic tract in the anorectal area. Air within the fistula can produce moving reverberation echoes confirming its presence. In contrast, an abscess appears as an irregular anechoic or hypoechoic area around the anorectum. Necrotic debris within the abscess cavity may create scattered echogenic foci. Endoluminal ultrasound was performed with rigid probes in 36 patients with Crohn's disease suspected of harboring an abscess or fistula. Thirty-two patients were found to have a fistula and an abscess associated with the fistula was seen in 29 of 32 (91%) patients. Seventeen of 32 patients (53%) underwent surgery and the EUS presence of an abscess

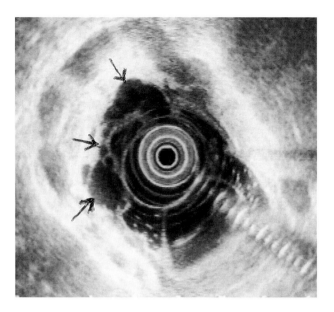

**Figure 12-11.** Endorectal ultrasound image of multiple rectal varices that appear as multiple anechoic structures within the submucosa (*arrows*).

or a fistula was confirmed in all cases (60). Interestingly, endoluminal ultrasound and digital examination have been found to be comparable in identifying inter-sphincteric and trans-sphincteric fistulous tracts (61). However, a digital examination will not delineate the course of a fistula and is unable to reveal the communication of the fistula with an abscess or an adjacent organ. A comparison has also been made between pelvic CT scan and endoluminal ultrasound for detection of fistulae and abscesses. Although endoluminal ultrasound and CT had an equal detection rate for abscesses, ultrasound detected the fistulae in 82% versus 24% by CT scan using operative findings as the gold standard (62).

The advantages of endoluminal ultrasound in rectal and perirectal disease are its efficacy, safety, simplicity, low cost, and lack of radiation (59). Future applications of endoluminal ultrasound certainly include ultrasound-guided trans-rectal drainage of perirectal abscesses.

## Endoscopic Ultrasound in Inflammatory Bowel Disease

Differentiation of ulcerative colitis and Crohn's disease is a clinical challenge and coventional transabdominal ultrasound has been of some help. The gut wall in ulcerative colitis is thickened and has decreased echogenicity, but the five-layer echo structure is maintained.

Ultrasonogram in Crohn's colitis, on the other hand, reveals a thickened and echo-poor gut wall, with loss of the five-layer stratification and differentiation (63). In-vitro data by Kimmey revealed that ultrasound was able to differentiate a normal (thickness < 3mm) colonic wall from an inflamed colon due to colitis which was thicker than 3 mm. However, differentiation between ulcerative colitis and Crohn's colitis was unreliable (64).

Experience in endosonography for inflammatory bowel disease is limited, but Shimizu et al. (65) have performed endosonography in patients with ulcerative colitis and Crohn's colitis. They have found progressive thickening of the mucosa and the submucosa and loss of distensibility of the colonic wall with increasing severity of ulcerative colitis. Five patterns of endosonographic findings in ulcerative colitis based on wall thickening and distensibility have been described (65, 66) but their clinical value is untested. The same group has found that intestinal thickening in Crohn's colitis is patchy and trans-mural, involving all layers (66).

In cases of indeterminate colitis, Hildebrandt et al. (67) have used EUS to determine whether the inflammation is mucosal or trans-mural, hypothesizing that patients with trans-mural disease are more likely to have Crohn's disease. They have then excluded the patients with trans-mural inflammation from surgical procedures requiring an ileal reservoir because there is a risk of recurrence of disease in the ileal pouch in patients with features of Crohn's disease in the spectrum of inflammatory bowel disease. Using this strategy, this group has found improved outcome in patients undergoing surgery for indeterminant colitis. However, EUS applications for inflammatory bowel disease are still limited due to lack of data.

## Interventional Endosonography in Colorectal Lesions

Trans-rectocolonic fine-needle aspiration may be performed by linear (rigid or flexible) endoluminal ultrasound probes with a biopsy channel. These probes allow visualization of a needle along its long axis. This technique has been utilized in sampling peri-rectal lymph nodes for detection of malignant invasion (17). Endosonographically guided FNA may also be useful in diagnosing colon cancer recurrence when no mucosal lesion is seen and a mass is seen deeper to the mucosa (25). Lesions causing submucosal compression may be punctured under EUS guidance to obtain tissue for diagnosis (Figure 12-12). Extrinsic lesions such as a teratoma, ovarian carcinoma, or abscess in close proximity to the rectum can also be punctured under EUS guidance to obtain a diagnostic aspirate (69).

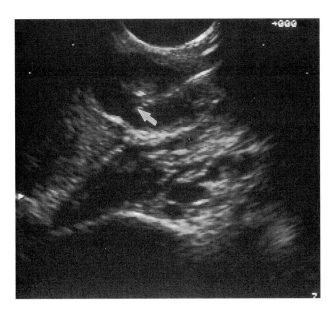

**Figure 12-12**. Hypoechoic, submucosal rectal mass undergoing trans-rectal EUS-guided fine-needle aspiration with a linear array echoendoscope (arrow = needle tip).

## Conclusion

In conclusion, endosonography is an extremely useful modality for management of ano-rectal lesions. Its role in defining and managing colonic disorders continues to rapidly evolve, but it is likely that EUS will play a significant role in colonic disorders, and minimally invasive surgical and endoscopic techniques will become the standard of care for many malignant and benign colorectal disorders.

### References

1. Wiersema MJ, Hawes RH. Normal colorectal anatomy and benign colon lesions. Gastrointest Endosc Clin N Am 1992;2:715–727.
2. Hulsmans FJH, Castelijns JA, Reeders JWAJ, Tytgat GNJ. Review of artifacts associated with transrectal ultrasound: understanding, recognition, and prevention of misinterpretation. J Clin Ultrasound 1995;23:483–494.
3. Bhutani MS, Nadella P. Utility of a side-viewing upper echoendoscope for endoscopic ultrasonography of malignant and benign conditions of the sigmoid colon and the rectum. Gastrointest Endosc 1998;47: AB95.
4. Konishi F, Ugajin, Ito K, et al. Endorectal ultrasonography with a 7.5 MHz linear array scanner for the assessment of invasion of rectal carcinoma. Int J Colorect Dis 1990;5:15–20.
5. Glaser F, Schlag P, Herfarth CH. Endorectal ultrasonography for the assessment of invasion of rectal tumors and lymph node involvement. Br J Surg 1990;77:883–887.
6. Hildebrandt U, Feifel G, Dhour G. The evaluation of the rectum by transrectal ultrasonography. Ultrasound Quart 1988;6:167–179.
7. Beynon J, Mortensen McC, Rigby HS. Rectal endosonography, a new technique for the preoperative staging of rectal carcinoma. Europ J Surg Oncol 1988;14:297–309.
8. Boyce GA, Sivak MV Jr., Lavery IC, et al. Endoscopic ultrasound in the pre-operative staging of rectal carcinoma. Gastrointest Endosc 1992;38:468–471.
9. Herzog U, Flue MV, Tondelli P, Schuppisser JP. How accurate is endorectal ultrasound in the preoperative staging of rectal cancer? Dis Colon Rectum 1993;36:127–134.
10. Hildebrandt U, Feifel G. Importance of endoscopic ultrasonography staging for treatment of rectal cancer. Gastrointest Endosc Clin N Am 1995;5:843–849.
11. Rifkin MD, Ehrlich SM, Marks G. Staging of rectal carcinomas: prospective comparison of endorectal US and CT. Radiology 1989;170:319–322.
12. Hulsmans FJ, Tio TL, Fockens P, et al. Assessment of tumor infiltration depth in rectal cancer with transrectal sonography: caution is necessary. Radiology 1994;190:715–720.
13. Maier AG, Barton PP, Neuhold NR, et al. Peritumoral tissue reaction at transrectal US as a possible cause of over staging in rectal cancer: histopathologic correlation. Radiology 1997;203:785–789.
14. Catalano MS, Sivak MV Jr, Rice T, et al. Endosonographic features predictive of lymph node metastases. Gastrointest Endosc 1994;40:442–446.
15. Bhutani MS, Hawes RH, Hoffman BJ. A comparison of the accuracy of echo features during endoscopic ultrasound (EUS) and EUS-guided fine-needle aspiration for diagnosis of malignant lymph node invasion. Gastrointest Endosc 1997;45:474–479.
16. Roubein LD, Lynch P, Glober G, Sinicrope FA. Interobserver variability in endoscopic ultrasonography; a prospective evaluation. Gastrointest Endosc 1996;44:573–577.
17. Milsom JW, Czyrko C, Hull TL, et al. Preoperative biopsy of pararectal lymph nodes in rectal cancer using endoluminal ultrasonography. Dis Colon Rectum 1994;37:364–368.
18. Winde G, Nottberg H, Keller R, et al. Surgical cure for early rectal carcinomas ($T_1$). Trans-anal endoscopic microsurgery vs. anterior resection. Dis Colon Rectum 1996;39:969–976.
19. Adams WJ, Wong WD. Endorectal ultrasonic detection of malignancy within rectal villous lesions. Dis Colon Rectum 1995;38:1093–1096.
20. Holzman MD, Eubanks S. Laparoscopic colectomy, prospects and problems. Gastrointest Endosc Clin N Am 1997;7:525–539.
21. Saitoh Y, Obara T, Einami K, et al. Efficacy of high-frequency ultrasound probes for the preoperative staging of invasion depth in flat and depressed colorectal tumors. Gastrointest Endosc 1996;44:34–39.
22. Yoshida M, Tsukamoto Y, Niwa Y, et al. Endoscopic assessment of invasion of colorectal tumors with a

new high-frequency ultrasound probe. Gastrointest Endosc 1994;41:587–592.

23. Matsunaga A, Mochizuki F, Fujita N, et al. Diagnosis of early colorectal cancer by endoscopic ultrasonography. Gastroenterol Endosc 1996;38:279–287.

24. Abulafi AM, Williams NS. Local recurrence of colorectal cancer: the problem, mechanisms, management and adjuvant therapy. Br J Surg 1994;81:7–19.

25. Romano G, Belli G, Rotondano G. Colorectal cancer: diagnosis of recurrence. Gastrointest Endosc Clin N Am 1995;5:831–841.

26. Charnley RM, Heywood MF, Hardcastle JD. Rectal endosonography for the visualization of the anastomosis after anterior resection and its relevance to local recurrence. Int J Colorect Dis 1990;5:127–129.

27. Romano G, Esercizio L, Santangelo M, et al. Trattamento chirurgico delle recidine dopo resezione per cancro del retto. Indicazioni e risultati, chirurgia 1991;4:446–450.

28. Ramano G, Esercizio L, Santangelo M, et al. Impact of computed tomography vs intrarectal ultrasound on the diagnosis, resectability and prognosis of locally recurrent rectal cancer. Dis Colon Rectum 1993;36: 261–265.

29. Hordijk ML. Restaging after radiotherapy and chemotherapy: value of endoscopic ultrasonography. Gastrointest Endosc Clin N Am 1995;5:601–608.

30. Kahn H, Alexander A, Rakinic J, et al. Preoperative staging of irradiated rectal cancers using digital rectal examination, computed tomography, endorectal ultrasound, and magnetic resonance imaging does not accurately predict to no pathology. Dis Colon Rectum 1997;40:140–144.

31. Achkar JP, Kassis ES, Luketich JD, et al. Endoscopic ultrasound determined maximal tumor thickness is an objective measure of tumor response to chemotherapy in esophageal cancer. Gastrointest Endosc 1997; 45:AB62.

32. Dumontier I, Roseau G, Palazzo L, et al. Endoscopic ultrasonography in rectal linitus plastica. Gastrointest Endosc 1997;46:532–536.

33. Wiersema MJ, Wiersema LM, Kochman ML. Primary linitis plastica of the colon. Gastrointest Endosc 1993;39:716–718.

34. Papp JP Jr, Levine EJ, Thomas FB. Primary linitis plastica carcinoma of the colon and rectum. Am J Gastroenterol 1995;90:141–145.

35. Law PJ, Bartram CI. Anal endosonography: technique and normal anatomy. Gastrointest Radiol 1989;14: 349–353.

36. Keating IP, Stewart PJ, Eyers AA, et al. Are special investigations of value in the management of patients with fecal incontinence? Dis Colon Rectum 1997;40: 896–901.

37. Law PJ, Kamm MA, Bartram CI. A comparison between electromyography and anal endosonography in mapping external anal sphincter defects. Dis Colon Rectum 1990;33:370–373.

38. Tjandra JJ, Milsom JW, Schroeder T, Fazio VW. Endoluminal ultrasound is preferable to electromyography

in mapping anal sphincteric defects. Dis Colon Rectum 1993;36:689–692.

39. Enck P, von Giesen HJ, Schäfer A, et al. Comparison of anal sonography with conventional needle electromyography in the evaluation of anal sphincter defects. Am J Gastroenterol 1996;91:2539–2543.

40. Solomon MJ, McLeod RS, Cohen EK, Cohen Z. Anal wall thickness under normal and inflammatory conditions of the anorectum as determined by endoluminal ultrasonography. Am J Gastroenterol 1995;90:574–578.

41. Nickl NJ, Bhutani MS, Catalano M, et al. Clinical implications of endoscopic ultrasound: the American Endosonography Club Study. Gastrointest Endosc 1996;44:371–377.

42. Wiersema MJ, Hawes RH. Normal colorectal anatomy and benign colorectal lesions. Gastrointest Endosc Clin N Am. 1992;2:715–727.

43. Chak A, Canto MI, Rösch T, et al. Endosonographic differentiation of benign and malignant stromal cell tumors. Gastrointest Endosc 1997;45:468–473.

44. Kameyama H, Niwa Y, Arisawa T, Goto H, Hayakawa T. Endoscopic ultrasonography in the diagnosis of submucosal lesions of the large intestine. Gastrointest Endosc 1997;46:406–411.

45. Nauheim KS, Zeitels J, Kaplan EL, et al. Rectal carcinoid tumors—treatment and prognosis. Surgery 1983; 94:670–676.

46. Orloff MJ. Carcinoid tumors of the rectum. Cancer 1971;28:175–180.

47. Bhutani MS. Curative endoscopic resection of a carcinoid tumor of the rectum (letter). Am J Gastroenterol 1994;89:645.

48. Matsumoto T, Iida M, Suekane H, et al. Endoscopic ultrasonography in rectal carcinoid tumors: contribution to selection of therapy. Gastrointest Endosc 1991;37:539–542.

49. Yoshikane H, Tsukamoto Y, Niwa Y, et al. Carcinoid tumors of the gastrointestinal tract: evaluation with endoscopic ultrasonography. Gastrointest Endosc 1993;39:375–383.

50. Hokama A, Oshiro J, Kinjof, Saito A. Utility of endoscopic ultrasonography in rectal carcinoid tumors (letter). Am J Gastroenterol 1996;91:1289–1290.

51. Hizawa K, Aoyagi K, Kurahara K, et al. Gastrointestinal lymph angioma: endosonographic demonstration and endoscopic removal. Gastrointest Endosc 1996; 43:620–624.

52. Fujimura Y, Nishishita C, Lida M, Kajihara Y. Lymphangioma of the colon diagnosed with an endoscopic ultrasound probe and dynamic CT. Gastrointest Endosc 1995;41:252–254.

53. Kochman ML, Wiersema MJ, Hawes RH, et al. Preoperative diagnosis of cystic lymphangioma of the colon by endoscopic ultrasound. Gastrointest Endosc 1997; 45:204–206.

54. Hulsmans FJH, Tio TL, Reeders JWAJ, Tytgat GNJ. Transrectal US in the diagnosis of localized colitis cystica profunda. Radiology 1991;181:201–203.

55. Petritsch W, Hinterleitner TA, Aichbichler B, et al. Endosonography in colitis cystica profunda and soli-

tary rectal ulcer syndrome. Gastrointest Endosc 1996; 44:746–751.

56. Bansal R, Bude R, Nostrant TT, Scheiman JM. Diagnosis of colonic pneumatosis cystoides intestinalis by endosonography. Gastrointest Endosc 1995;43:90–93.

57. Yoshida M, Kawabata K, Kutsumi H, et al. Polypoid prolapsing mucosal folds associated with diverticular disease in the sigmoid colon: usefulness of colonoscopy and endoscopic ultrasonography for the diagnosis. Gastrointest Endosc 1996;44:489–491.

58. Dhiman RK, Choudhri G, Saraswat VA, et al. Endoscopic ultrasonographic evaluation of the rectum in cirrhotic portal hypertension. Gastrointest Endosc 1993;39:635–640.

59. Bhutani MS, Hawes RH. Endoluminal ultrasound. In: Allan RN, Rhodes JM, Hanauer SB, et al., eds. Inflammatory bowel diseases. Edinburgh: Churchill-Livingstone, 1997.

60. Tio TL, Mulder CJJ, Wijers OB, et al. Endosonography of peri-anal and peri-colorectal fistula and/or abscess in Crohn's disease. Gastrointest Endosc 1990;36:331–336.

61. Choen S, Burnett S, Bartram CI, Nicholls RJ. Comparison between anal endosonography and digital examination in the evaluation of anal fistulae. Br J Surgery 1991;78:445–447.

62. Schratter-Sehn AU, Locks H, Vogelsang H, et al. Endoscopic ultrasonography versus computed tomography in the differential diagnosis of perianorectal complications in Crohn's disease. Endoscopy 1993;25:582–586.

63. Limberg B. Diagnosis of acute ulcerative colitis and colonic Crohn's disease by colonic sonography. J Clin Ultrasound 1989;17:25–31.

64. Kimmey MB, Wang KY, Haggit RC, et al. Diagnosis of inflammatory bowel disease with ultrasound. Invest Radiol 1990;25:1085–1090.

65. Shimizu S, Tada M, Kawai K. Value of endoscopic ultrasonography in the assessment of inflammatory bowel diseases. Endoscopy 1992;24 (suppl): 354–358.

66. Shimizu S, Tada M, Kawai K. Endoscopic ultrasonography in inflammatory bowel diseases. Gastrointest Endosc Clin N Am 1995;5:851–859.

67. Hildebrandt U, Kraus J, Ecker KW, et al. Endosonographic differentiation of mucosal and transmural nonspecific inflammatory bowel disease. Endoscopy 1992;24 (suppl 1): 359–363.

68. Hoffman BJ, Bhutani MS, Aabakken L, et al. Endoscopic ultrasound guided fine needle aspiration in the evaluation of extra-rectal pelvic masses. Gastrointest Endosc 1996;43:423.

# 13

# Endoscopic Ultrasound-Guided Fine-Needle Aspiration Biopsy

## Ian D. Norton
## Maurits J. Wiersema

*There is no structure in the human body that can't be reached with a strong arm and a 14-gauge needle*
Samuel Shem

The evolution of endoscopic ultrasound witnessed by gastroenterologists and surgeons has very much mirrored the history of transabdominal ultrasound. Transabdominal ultrasound initially was pioneered as a method for obtaining detailed imaging without the use of ionizing radiation. The test soon matured into one that was also used for more invasive diagnostic and therapeutic interventions. There has been a parallel trend with endoscopic ultrasound. With the introduction of linear scanning instruments, it is now possible to place devices into the ultrasound plane of view and permit various diagnostic and therapeutic maneuvers to be performed. The addition of biopsy capability has firmly rooted EUS in the gastroenterologists' armamentarium for diagnostic testing. Although computed tomography and magnetic resonance imaging permit detailed anatomic information to be obtained, EUS still appears to have a unique advantage by allowing placement of a biopsy needle into lesions that are often too small to be identified by these complementary imaging techniques or too well encased by surrounding vascular structures to allow percutaneous biopsy methods to be used safely. For these reasons EUS will certainly continue to be employed for procurement of a tissue diagnosis in a minimally invasive fashion.

The added complexity and the increased risk of performing EUS-guided fine-needle aspiration biopsy necessitates additional training for individuals planning to perform this procedure. Specialized equipment is also needed for EUS FNA. Both factors have played a role in limiting the availability of this technique, except in the setting of larger community or academic-based referral centers. However, as we have seen with transabdominal ultrasound, greater clinical experience, improvements in technology, and lower equipment costs will undoubtedly expand the availability of

EUS-guided FNA for clinical decision making in everyday practice. Procedures that safely provide more accurate diagnostic information and enhance our efficiency in patient care will ultimately decrease costs. EUS FNA appears well suited to this task.

To date, the main application of this technology has been fine-needle aspiration biopsy of mucosal and submucosal lesions and peri-intestinal structures including lymph nodes, as well as masses arising in the pancreas, liver, adrenal gland, and bile duct. The technique has also been used to aspirate peritoneal and pleural fluid. Recently, the equipment has also been employed for endoscopic drainage of pancreatic pseudocysts (1,2), celiac ganglion neurolysis (3), and even retrograde cholangiopancreatography (4). Other innovative methods, such as the successful delivery of antitumor agents to malignant masses via fine-needle injection, suggest that EUS FNA will continue its rapid evolution.

The review that follows attempts to cover the large body of English-language literature that has been published concerning EUS FNA. Most of the literature published to date has been based on large, single-center studies with their inherent limitations. However, based on these results, and as EUS FNA has matured, it is now possible to initiate more critical analysis of how this technology may influence patient care now and in the future. This chapter will outline the equipment and techniques used for EUS FNA and review the indications, efficacy, and safety of the procedure.

## Equipment

The optimal instrument for performing EUS FNA is the electronic curved linear array echoendoscope, which

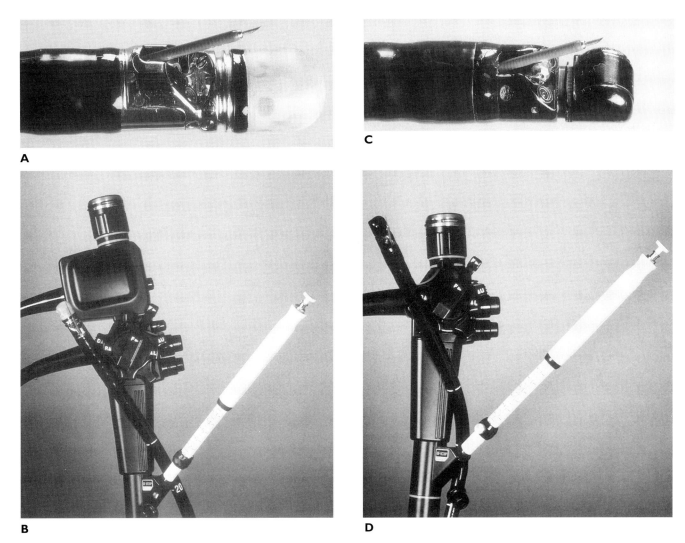

**Figure 13-1.** Several echoendoscopes are available for performing EUS-guided fine-needle aspiration biopsy. The mechanical linear scanning probe ((A) and (B), GF-UM30P, Olympus Corporation, Melville, NY) is shown with the needle aspiration catheter protruding from the biopsy port (Wilson-Cook, Winston-Salem, NC). The balloon has not been placed over the probe tip, allowing a more detailed view. An electronic curved linear array echoprobe is shown ((C) and (D), GF-UC30P, Olympus Corporation, Melville, NY) with the needle aspiration catheter protruding through its biopsy port.

permits real-time visualization of the needle as it is advanced into the periluminal space. Although EUS FNA has been described using the radial scanning probe, the needle cannot be tracked throughout its entire course with this instrument and serious complications have been described (5). For this reason, the radial scanning guided technique should probably be abandoned. A mechanical linear scanning probe (GF-UM30P, Olympus Corporation, Melville, NY) has been introduced, which has the advantage that it can be used with the same processor as the radial scanning probes (Figures 13-1.A, 13-1.B, 13-1.C, 13-1.D). The probe is a fiberoptic instrument and uses a rotating mirror system to allow scanning oriented in the long axis of the endoscope and thereby provide a linear view. A needle

catheter may be passed through the imaging plane permitting biopsy of lesions within or adjacent to the gastrointestinal tract. Sufficient experience has not yet been obtained with this product to assess its durability or applicability to a variety of lesions.

Currently there are two manufacturers marketing electronic curved linear echoendoscopes in the United States (GF-UC30P, Olympus Corporation; FG-36UA, FG-32UX, Pentax Precision Instruments, Inc., Orangeburg, NY). Both of these instruments have biopsy channels with an elevator, which provides some additional control when attempting to direct the needle into a lesion. Additionally, the biopsy channel is of a sufficient size to permit passage of 6 or 7 French-size stents. A comparison of the features of all of these different types

**Table 13-1.** Linear scanning echoendoscopes currently available in the United States.

|  | GF-UM30P | GF-UC30P | FG-36UX |
|---|---|---|---|
| US scanning orientation | Linear/Mechanical | Linear/Electronic | Linear/Electronic |
| Endoscopic image | Fiberoptic oblique forward | Fiberoptic oblique forward | Fiberoptic or video oblique forward |
| Biopsy channel size | 2.8 mm | 2.8 mm | 2.4 mm |
| Elevator | Yes | Yes | Yes |
| Doppler/Color Doppler | No | Yes | Yes |
| Color Angio® | No | No | Yes |

of equipment is provided in Table 13-1. One technical point deserves particular emphasis: the importance of Doppler capability with the electronic instruments, which is not available with the mechanical types of probes. Although evidence has not been provided that proves that Doppler improves the safety of performing EUS FNA, common sense suggests that this feature should aid efficiency and also permit avoidance of structures or lesions that may be vascular in nature. The processor employed with the GF=UM30P (AI Envision Plus, Dornier Surgical Products, Phoenix, AZ) does not have power Doppler capability, but the gray-scale resolution in the near field is exceptional. In contrast, the Pentax probe (FG-32UA or FG-36 UX, Pentax Precision Instruments, Inc., Orangeburg, NY) when used in conjunction with the Hitachi 525 processor (Hitachi, Tokyo, Japan), provides a full spectrum of Doppler capabilities including Color Angio® (Diasonics, United States) with adequate gray-scale resolution and depth of penetration. To date, a direct comparison between these two instruments has not been performed.

An initial stumbling point for performing EUS FNA was the development of a needle that could be reliably employed without damaging the instrument. In essence, this has been accomplished by developing a needle system that is ensheathed by a wire spiral with or without a catheter (Wilson-Cook, Winston Salem, NC; GIP Mediglobe, Tempe, AZ; Olympus Corporation, Melville, NY). All types of needles use a handle mechanism, which secures to the luer lock adaptor on the ultrasound endoscope. Due to the slightly different configuration of the biopsy channels and their respective lengths among different brands of echoprobes, short spacers may need to be used when employing the Wilson-Cook needle with the Pentax product. Needle sizes available range from 19 to 22 gauge with a depth of penetration of up to 10 cm. All needles are available with a central stylet beveled to match the needle tip, thereby enhancing the sharpness of the device. A Tru-Cut biopsy needle device has not been made commercially available although one manufacturer (GIP Mediglobe) has developed a prototype with a 15-gauge

needle providing a 10-mm length core of tissue (6). Preliminary testing in animals suggests that the device functions as expected and can be used with echoendoscopes incorporating a larger caliber biopsy channel.

## Technique

Performance of EUS FNA necessitates a team approach to patient care, with nurses specifically trained in the procedure and on-site cytotechnology support. Although gastroenterologists routinely perform procedures involving needle-type devices for other indications (for example, injection-assisted polypectomy or sclerotherapy), the devices employed for EUS FNA are substantially different and therefore some degree of specialized training is needed for endoscopy assistants. Gastrointestinal assistants should become thoroughly familiar with the EUS FNA system by reviewing its functioning outside of the patient as well as by passing the needle device through the echoendoscope with the tip of the instrument sitting in a beaker of water. The latter exercise is helpful for allowing the nursing staff to visualize the movement of the needle relative to the handle mechanism.

Identification of the biopsy site is the first step in performing the procedure. A consistent strategy should be employed in this regard. Specifically, if a malignancy is being staged, the site that would provide the most advanced stage of the disease should be selected (e.g. celiac nodes and not mediastinal lymph nodes in a patient with primary esophageal carcinoma). Once this has been determined, the needle catheter device with the stylet in place can be advanced through the biopsy channel. The handle mechanism is secured to the luer lock. To facilitate passage of the needle catheter through the very distal aspect of the instrument, the elevator should be fully released or in the down position. The optimal degree of balloon inflation that should be present when performing the procedure remains unclear. Due to the nature of the linear probe, the balloon is typically left inflated, with the vertical control of the elevator in the "up" position to displace the balloon behind

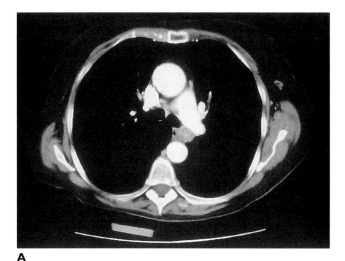

A

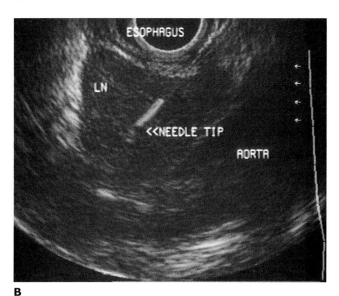

B

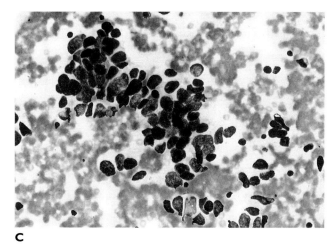

C

**Figure 13-2.** A 68-year-old female with a history of heavy tobacco use presented with three months of lethargy and progressive weight loss. Physical examination was unremarkable. Upon evaluation, a chest CT scan was performed to look for an occult malignancy despite an unremarkable chest x-ray. As shown (A), left posterior periesophageal mediastinal lymphadenopathy was identified. Endoscopic ultrasound with FNA was requested. The needle tip can be seen entering the lymph node (*LN*) with the aorta adjacent to the biopsied lymph node (B). Cytology demonstrated metastatic small cell carcinoma (C), Diff-Quik stain, American Scientific Products, McGraw Park, IL, original magnification 150×).

the transducer. Unfortunately, if some of the balloon is interposed between the transducer and the intestinal wall, the needle will puncture the balloon. Nevertheless, leaving the balloon inflated optimizes acoustic contact. Advancement and locking of the catheter assembly will push the luminal mucosa away from the transducer and therefore reduce the US view. This can be overcome by periodically applying suction to the biopsy port, which will remove a small air pocket.

When performing linear EUS the image is oriented so that the cranial aspect is toward the right and the caudal aspect is toward the left of the image. This implies that the needle will enter from the right side of the image and traverse toward the bottom left-hand corner of the field of view (Figures 13-2.A, 13-2.B, 13-2.C). However, a variety of different orientations are often used by both European and US-based ultrasonographers.

Occasionally, maintaining the position of the ultrasound probe adjacent to the site where the biopsy will

be performed can be rather difficult. This problem is particularly apparent when attempting to biopsy a mass in the head of the pancreas with the probe in the second portion of the duodenum. Usually, position will be lost when the scope has been reduced to the "short" position because the probe will tend to rotate anteriorly during the manuever. To return the instrument to the correct orientation it must be rotated counterclockwise, often resulting in the probe falling back into the stomach. This problem is analogous to reducing the duodenoscope into a short scope position for cannulation during endoscopic retrograde cholangiopancreatography. For these reasons, when performing EUS FNA of a pancreatic head mass a "long" scope position may be unavoidable. In some cases inflating the balloon to a moderate degree helps to stabilize the tip of the scope and allow consistent imaging.

Once the target lesion has been identified with EUS, the needle is gradually advanced until it can be seen within the ultrasound plane of view. With the Olympus needle a separate adjustment is made for the protective sheath length prior to advancing the needle. Traversal of the muscularis propria can sometimes be difficult, and occasionally a swift jabbing motion is necessary. Similarly, advancement into pancreatic neoplasms may require some force and necessitate rapid needle advancement. When the needle has entered the

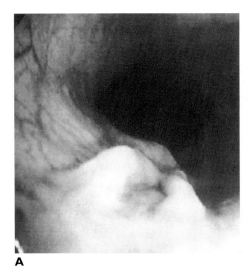

A

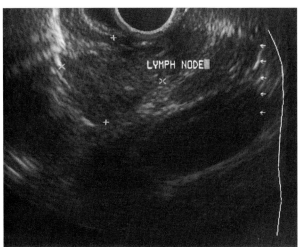

B

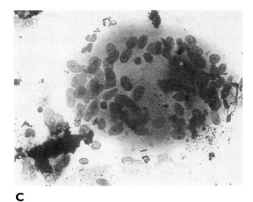

C

**Figure 13-3.** A 47-year-old female with a remotely positive PPD presented with several months of odynophagia. Endoscopy demonstrated an ulcerated area in the proximal esophagus, which on biopsy demonstrated acute and chronic inflammation (A). EUS revealed an inhomogenous peri-esophageal lymph node with a fistula tract to the esophagus (B). EUS FNA was done with cytology demonstrating multinucleated giant cells with non-caseating granulomatous inflammation (C), Diff Quik stain original magnification 150×. Lymph node cultures and serum fungal titers were negative. Antituberculosis therapy was recommended.

lesion of interest, the stylet is removed and negative pressure is applied with a 10-ml syringe. Application of negative pressure can be simplified by using a short extension tubing or a syringe lock (available with the Wilson-Cook product). The degree of negative pressure may be of importance. In vascular tumors (for example, neuroendocrine) or in lymph nodes, limited or no negative pressure results in a less bloody aspirate and a specimen that is more easily examined by the pathologist. With an on-site cytotechnologist present, adjustments in negative pressure to obtain an optimal specimen can be made during the examination. Typically, five to ten gradual to and fro movements of the needle are made within the lesion. The needle should not be fully withdrawn outside of the lesion into the intestinal lumen to avoid contamination of the specimen by luminal contents and epithelium. Prior to removing the needle, the negative pressure is released by releasing the plunger on the syringe. For the Wilson-Cook needle the needle lock is manually secured so that the needle cannot be inadvertently advanced. With the GIP and Olympus device this is done automatically. The needle handle is then unscrewed from the endoscope and the entire assembly brought over to a work surface for slide preparation. With solid lesions the aspirate is sprayed onto labeled glass slides. One slide is air dried for on-site interpretation and the other slide is ethanol or spray fixed. In cases where lymphoma is in the differential, additional material is collected in a preservative solution that permits flow cytometric analysis. Additionally, in patients in whom an infectious etiology is suspected culture media can also be employed (Figures 13-3.A, 13-3.B, 13-3.C). After the material has been sprayed out onto the glass slides, a saline wash is performed through the needle, and this material is also collected to be made into a cell block. The stylet is then wiped off to remove any remaining blood. The needle is purged of any remaining fluid, using air, and the entire needle device is reassembled for further use.

Several technical points merit further comment. When aspirating cystic lesions, only a single pass should be performed and the lesion should be drained completely, if possible. As will be discussed later, cyst aspiration may result in infectious complications and routine antibiotic prophylaxis administered prior to the procedure and continuing for 48 hours afterwards is a wise precaution. Cystic lesions of the pancreas can contain very viscous fluid and it may take some time to completely drain the material.

EUS has several advantages over standard radiographic-guided techniques for sampling lymph nodes. Unlike computed tomography, in which lymph nodes typically have a fairly uniform x-ray density, ultrasound can document subtle tissue differences identified within a lymph node. Therefore, the EUS operator can target those areas that have echo characteristics

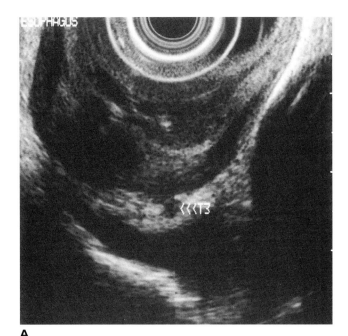

**A**

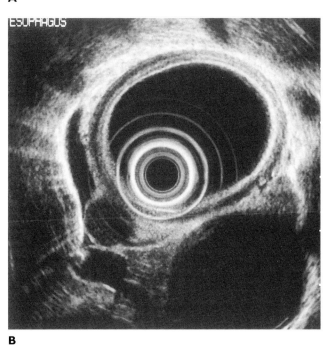

**B**

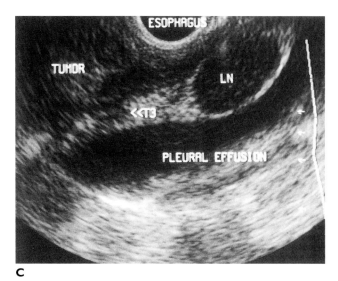

**C**

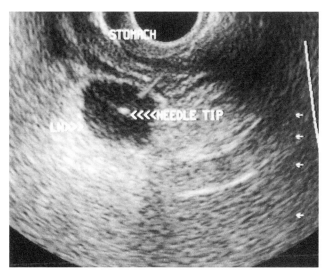

**D**

**Figure 13-4.** A 47-year-old male with progressive dysphagia was found to have an exophytic mass lesion in his distal esophagus, which on biopsy confirmed an adenocarcinoma. EUS with the radial scanning probe (A), (B) demonstrates transmural invasion (*T3*), regional lymphadenopathy and a right pleural effusion. The electronic linear scanning probe also demonstrated a T3N1 tumor (C) (LN-lymph node), (D). Perigastric lymphadenopathy underwent EUS FNA and demonstrated metastatic adenocarcinoma. Note that the needle traverses normal gastric wall uninvolved with tumor.

similarly to that seen in the primary tumor (Figures 13-4.A, 13-4.B, 13-4.C, 13-4.D). If on-site cytological study identifies only necrosis, the operator should be suspicious that the node contains malignancy. To obtain diagnostic tissue, sampling should occur from the periphery of the lesion or areas that do not have the same echo texture as the region from which the necrotic tissue was first aspirated. Some have suggested that the use of Tru-Cut needles would resolve these difficulties. Though this may be true for certain tumor types such as lymphomas, cytological aspirates can sample a very large area by moving the needle within the lesion. Also, the small-gauge needles used for FNA are safer than the larger Tru-Cut needle.

The number of needle passes needed for an adequate specimen is lesion dependent. For lymph nodes five passes or less is typically enough, but for pancreatic masses, obtaining adequate tissue may require ten or more passes with the biopsy needle (7). Part of this difficulty in obtaining adequate tissue rests on the degree of differentiation of the tumor. In well-differentiated pancreatic malignancies the pathologist may have a more difficult time confirming malignancy. Additionally, some pancreatic neoplasms have a significant degree of fibrosis, and therefore do not provide very cellular samples when biopsied with EUS FNA. When planning a therapeutic procedure such as celiac plexus neurolysis, it is usually appropriate to obtain a final diagnosis on site in order to avoid performing procedures on patients with benign disease. In this setting, obtaining the proper diagnosis with rapid cytologic analysis may require a larger number of passes.

When EUS FNA is performed on solid lesions, an echo-poor zone sometimes forms adjacent to the biopsied mass leading to physical separation of the mass and the intestinal wall. This is due to hemorrhage and can be treated by applying pressure with the endoscope tip. The bleeding site is monitored for five to ten minutes to make sure that the hemorrhage is self-limited Minor intraluminal bleeding may occur after EUS FNA. To date, no clinically significant intraluminal hemorrhage has been described with the technique.

The optimal route for biopsying lesions should be carefully considered. Specifically, pancreatic lesions that can be visualized from both the stomach and duodenum are usually more easily biopsied from within the stomach due to less scope flexion and a more stable position. When vascular structures interfere with the ability to reach a particular lesion, a different site should be considered. The consequences of traversing vascular structures to permit a biopsy (that is, placing the needle through a vessel in order to biopsy a mass lesion behind the vessel) has not been explored. Occasionally, the needle may inadvertently puncture an adjacent vascular structure. Fortunately, the small-gauge needles that are usually used for EUS FNA have not produced any clinically recognized complications from accidental puncture of vascular structures.

With the recent introduction of instruments possessing an elevator on the biopsy channel, occasional problems have been reported with loss of the elevator function due to stretching or breaking of the cable. This is due to use of excessive force. Additionally, once the needle has entered into the lesion, it may be best to release the elevator slightly because the needle entry into the lesion should stabilize the scope position. This technique minimizes pressure on the elevator as the needle is moved in and out of the target.

A technical concern that has been raised centers on biopsying periluminal lymph nodes through an area of the gastrointestinal tract that is involved by a neoplastic process. Although these needles have a stylet, we have identified contamination of the asperate with normal gastrointestinal mucosal cells. In fact, on occasion we can identify benign squamous cells in aspirates obtained from the liver or periesophageal lymph nodes (7). Recognizing this, the reliability of biopsying through tumor to stage lymph nodes is of questionable merit.

The expanding role of EUS FNA in patients with mediastinal lymphadenopathy merits comment in regards to technical aspects of performing this procedure. Occasionally, when sampling lesions that invade the bronchus or trachea, the patient may start coughing due to the traversal of the needle through the airway. This can be easily overcome by redirecting the needle.

Direct endoscopic visualization of the needle device is rarely of benefit during EUS FNA. Ultrasound visualization is almost always sufficient to guide the needle and perform the biopsy. Occasionally, a patient may present with a small, subepithelial mass lesion that may be difficult to identify initially with ultrasound visualization alone. In this setting, the echo-probe can be placed directly over the lesion with direct endoscopic visualization and the biopsy can proceed as previously described.

The benefit of antibiotic prophylaxis for EUS FNA has not been well studied. Some authors recommend that all patients undergoing biopsy of a perirectal lesion or any type of cystic lesion receive an oral quinolone for prophylaxis before the procedure, with antibiotic therapy continued for 48 hours post-procedure. This approach is supported by a recent abstract reporting a 19% incidence of bacteremia with EUS FNA of solid lesions (8). Whether antibiotic prophylaxis should be used in all patients is unknown.

## Pancreatic Masses

Endoscopic ultrasound affords excellent views of the entire pancreas, permitting biopsy of lesions in any part of the gland. Furthermore, biopsy from the stomach or proximal duodenum avoids a needle tract traversing the peritoneum, negating the small risk of tumor seeding. There are several indications for pancreatic mass biopsy:

1. *Definitive diagnosis*: Not all pancreatic masses are adenocarcinoma (Figures 13-5.A, 13-5.B). Biopsy may help differentiate adenocarcinoma from other lesions such as lymphoma, nonfunctional neuroendocrine tumor, and mixed solid and cystic papillary neoplasm. Although focal pancreatitis (pseudotumorous pancreatitis) is difficult to differentiate from adenocarcinoma prior to formal resection (9, 10), the specificity of biopsies obtained for suspected adenocarcinoma makes a positive biopsy for malignancy useful in this setting. Furthermore, a definitive diagnosis is often desired by patients and their physicians even if therapeutic interventions are not being considered.
2. *Before chemotherapy/radiation therapy*: Confirmation of a tissue diagnosis of adenocarcinoma is required by essentially all medical and radiation oncologists before beginning treatment.

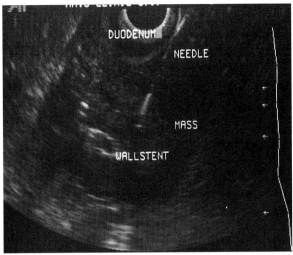

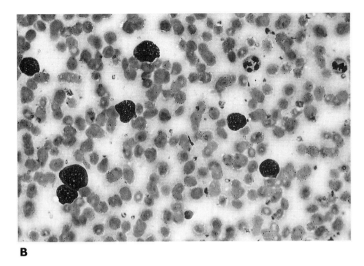

**Figure 13-5.** A 60-year-old male with a history of treated Burkitt's lymphoma in remission presented with painless jaundice. CT scan demonstrated extrahepatic biliary dilatation but was otherwise normal. ERCP at another institution revealed a distal common bile duct stricture. A wall stent was placed and brushings from the bile duct were negative. EUS demonstrated a 3-cm mass in the periduodenal space encasing the bile duct. Fine-needle aspiration biopsy was performed (A) that demonstrated recurrence of the lymphoma ((B), Diff-Quik stain, original magnification 150×).

**Table 13-2.** Diagnostic characteristics of EUS FNA for pancreatic mass lesions.

|  | n | Sensitivity (%) | Specificity (%) | Accuracy (%) |
|---|---|---|---|---|
| Chang (32) |  | 91 | 100 | 87 |
| Giovannini (33) | 43 | 75 | 100 | 79 |
| Cahn (34) | 50 | 88 | 100 | 87 |
| Bhutani (35) | 47 | 64 | 100 | 72 |
| Chang (36) | 44 | 92 | 100 | 95 |
| Erickson (37) | 28 | - | - | 96 |
| Faigel (38) | 45 | 72 | 100 | 75 |
| Gress (5) (Linear) | 95 | - | - | 86 |
| Gress (5) (Radial) | 26 | - | - | 81 |
| Wiersema (7) | 124 | 87 | 100 | 88 |
| Binmoeller (12) | 58 | 76 | 100 | 92 |
| Binmoeller* (12) | 45 | 87 | 100 | 91 |

*used the GF UM 30P scope

3. *Before celiac plexus neurolysis*: The diagnosis of adenocarcinoma in an unresectable lesion provides an opportunity for celiac plexus neurolysis during the same EUS procedure. This setting requires cytopathological examination of the aspirate *during* the procedure.

4. *Before surgical resection of adenocarcinoma*: The importance of tissue diagnosis in this setting is debated, and therefore the indication for FNA in this setting relies somewhat on the surgeon involved. Many surgeons will embark upon resection of a mass when biopsy is negative for malignancy (11). Furthermore, although rare, hemorrhage and pancreatitis that may follow multiple passes with the needle can make resection more difficult. It is not our practice to routinely biopsy presumed pancreatic malignancies prior to resection.

Data have rapidly accumulated over the past three years regarding the usefulness of EUS FNA in the setting of a pancreatic mass. Compared to other modalities, the results of EUS FNA of pancreatic masses are excellent, with a sensitivity of about 85% to 90% and a specificity of 100% (see Table 13-2). A recent publication suggests a slight increment in diagnostic accuracy can be achieved by using a larger needle that permits cores of tissue rather than aspirates to be obtained for histopathological examination (12). Table 13-2 summarizes available data from peer-reviewed publications on the diagnostic characteristics of EUS FNA of pancreatic mass lesions.

**Table 13-3a.** Detection of malignancy at EUS-guided aspiration of pancreatic cystic lesions.

|  | Sensitivity (%) | Specificity (%) | Accuracy (%) |
|---|---|---|---|
| Cytology | 57 | 100 | 80 |
| CA 125 (>60 units) | 67 | 88 | 76 |
| TPA* (>100000 units) | 43 | 100 | 73 |
| CA 19-9 (>50000 units) | 30 | 50 | 39 |

*Proliferation tissue polypeptide antigen
(n = 45)
Reprinted with permission from reference 39.

**Table 13-3b.** Detection of mucinous lesions at EUS-guided aspiration of pancreatic cystic lesions.

|  | Sensitivity (%) | Specificity (%) | Accuracy (%) |
|---|---|---|---|
| Cytology or Mucin Stain Positive | 75 | 80 | 77 |
| CEA (>50 units) | 92 | 80 | 88 |
| Mucin Panel | 100 | 60 | 86 |

(n = 45)
Reprinted with permission from reference 39.

## Pancreatic Cystic Lesions

A review of the radiological literature indicates that simple needle drainage of pancreatic pseudocysts does not offer long-term benefits, with a one-year recurrence rate of 75% (13). Therefore, the benefits of EUS-guided aspiration of pancreatic and peripancreatic cystic lesions lie not primarily in removal of cystic fluid, but as a diagnostic tool for cyst fluid analysis. Up to 10 percent of pancreatic cystic lesions are neoplastic (14), many of which are initially misdiagnosed as pseudocysts. Some pancreatic cystic tumors are malignant (cystadenocarcinoma) or have malignant potential (for example, mucinous cystadenoma, intraductal papillary mucinous tumor (IPMT)), whereas others have little or no malignant potential (such as serous cystadenoma, retention cyst) (14). Therefore, accurate diagnosis is essential for appropriate patient care. In addition to routine cytology, several studies have addressed the usefulness of biochemical and genetic indices of cyst fluid in the differentiation of malignant from benign cystic neoplasms. A panel of tumor antigens has been proposed to be helpful in defining the malignant potential of mucinous lesions and cyst fluid. These results are summarized in Tables 13-3a and 13-3b. In another study, high CA19-9 levels helped discriminate mucinous from other cystic lesions and low CEA values helped distinguish serious from other morphologic subtypes (15). The presence of mucin containing goblet cells or a positive mucin stain strongly suggests IPMT, mucinous cystadenoma, or mucinous cystadenocarcinoma (14,16). In one small study, K-ras mutations were absent in all cases of serous cystadenomas and present in all cases of cystadenocarcinoma (17). High amylase concentrations in aspirated cyst fluid suggest pseudocyst or retention cyst (14), although there are case reports of elevated amylase levels in cystic tumors (18).

The number of cysts analyzed in most studies is too small to make confident sensitivity and specificity measures of any of these markers with respect to malignant potential. There is a paucity of literature regarding the utility of EUS-guided aspiration of pancreatic cystic lesions. Endoscopic ultrasound may be well suited to this purpose, because the entire pancreas is easily accessible to EUS-guided drainage. However, there is a theoretical risk of introducing infection to the cyst cavity, because the needle traverses a nonsterile channel and gut surface. This infective risk is less of an issue with the percutaneous approach if the bowel is avoided. The magnitude of this risk remains to be determined. However, it would seem prudent that EUS-guided cyst drainage be performed with antibiotic prophylaxis.

## Peri-Intestinal Lymphadenopathy

The demonstration and biopsy of regional and distant lymphadenopathy is important in many situations. Although the EUS appearance of lymph nodes may be suggestive of malignant involvement, this alone has been shown to have limited accuracy in a recent series (19). However EUS FNA appears to enhance lymph node staging accuracy, which may influence the choice of therapy (7). For example, in esophageal malignancy, the presence of celiac lymphadenopathy designates the

**Table 13-4.** Diagnostic characteristics of EUS FNA for peri-intestinal lymph nodes.

| | n | Sensitivity (%) | Specificity (%) | Accuracy (%) |
|---|---|---|---|---|
| Bhutani (39) | 22 | 100 | 100 | 100 |
| Chang (36) | 14 | 83 | 100 | 88 |
| Erickson (37) | 14 | 100 | 100 | 100 |
| Gress (5) | 56 | - | - | 93 |
| Wiersema (7) | 192 | 92 | 93 | 92 |
| Binmoeller (40) | 43 | 91 | 100 | 95 |
| Reed (21) | 57 | 72 | 97 | 86 |

lesion as M1a, implying that the lesion is not resectable with curative intent. In one study, patients with esophageal cancer and celiac node involvement had a median survival of 3 months compared to 28 months in those without celiac involvement (20). Reed et al. demonstrated that EUS FNA was an accurate method for providing celiac lymph node staging in the setting of esophageal carcinoma considered resectable by CT (21). In 59 of 62 patients (95%) the celiac region was evaluated by EUS (three patients had obstructing tumors precluding endoscope passage into the stomach). Suspicious celiac lymph nodes were identified by EUS in 19, with the remaining 40 patients being EUS negative. Twenty-six patients were ultimately identified to have metastatic celiac lymph nodes. EUS FNA, when compared to CT, demonstrated superior sensitivity (72% versus 8%) and similar specificity (97% versus 100%). These findings support the conclusion that EUS FNA documentation of celiac lymph node metastases may be helpful in guiding therapy in patients with distal esophageal adenocarcinoma.

From a technical standpoint, lymph node biopsy may be easier than biopsy of the primary lesion. This is particularly true of pancreatic adenocarcinoma, in which the primary lesion is often associated with a dense desmoplastic reaction, resulting in a relative paucity of malignant cells to sample as well as rendering the lesion firm and technically difficult to puncture. Table 13-4 demonstrates the accuracy of peri-intestinal lymph node biopsy using EUS FNA.

Peri-intestinal and peri-esophageal lymph node biopsies have also been useful in the diagnosis of non-Hodgkin's lymphoma (22,23). The type of non-Hodgkin's lymphoma may influence the diagnostic capability of EUS FNA. Using percutaneous fine-needle biopsy, high-grade non-Hodgkin's lymphomas are more accurately diagnosed than are low-grade lymphomas (24). Further study is needed in this area to determine the benefits of EUS FNA in this setting, as well as the role of flow cytometry and possibly core biopsies to enhance diagnosis (22).

The importance of EUS FNA in the setting of rectal carcinoma is dependent on whether the presence of local extraluminal disease would alter patient management. These situations include:

1. Determination of local node status
2. Demonstration of peritoneal seeding
3. Suspicion of local recurrence with negative endoscopic biopsy

The determination of peri-rectal involvement preoperatively could lead to identification of patients in whom neo-adjuvant chemo-radiation may be beneficial. Patients with T3N1 rectal lesions have been shown to have a 20% local recurrence following surgical therapy alone. This risk of pelvic recurrence has been shown to be reduced through the use of neo-adjuvant radiation. Furthermore, preoperative radiation may be less morbid than postoperative therapy. Hence, there is a rational basis for the use of EUS FNA to determine local lymph node status before resection. Biopsy proven peritoneal seeding or malignant ascites would identify patients in whom surgical intervention with curative intent would not be possible.

Limited literature is available regarding the efficacy of EUS FNA in the setting of primary or recurrent colorectal neoplasia. In a recent study, EUS FNA was reported in 70 patients with a peri-rectal or peri-colonic lesion (25). The indication and result of EUS FNA in this series were as follows:

- Suspected local recurrence of disease with negative mucosal biopsies in 38 patients. EUS FNA confirmed the clinical suspicion in 31 cases (82%). Three cases were biopsy negative and remain so 36 months later. In four cases no diagnostic tissue was obtained and all had recurrence at laparotomy.
- Suspected recurrence of anal SCC following chemo-radiation therapy in eight patients. This was confirmed in six cases. The two patients with negative EUS FNA remain disease free at 13 months.
- Suspicious peri-rectal nodes in association with T2 tumors in seven patients. All have confirmation of nodal spread at EUS FNA.
- Suspected peritoneal carcinomatosis in seven cases. This was confirmed by EUS FNA in all cases.
- Extrinsic compression of the bowel in 10 cases. EUS FNA provided a diagnosis in eight patients: sarcoma in three, mesothelioma in two, and one of each of the following: abscess, recurrent adenocarcinoma,

**Table 13-5.** Diagnostic characteristics of EUS FNA for mediastinal lymphadenopathy.

| | n | Sensitivity (%) | Specificity (%) | Accuracy (%) |
|---|---|---|---|---|
| Giovannini (33) | 24 | 81 | 100 | 83 |
| Silvestri (41) | 26 | 89 | 100 | 92 |
| Gress (26) | 24 | 93 | 100 | 96 |
| Hunerbein (42) | 25 | 89 | 83 | – |
| Janssen (43) | 35 | - | - | 91 |
| Serna (44) | 7 | 86 | 100 | 86 |
| Wiersema (27) | 48 | 88 | 100 | 90 |

**Table 13-6.** Gastrointestinal wall lesions.

| | n | Sensitivity (%) | Specificity (%) | Accuracy (%) |
|---|---|---|---|---|
| Giovannini (33) | 7 | 60 | 100 | 72 |
| Gress (26) | 27 | – | – | 81 |
| Wiersema (7) | 103 | 61 | 79 | 67 |

and hemangiopericytoma. The two patients with negative EUS FNA had sarcoma diagnosed at laparotomy.

Overall, the sensitivity, specificity and diagnostic accuracy of EUS FNA for peri-colonic and peri-rectal lesions were 83%, 100%, and 95%, respectively.

## Mediastinal Lymphadenopathy

The esophagus provides a convenient conduit to the posterior mediastinum. Lymph nodes in the subcarinal, aortopulmonic, and peri-esophageal regions are readily biopsied with EUS. This is of particular relevance with regard to nonsmall cell carcinoma of the lung. Contralateral mediastinal lymph node metastases render the lesion unresectable with curative intent. Furthermore, ipsilateral mediastinal lymph node staging is important prognostically and may be helpful in the stratification of patients for neo-adjuvant trials. The actual costs of EUS FNA, mediastinoscopy, and staging thoracotomy have been calculated to be $1975, $7759, and $26,028, respectively (26). These differences in cost are largely based on the hospital stay and operating room costs incurred with each of these procedures. EUS FNA is the least expensive because it is performed as an outpatient procedure using conscious sedation.

Complications from EUS FNA of mediastinal lesions are infrequent and rarely severe. In recently published series by Gress (26) and Wiersema (27) there were no complications. Table 13-5 summarizes the diagnostic characteristics of EUS FNA for mediastinal lymphadenopathy. EUS FNA may also be useful in the diagnosis of other mediastinal mass lesions such as tuberculosis, sarcoid, and non-Hodgkin's lymphoma.

## Mucosal and Submucosal Lesions

In the largest series to date (7), EUS FNA was performed on 103 lesions arising from the gastrointestinal wall (excluding stromal tumors). Sensitivity varied with the type of lesion (89% for non-Hodgkin's lymphoma, 40% for gastric adenocarcinoma). The accuracy of EUS FNA was 69% for esophageal lesions, 62% for gastric, 69% for duodenal, and 100% for rectal lesions. EUS FNA of a gastrointestinal wall lesion was correct in 24 of 36 cases (33%) where endoscopic biopsies had been nondiagnostic. Neverless, there is still insufficient data to define the role of EUS FNA in helping differentiate benign from malignant stromal lesions of the gastrointestinal tract. The results of EUS FNA of gastrointestinal wall lesions are summarized in Table 13-6.

## Miscellaneous

Since, the gastrointestinal tract is in close proximity to many mediastinal and abdominal structures, the possible benefits of EUS-guided FNA of tissues other than those previously described may be substantial. This raises the possibility of EUS-guided FNA of many tissues other than those previously described. The demonstration of malignant involvement of serosal fluid precludes curative surgery for both pulmonary and gastrointestinal adenocarcinomas. Although restricted to case reports (28,29), the drainage of pleural or ascitic fluid at the time of EUS is technically simple and if the cytology is malignant, can dramatically alter medical and surgical treatment. Similarly, biopsy of suspected hepatic metastases, which can be done easily with EUS through the stomach under real-time control, can be of great importance in patient management. A single case report of EUS-guided FNA of an adrenal mass has been published (30). The authors could demonstrate the left adrenal in 30 of 31 examinations (97%) and were able to confirm metastatic disease to the left adrenal in one patient in whom CT-guided FNA had been unsuccessful.

## Safety

Complications with EUS FNA are infrequent and usually minor. In the largest series published to date, there were five complications in 554 consecutive mass or lymph node biopsies (7) and none was fatal. Two patients had endoscope-induced perforation, two patients had febrile episodes following aspiration of cystic lesions, and one patient had hemorrhage from the wall of a pseudocyst. Complications are usually mild and comprise mild pancreatitis, self-limiting hemorrhage, and fever. Pneumoperitoneum has been reported when endoscopy closely followed EUS FNA (31), suggesting that gut insufflation should be minimized or avoided for a short period after EUS FNA.

## Summary

EUS FNA is a sensitive and accurate tool for establishing a tissue diagnosis for luminal and periluminal lesions when other techniques have failed or are not possible. The safe performance of EUS FNA requires the use of a linear scanning echoprobe with a small-gauge needle to biopsy solid lesions. The major limitation in the widespread application of EUS FNA has been the expense associated with the equipment and a shortage of individuals trained in performing the procedure. However, as the method gains widespread acceptance and with technological advancements, EUS FNA will undoubtedly become part of the standard evaluation of patients presenting with mass lesions.

### References

1. Pfaffenbach B, Langer M, Stabenow-Lohbauer U, Lux G. [Endosonography-controlled transgastric drainage of pancreatic pseudocysts]. Deutsche Medizinische Wochenschrift 1998;123:1439–1442.
2. Giovannini M, Bernardini D, Seitz JF. Cystogastrostomy entirely performed under endosonography guidance for pancreatic pseudocyst: results in six patients [see comments]. Gastrointest Endosc 1998;48:200–203.
3. Wiersema MJ, Wiersema LM. Endosonography-guided celiac plexus neurolysis. Gastrointest Endosc 1996; 44:656–662.
4. Wiersema MJ, Sandusky D, Carr R, et al. Endosonography-guided cholangiopancreatography. Gastrointest Endosc 1996;43:102–106.
5. Gress FG, Hawes RH, Savides TJ, et al. Endoscopic ultrasound-guided fine-needle aspiration biopsy using linear array and radial scanning endosonography [see comments]. Gastrointest Endosc 1997;45:243–250.
6. Karler B. Personal communication. GIP Mediglobe, Tempe, Arizona 1999.
7. Wiersema MJ, Vilmann P, Giovannini M, et al. Endosonography-guided fine-needle aspiration biopsy: diagnostic accuracy and complication assessment. Gastroenterology 1997;112:1087–1095.
8. Van de Mierop F, Buorgeois S, Hiel M, et al. Bacteremia after EUS guided puncture: a prospective analysis. Gastrointest Endosc 1999;49:A13100. Abstract.
9. Rosch T, Lorenz R, Braig C, et al. Endoscopic ultrasound in pancreatic tumor diagnosis. Gastrointest Endosc 1991;37:347–352.
10. Hayashi Y, Nakazawa S, Kimoto E, et al. Clinicopathologic analysis of endoscopic ultrasonograms in pancreatic mass lesions. Endoscopy 1989;21:121–125.
11. Tillou A, Schwartz MR, Jordan PH Jr. Percutaneous needle biopsy of the pancreas: when should it be performed? World J Surg 1996;20:283–286.
12. Binmoeller KF, Thul R, Rathod V, et al. Endoscopic ultrasound-guided, 18-gauge, fine needle aspiration biopsy of the pancreas using a 2.8 mm channel convex array echoendoscope. Gastrointest Endosc 1998; 47:121–127.
13. Hanke S, Petersen J. Percutaneous puncture of pancreatic cysts guided by ultrasound. Surg Gyn Ob 1976;142:551–552.
14. Warshaw AL, Compton CC, Lewandrowski K, et al. Cystic tumors of the pancreas. New clinical, radiologic, and pathologic observations in 67 patients. Ann Surg 1990;212:432–443.
15. Hammel P, Levy P, Voitot H, et al. Preoperative cyst fluid analysis is useful for the differential diagnosis of cystic lesions of the pancreas. Gastroenterology 1995; 108:1230–1235.
16. Hammel PR, Forgue-Lafitte ME, Levy P, et al. Detection of gastric mucins (M1 antigens) in cyst fluid for the diagnosis of cystic lesions of the pancreas. Int J Cancer 1997;74:286–290.
17. Bartsch D, Bastian D, Barth P, et al. K-ras oncogene mutations indicate malignancy in cystic tumors of the pancreas. Ann Surg 1998;228:79–86.
18. Lumsden A, Bradley EL. Pseudocyst or cystic neoplasm? Differential diagnosis and initial management of cystic pancreatic lesions. Hepato-gastroent 1989; 36:462–466.
19. Bhutani MS, Hawes RH, Hoffman BJ. A comparison of the accuracy of echo features during endoscopic ultrasound (EUS) and EUS-guided fine needle aspiration for diagnosis of malignant lymph node invasion. Gastrointest Endosc 1996;45:474–479.
20. Hiele M, De Leyn P, Schurmans P, et al. Relation between endoscopic ultrasound findings and outcome of patients with tumors of the esophagus or esophagogastric junction. Gastrointest Endosc 1997;45:381–386.

21. Reed CE, Mishra G, Sahai A, et al. Esophageal cancer staging: improved accuracy by endoscopic ultrasound of celiac lymph nodes. Ann Thor Surg 1999;67:319–321.

22. Wiersema MJ, Gatzimos K, Nisi R, Wiersema LM. Staging of non-Hodgkin's gastric lymphoma with endosonography-guided fine-needle aspiration biopsy and flow cytometry. Gastrointest Endosc 1996;44:734–736.

23. Lewis JD, Faigel DO, Dowdy Y, et al. Hodgkin's disease diagnosed by endoscopic ultrasound-guided fine needle aspiration of a periduodenal lymph node. Am J Gastroent 1998;93:834–836.

24. Pilotti S, Di Palma S, Alasio L, et al. Diagnostic assessment of enlarged superficial lymph nodes by fine needle aspiration. Acta Cytologica 1993;37:853–866.

25. Giovannini M, Bernardini D. Endosonography guided biopsy of rectal and colic area lesions. Acta Endoscopica 1998;28:45–51.

26. Gress FG, Savides TJ, Sandler A, et al. Endoscopic ultrasonography, fine-needle aspiration biopsy guided by endoscopic ultrasonography, and computed tomography in the preoperative staging of non-small-cell lung cancer: a comparison study [see comments]. Ann Int Med 1997;127:604–612.

27. Wiersema MJ, Harada N, Daiehagh P, et al. Evaluation of mediastinal lymphadenopathy with transesophageal endosonography guided fine needle aspiration biopsy. Acta Endoscopica 1998;28:7–19.

28. Chang KJ, Albers CG, Nguyen P. Endoscopic ultrasound-guided fine needle aspiration of pleural and ascitic fluid. Am J Gastroent 1995;90:148–150.

29. Mizutani S, Ohhashi K, Yamao K, et al. [Usefulness for choice of treatment by endoscopic ultrasound (EUS) guided fine needle aspiration (FNA) cytology of ascites—report of two cases]. Jap J Gastroent 1998;95:1047–1051.

30. Chang KJ, Erickson RA, Nguyen P. Endoscopic ultrasound (EUS) and EUS-guided fine-needle aspiration of the left adrenal gland. Gastrointest Endosc 1996;44:568–572.

31. Mergener K, Jowell PS, Branch MS, Baillie J. Pneumoperitoneum complicating ERCP performed immediately after EUS-guided fine needle aspiration. Gastrointest Endosc 1998;47:541–542.

# 14

# Over-the-Guide-Wire Ultrasonic Esophagoprobe and Catheter Miniprobe for Stenosing Tumors

## Kenneth F. Binmoeller

Gastrointestinal tumors usually do not become symptomatic until late in the course of disease when exophytic growth has resulted in significant stenosis. The inability to safely pass endoscopes into and through the stenotic lumen with conventional radial scanning echoendoscopes has been a significant problem in all of the studies that have evaluated the usefulness of EUS for tumor staging in these situations. In fact, up to one-half of patients with esophageal cancers referred for staging EUS cannot be adequately examined with the conventional echoendoscope because of tumor-associated stenosis (1–4). This chapter discusses the problem of the nontraversable stenosis using conventional echoendoscopes and two instruments that have been developed to resolve this limitation: the ultrasonic esophagoprobe and the catheter miniprobe.

## Strategies for Endosonographic Evaluation of High-Grade Stenoses

Various strategies can be employed to enable endosonographic evaluation of patients with high-grade stenosing malignancies. The most obvious solution is to dilate the stricture to allow passage of the echoendoscope. The concern about this approach is the risk of perforation. Because conventional echoendoscopes have an outer shaft diameter of around 13 mm, fairly aggressive dilatation to 46 French or more is necessary to enable passage of the echoendoscope. Dilatation carries an inherent risk of perforation, and passage of the echoendoscope after dilatation harbors an additional risk. Echoendoscopes have oblique viewing optics, so passage through a stenosis is "blind." Furthermore, the distal tip of the instrument contains a rigid 4-cm long

transducer. The risk of perforation is even greater if tortuosity or angulation of the lumen is present, as is often the case at the gastric cardia.

The high risk of perforation when dilatation is performed prior to the passage of the echoendoscope was documented in a study by Van Dam et al. (2). In a series of 79 patients with esophageal carcinoma, 21 (26.6%) presented with high-grade malignant strictures defined as a tumor obstruction precluding passage of an echoendoscope without prior dilatation. These authors found it necessary to dilate strictures to 16 to 17 mm (and rarely to 18 mm) to pass the conventional echoendoscope. Dilatation resulted in esophageal perforation in five patients (24%), either secondary to dilation or during passage of the echoendoscope. The authors recommended that esophageal strictures should not be dilated for the purpose of performing EUS.

Catalano et al. (5) have similarly reported a high perforation rate associated with EUS in stenosing esophageal carcinoma. Despite dilatation in 21 patients prior to EUS, passage of the echoendoscope was possible in only seven patients. Perforation occurred in 5 of the 21 patients (24%) during attempts to pass the echoendoscope, a rate identical to that of the study by Van Dam et al. (2).

An alternative approach to the nontraversable stenosis is to image the tumor either above or—if partial cannulation is possible—within the tumor. Staging a tumor above the stenosis has the obvious problem of potential understaging, because the tumor may be of a more advanced stage distal to the position of the transducer (Figure 14-1.A.). Furthermore, celiac axis imaging is not possible, which precludes the M-staging of esophageal carcinoma. Accuracy rates usually have been less than 50% (2,6). In 21 patients with high-grade malignant esophageal strictures, Van Dam et al. (2)

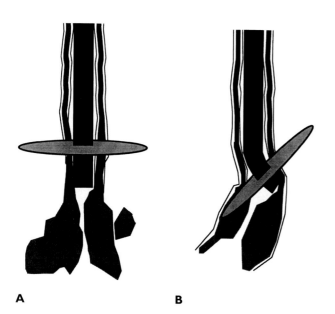

**A**                    **B**

**Figure 14-1.** Endosonographic examination of a nontraversable stenosing esophageal malignancy. (A) Scanning from the proximal tumor border understages the tumor. (B) Scanning within the tumor stenosis may overstage the tumor due to oblique scanning.

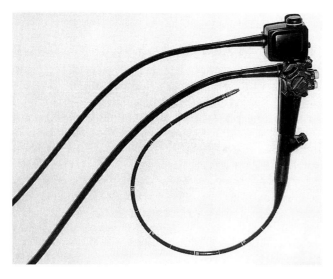

**Figure 14-2.** Overview of the ultrasonic esophagoprobe. The instrument resembles a conventional echoendoscope, but lacks an optical component.

found the accuracy of EUS staging from the proximal margin to be 33% for the T-stage and 10% for the N-stage. Staging can be considered to be reliable only when maximal T-stage is present at the proximal tumor pole (i.e., infiltration of neighboring organs (T4 stage)).

Staging from within the tumor is not only subject to the limitation of potential understaging, but also to overstaging because the transducer may assume an an-

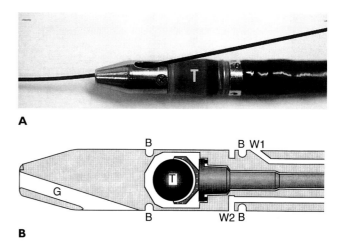

**A**

**B**

**Figure 14-3.** Distal end of the ultrasonic esophagoprobe. (A) Photograph shows how the guide wire enters at the tip and exits along the side T = transducer. (B) Schematic drawing shows the internal components (R = ridge for balloon, G = guide wire channel, W1 = water channel for lumen filling, W2 = water channel for balloon filling, B = groove for balloon, T = transducer).

gulated or wedged position in the stenosis and produce oblique or tangential scanning artifact in the form of accentuated tumor infiltration (Figure 14-1,B). Hordijk et al. (6) found that overstaging occurred in 54% of patients with highly stenotic esophageal tumors, resulting in an accuracy rate of only 46%.

## Ultrasonic Esophagoprobe

To resolve the difficulties associated with imaging of stenotic tumors, the ultrasonic esophagoprobe was developed by the author and coworkers at the University Hospital Eppendorf in Hamburg, Germany, in collaboration with the Olympus Corporation.

### Principle Elements of Design

The ultrasonic esophagoprobe (Figures 14-2 and 14-3) was designed to enable easy and safe insertion of an endosonographic instrument through a stenotic esophageal or cardia carcinoma for complete T-, N-, and celiac axis lymph node staging. Three fundamental principles were integrated into the conception of the instrument:

1. Thin shaft diameter
2. Insertion over a previously placed guide wire
3. Tapered (cone-shaped) instrument tip

The outer shaft diameter of the esophagoprobe is 7.8 mm, which is identical to that of the Olympus XP-20 pediatric gastroscope. This diameter was selected because the majority of esophageal tumors will allow passage of the pediatric gastroscope. If passage fails, preliminary bougienage to a 33 French diameter (11 mm) will usually permit subsequent passage of the pediatric gastroscope.

From a technical standpoint, the reduction of the diameter of the esophagoprobe from 13 mm (conventional echoendoscopes) to 7.8 mm required the elimination of two components: the fiber-optics and the instrumentation channel. The fiber-optics are dispensable because the probe is inserted over a guide wire. Furthermore, orientation within the esophagus can be guided by the sonographic image. The instrumentation channel is also dispensable.

Insertion of the esophagoprobe over a guide wire not only eliminates the need for fiber-optics, but also establishes a path through the stricture for easier and possibly safer insertion. The guide wire enters at the very tip of the instrument and exits through a side port about 1 cm away from the tip (Figure 14-3.A). This design was necessary because it is not technically possible for the guide wire to pass through the transducer. It also avoids the need for an additional working channel for the guide wire.

Analogous to bougies used for dilatation of esophageal stenoses, the esophagoprobe is equipped with a tapered metal tip to enable graduated passage through a stricture. The metal tip measures 1.7 cm and is incorporated just distal to the transducer.

## Technical Specifications of the Esophagoprobe

The technical specifications of the ultrasound transducer are nearly identical to that of existing mechanical radial scanning echoendoscopes. The 7.5-MHz transducer consists of a single piezoelectric element transducer that mechanically rotates at a speed of 10 rotations/second to produce a 360-degree radial sector scan of the examined area. The scanning plane is perpendicular to the axis of the shaft. The focus point is fixed at 20 mm, which is 10 mm shorter than that of the conventional 7.5-MHz mechanical radial scanning echoendoscope. The transducer length measures 2.0 cm.

An acoustic interface between the transducer and bowel wall is provided by water filling of a latex balloon that covers the transducer (Figure 14-4). The balloon fits into grooves at the proximal and distal ends of the transducer. A separate channel feeds water into the balloon. Similar to the conventional echoendoscope, balloon filling is activated by depressing the distal valve at the instrument handle. Water is evacuated from the balloon by depressing the proximal valve.

The esophagoprobe has the standard up-down and right-left dials for four-way tip deflection. The range of tip deflection is similar to that of the conventional echoendoscope.

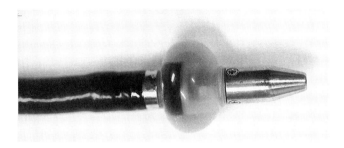

**Figure 14-4.** Latex balloon filled with water mounted over transducer of the ultrasonic esophagoprobe.

Because water filling of the bowel lumen may be required to improve acoustic coupling, a separate channel was integrated into the instrument for this purpose (Figure 14-3.B). Water is instilled using a 50-ml syringe or water pump through a side port at the handle. The water exits through four tiny holes, each 0.85 mm in diameter, located just proximal to the transducer.

Additional features of the esophagoprobe include a motor drive switch to activate rotation of the transducer, and a freeze button at the instrument handle, analogous to the conventional Olympus UM-20 and UM-130 echoendoscopes. The esophagoprobe is connected to the standard Olympus image processors (EUM-20 and M-30) used with the conventional radial scanning echoendoscopes.

## Procedure

The patient is placed in the left lateral decubitus position for endoscopic examination and intravenous sedation is administered. The tumor stenosis is first intubated with a thin diameter (e.g. pediatric) gastroscope. If passage fails, preliminary bougienage of the stenosis to 11 mm (33 Fr) is performed using the over-the-guide-wire technique. After bougienage, the gastroscope is negotiated through the stricture and advanced into the stomach. A hydrophilic guide wire is then inserted into the gastric antrum and the gastroscope is withdrawn, leaving the guide wire in place. The esophagoprobe is threaded over the guide wire and advanced through the esophagus. The guide wire is usually removed after the esophagoprobe enters the stomach, because the wire causes artifact in the scanning field. However, leaving the guide wire in place does have the advantage in that it provides a method for easy reinsertion of the instrument.

The endosonographic examination begins in the upper stomach, searching for metastatic perigastric lymph nodes and lymph nodes in the region of the celiac axis. Acoustic coupling with the wall of the stomach is achieved by filling the balloon with water. If additional acoustic coupling is necessary, the stomach

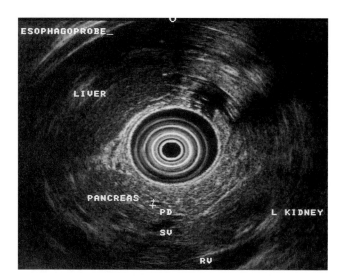

**Figure 14-5.** Endosonographic "four-organ" view from the upper stomach: the liver (left lobe), the pancreas (body and tail), the left kidney, and the spleen. The pancreatic duct (*PD*) is seen coursing though the pancreas. Dorsal to the pancreas, the splenic vein (*SV*) is seen in longitudinal section. The left kidney is seen inferior to the pancreatic tail and to the left of the spleen. The renal vein (*RV*) is seen entering the kidney hilum.

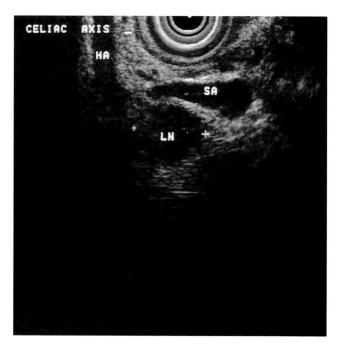

**Figure 14-7.** Metastatic lymph node (*LN*) in the region of the celiac axis. (*SA* = splenic artery, *HA* = hepatic artery).

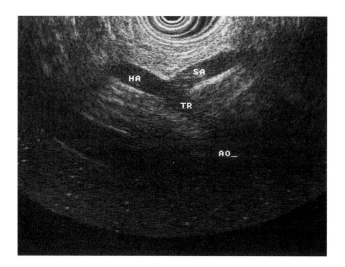

**Figure 14-6.** Celiac axis dividing into two arched hypoechoic tubular structures, the splenic (*SA*) and hepatic (*HA*) arteries. No metastatic lymph nodes are seen. (*AO* = descending abdominal aorta, *TR* = trunk).

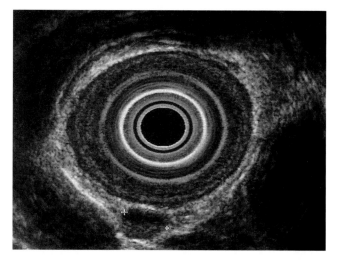

**Figure 14-8.** Endosonographic image of T2 esophageal tumor involving the entire circumference of the esophageal wall. The outer margins of the tumor growth are sharply demarcated. A metastatic lymph node is seen adjacent to the tumor.

lumen can be filled with 100 to 150 ml of deaerated water. Neighboring organs, including the left lobe of the liver, the pancreatic body and tail, the left kidney, and the spleen, are well visualized using the esophagoprobe (Figure 14-5). The celiac axis is located by either following the splenic artery to its emergence from the celiac trunk or by following the abdominal aorta until the takeoff of the celiac trunk is visualized (Figure 14-

6). This area is carefully inspected for metastatic lymph nodes. If present (Figure 14-7), metastatic celiac nodes qualify an esophageal cancer as M1 stage (7). The esophagoprobe is slowly withdrawn into the esophagus for T- and N-staging of the cancer (Figures 14-8 through 14-11). The balloon will usually need to be deflated to enable passage of the instrument through the stenosis.

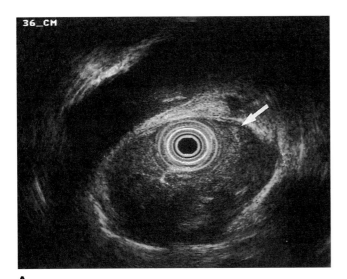

A

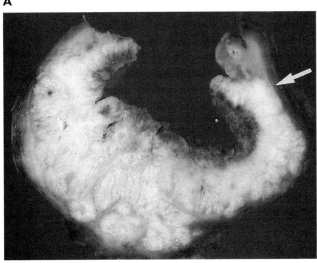

B

**Figure 14-9.** (A) Endosonographic image of a T3 esophageal tumor. *Arrow* indicates muscularis propria layer. (B) Corresponding gross surgical specimen showing tumor infiltration into the peri-esophageal fatty tissue. *Arrow* indicates muscularis propria layer.

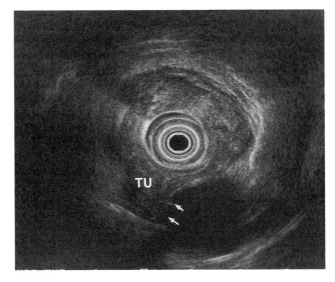

**Figure 14-10.** Endosonographic images of T4 tumor invading the aorta.

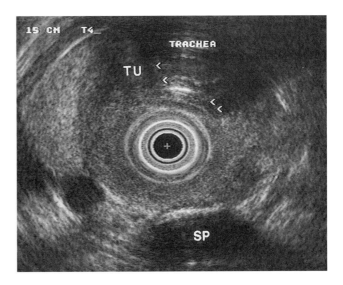

**Figure 14-11.** Endosonographic images of T4 tumor invading the trachea (*arrows* show interruption of interface plane).

## Experience with the Ultrasonic Esophagoprobe

Over a 4.5-year period, the esophagoprobe was used by the author and his coworkers at the University Hospital Hamburg in 221 consecutive patients with stenosing esophageal carcinomas. The stenosis was negotiated in all patients; only 8% of patients had highly stenosing tumors that required preliminary bougienage up to a 33 French diameter. The celiac axis region was adequately visualized in 94% of patients. No complications occurred.

The majority (87%) of patients with stenosing carcinomas were found to have T3 or T4 esophageal can-

cers. Nonetheless, a sizeable number of patients (13%) were found to have T2 tumors at endosonographic staging. Among the subgroup of patients who underwent resective surgery, approximately one-third were found to have T2 tumors. T4-stage cancers invading adjacent organs were diagnosed in 21% of patients.

Ninety-one patients (41%) underwent surgery as the primary treatment after endosonographic staging. Except for tumors that were found to invade neighboring organs at surgery (operative T4 stage), the pathological TNM stage served as the parameter for statistical correlation with the endosonographic TNM stage. The overall accuracy rates for TNM staging were found to

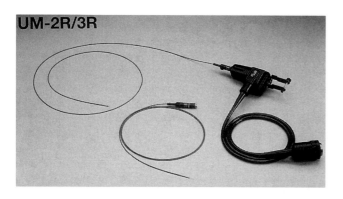

**Figure 14-12.** Photograph of the Olympus UM-2R and UM-3R catheter miniprobes.

be 84%, 78%, and 83% for stages T1, T2 and T3, respectively. These results are similar to results that have been reported in the literature for esophageal tumor staging using conventional echoendoscopes.

Erroneous T-staging was due to both overstaging (9% of patients) and understaging (7% of patients). The predominant cause of overstaging was tumor-associated inflammation and fibrosis that resembled extension of the tumor beyond the muscle layer into the surrounding peri-esophageal fatty tissue. The other cause was the inherent limitation of ultrasound imaging to precisely differentiate the line of demarcation between the outer margin of the muscularis propria and the surrounding fatty tissue. Oblique or tangential scanning may cause the outer margin of the muscularis propria to appear irregular. The cardia is particularly susceptible to this artifact. Understaging of T3 tumors was due to microscopic invasion of tumor into the adventitial tissue. Esophageal cancers are particularly prone to microscopic invasion beyond the esophageal wall because there is no anatomical barrier to tumor spread analogous to the serosa found in the stomach and intestines.

Cancers of the gastric cardia deserve special mention, as they may be classified as primary esophageal or gastric cancers. This may give rise to discrepancies in endosonographic, intraoperative, and pathological staging. The controversy as to whether a tumor of the cardia should be classified as gastric or esophageal in origin is not yet resolved. According to the TNM classification guidelines (supplement 1993), tumors involving more than 50% of the esophagus are classified as esophageal carcinoma and those involving more than 50% as stomach, including those equally distributed over esophagus and stomach (8).

In spite of the significantly reduced outer diameter of the esophagoprobe transducer, the quality of endosonographic imaging is equivalent to that of the standard Olympus mechanical radial scanning echoendoscope at 7.5 MHz. The esophagoprobe produces clear images with excellent resolution and an adequate depth of ultrasound penetration for complete T- and N-staging. The capability for full four-way deflection of the instrument tip is important because this enables visualization of the celiac axis for M-staging. Tip deflection is also necessary to appreciate the full extent of tumor infiltration of the subcardial region in carcinomas of the gastric cardia.

## Ultrasonic Catheterprobes

The miniature catheterprobe (miniprobe) is a new alternative to the esophagoprobe for staging stenosing esophageal carcinomas. The miniprobe can be passed through the instrumentation channel of a standard gastroscope (9–15). The first radial scanning ultrasonic probe was developed by Olympus Corporation in 1989 and had a transducer scanning at 7 MHz with an outer diameter of 3.4 mm (12). Since then, miniprobes have acquired higher-frequency transducers (12 MHz and higher) and smaller diameters. The latest Olympus models that are commercially available are the UM 2R and 3R (scanning at 12 and 20 MHz, respectively) (Figure 14-12). Both models have an outer diameter of 2.4 mm, a working length of 205 cm, and can be easily passed through a diagnostic gastroscope which has a biopsy channel diameter of 2.8 mm. The transducer technology is mechanical radial scanning, analogous to the conventional echoendoscope.

Miniprobes have the significant advantage that they can be guided into a stricture under direct vision during diagnostic endoscopy. Thus, staging can be performed quickly and efficiently without a need for an exchange of instruments. However, experience with catheter miniprobes has shown that they have several technical shortcomings when used for the staging of stenosing esophageal lesions. The penetration depth is limited to 2 to 3 centimeters, which is often the approximate thickness of a stenosing tumor. This limits the ability to accurately stage the depth of tumor infiltration. This limited depth of penetration is compounded by the short focal point distance of 5 to 10 mm, causing structures that lie outside of the focal point to appear fuzzy. Blurring of the outer tumor margins makes it difficult to accurately differentiate between a T2 and a T3 lesion (Figure 14-13). Also, regional lymph nodes are either not adequately visualized, or seen as blurred hypoechoic structures.

The miniprobe also lacks active tip control. Tip deflection is not required in the tubular esophagus, but it is essential to image the celiac axis region when viewed from the proximal stomach. The ultrasonic esophagoprobe is equipped with active tip deflection in large part to enable visualization of the celiac axis and the paragastric regions and allow more precise celiac axis imaging.

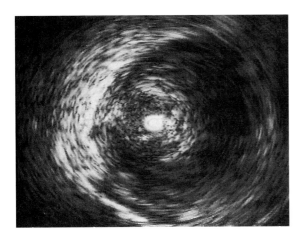

**Figure 14-13.** Miniprobe endosonographic image of a stenosing esophageal carcinoma. Precise T- and N-staging is hindered by the limited ultrasound penetration depth and short focal point distance.

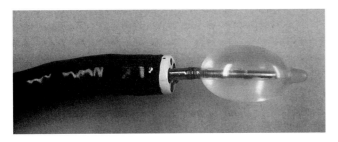

**Figure 14-14.** Miniprobe with balloon sheath (Olympus MH-246) filled with water. The miniprobe is inserted through and exits at the distal tip of a 2.8-mm channel gastroscope.

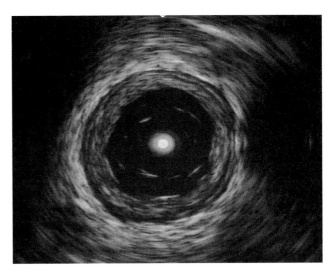

**Figure 14-15.** Miniprobe (Olympus UM-3R) endosonographic image of the esophageal wall showing detailed resolution of the wall layers.

Unlike conventional echoendoscopes and the ultrasonic esophagoprobe, the miniprobe is not equipped with a mounted balloon for water filling. This is a drawback when air surrounds the transducer and impedes acoustic coupling with the bowel wall. A special balloon sheath (MH-246 R) (Figure 14-14) has been recently developed for the miniprobe to overcome this limitation. The sheath works well but additional time is required to completely remove all air bubbles from the ballon. The balloon sheath increases the outer diameter of the miniprobe and therefore requires a larger channel gastroscope with at least a 3.2-mm diameter channel. Fockens et al. (16) used a balloon-fitted miniprobe to stage highly stenotic esophageal carcinomas in four patients and reported complete T- and N-staging. However, imaging of the celiac axis was not possible despite the use of the water-filled balloon sheath. In the author's opinion, compared with the esophagoprobe, there is no advantage to using a balloon-fitted miniprobe for staging stenosing esophageal lesions.

Several investigators have examined the accuracy rates of the miniprobe for gastrointestinal tumor stag-

ing. Maruta et al. (10) used different miniprobe models to stage tumors of the upper gastrointestinal tract, including seven esophageal cancers. For tumors extending beyond the submucosa, the accuracy rate was found to be only 33%, reflecting the technical limitations previously mentioned. Chak et al. (13) used the UM-2R and UM-3R miniprobes to stage esophageal malignancies in 13 patients, and compared results with the conventional echoendoscope. The miniprobe understaged esophageal tumors in 23% of patients because of inadequate imaging of the extraluminal border. In two patients whose tumors were T4 by conventional endosonography (one with pleural invasion and one with aortic invasion), miniprobe-based staging was only T3 and T2; in one patient found to have a T3 lesion by conventional endosonography, the miniprobe-based staging was only T2. Overall, endosonography using conventional echoendoscopes was preferred in 92% of patients because of the superior images obtained of the extraluminal tumor margins and regional lymph nodes as compared to results obtained with the miniprobe.

Catheter miniprobes are ideally suited for endosonographic imaging of superficial cancers. The use of a high-frequency transducer with a short focal distance produces high-resolution images of the layers of the esophagus (Figure 14-15). Whereas conventional echoendoscopes and the ultrasonic esophagoprobe will typically visualize the esophageal wall as a five-layer structure, miniprobes will depict seven to nine layers and may resolve the muscularis propria layer (10). Hasegawa et al. (14) compared the accuracy rates of the conventional echoendoscope (GF-UM 20) with a 15-MHz miniprobe in 22 patients with superficial esophageal carcinoma and found the accuracy of the miniprobe to be uniformly superior to the conventional instrument for T-staging (92% versus 76%, respectively). Accurate differentiation between T1-mucosa and T1-submucosa lesions is important because this may impact on the treatment of early cancers. Tumors limited to the T1-mucosa have been shown to be associated with a negligible risk of lymphatic spread and may therefore be candidates for curative endoscopic resection (endoscopic mucosectomy) (17).

## Conclusion

The preoperative staging of stenosing upper gastrointestinal carcinomas is difficult and hazardous using conventional echoendocopes. The ultrasonic esophagoprobe was developed to enable easy and safe endosonographic staging of stenosing lesions. Using the ultrasonic esophagoprobe in over 200 patients with stenosing esophageal cancers over a five-year period, the author was able to traverse the stenosis for complete T- and N-staging in all cases with no complications. Highly stenosing tumors that could not be passed even with the pediatric gastroscope were traversable after minimal dilatation of the stenosis to an 11-mm (33 Fr) diameter. Visualization of the celiac axis was possible in most cases, and the accuracy rates for TNM staging of esophageal cancers was found by the author to be similar to those reported in the literature for the conventional echoendoscope. The quality of endosonographic imaging was practically indistinguishable from that of the conventional echoendoscope.

Catheter miniprobes can be passed under direct vision through a stenosis, but their limited depth of penetration makes it difficult to accurately stage stenosing esophageal cancers. Furthermore, miniprobes lack tip deflection and are therefore unable to visualize the celiac axis region for M-staging of esophagal cancers. The higher resolution of the wall layers of the esophagus afforded by miniprobes makes this instrument more suitable for the endosonographic staging of superficial esophageal cancers.

### References

1. Grimm H, Binmoeller KF, Hamper K, et al. Endosonography for preoperative locoregional staging of esophageal and gastric cancer. Endoscopy 1993;25: 224–230.

2. Van Dam J, Rice TW, Catalano MF, et al. High-grade malignant stricture is predictive of esophageal tumor stage: risks of endosonographic evaluation. Cancer 1993;71:2910–2917.

3. Heyder N, Lux G. Malignant lesions of the upper gastrointestinal tract. Scand J Gastroenterol Suppl 1986;123.

4. Dancygier H, Classen M. Endoscopic ultrasonography in esophageal diseases. Gastrointest Endosc 1989; 35:220–225.

5. Catalano MF, Van DJ, Sivak MJ. Malignant esophageal strictures: staging accuracy of endoscopic ultrasonography. Gastrointest Endosc 1995;41:535–539.

6. Hordijk ML, Kok TC, Wilson J, Mulder AH. Assessment of response of esophageal carcinoma to induction chemotherapy. Endoscopy 1993;25:592–596.

7. American Joint Committee on Cancer. Manual of staging of cancer. 5th ed. Philadelphia: Lippincott-Raven, 1997.

8. Hermanek P. pTNM and residual tumor classifications: problems of assessment and prognostic significance. World J Surg 1995;19:184–190.

9. Rosch TH, Classen M. A new ultrasonic probe for endosonographic imaging of the upper GI tract. Preliminary observations. Endoscopy 1990; 22:41–46.

10. Maruta S, Tsukamoto Y, Niwa Y, et al. Evaluation of upper gastrointestinal tumors with a new endoscopic ultrasound probe. Gastrointest Endosc 1994;40:603–608.

11. Frank N, Grieshammer B, Zimmermann W. A new miniature ultrasonic probe for gastrointestinal scanning: feasibility and preliminary results. Endoscopy 1994;26:603–608.

12. Yasuda K. Development and clinical use of ultrasonic probes. Endoscopy 1994;26:816–817.

13. Chak A, Canto M, Stenvens P, et al. Clinical applications of a new through-the-scope ultrasound probe: prospective comparison with an ultrasound endoscope. Gastroint Endoscopy 1997;45:291–295.

14. Hasegawa N, Niwa Y, Arisawa T, et al. Preoperative staging of superficial esophageal carcinoma: comparison of an ultrasound probe and standard endoscopic ultrasonography. Gastrointest Endosc 1996;44:388–393.

15. Yanai H, Yoshida T, Harada T, et al. Endoscopic ultrasonography of superficial esophageal cancers using a thin ultrasound probe system equipped with switchable radial and linear scanning modes. Gastrointest Endosc 1996;44:578–582.

16. Fockens P, Van DH, Tytgat G. Endosonography of stenotic esophageal carcinomas: preliminary experience with an ultra-thin, balloon-fitted ultrasound probe in four patients. Gastrointest Endosc 1994;40: 226–228.

17. Makuuchi, H. Endoscopic mucosal resection for early esophageal cancer. Dig Endosc 1996;8:175–179.

# 15

# Future Directions for Endoscopic Ultrasound: Interventional EUS

## Peter Vilmann
## Michael Bau Mortensen

The introduction of curved array echoendoscopes enabling direct ultrasonographic monitoring of instruments introduced through the working channel, has further stimulated the interest in interventional EUS. The use of endoscopic ultrasonography-guided fine-needle aspiration biopsy is now recognised as an integral part of the EUS examination in many clinical situations (1). Recently, instruments with larger instrument channels and an elevator for manipulation of accessories introduced via the instrument channel have become available (Figure 15-1). These instruments enable direct EUS monitoring of therapeutic procedures that use accessories other than biopsy needles. It is the aim of this chapter to describe the current status of interventional EUS procedures and to give some hints about future directions and applications of interventional EUS.

## Definitions

So far, there has been no specific attempt to define interventional EUS. However, to assess the different ways EUS can interact with various interventional procedures, it is helpful to define some of the terms used in conjunction with EUS-guided interventions.

*Interventional EUS* may be defined as a procedure where EUS, directly or indirectly, is used for monitoring of an invasive (interventional) procedure. An interventional EUS procedure can be either an *interventional diagnostic* procedure or an *interventional therapeutic* procedure (Table 15-1). *Directed, assisted, guided* and *aided* are some of the terms that have been used in conjunction with different interventional EUS procedures. However, these descriptions have been used independently whether the interventional procedure was di-

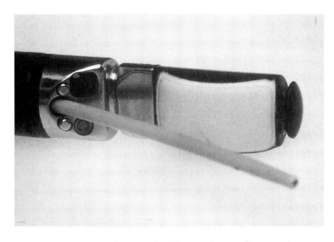

**Figure 15-1.** Distal end of a large channel curved array echoendoscope (Pentax FG-38 UA) with an endosprosthesis introduced via the biopsy channel. The working channel is 3.2 mm in diameter.

**Table 15-1.** Interventional endoscopic ultrasound

| | |
|---|---|
| 1. Diagnostic EUS | Fine-needle aspiration biopsy<br>Histological needle biopsy<br>Injection for diagnosis<br>Aspiration of fluid |
| 2. Therapeutic EUS | Injection<br>Drainage procedures<br>Resection of lesions<br>Tumor therapy |

rectly monitored on the ultrasound real-time image or whether EUS was performed in order to assist the interventional procedure without being able to monitor or visualize the procedure itself. Therefore, it seems reasonable to define two different ways of performing an EUS-guided intervention:

**Table 15-2.** Diagnostic endoscopic ultrasound intervention.

| | |
|---|---|
| 1. EUS-guided fine-needle aspiration biopsy | GI-tract lesions |
| | Lesions in extraluminal organs |
| | Lymph nodes |
| 2. EUS-guided histological needle biopsy | GI-tract lesions, extraluminal organs, lymph nodes |
| 3. EUS-guided injection for diagnosis | Cholangio-pancreatography, lymphography |
| 4. EUS-guided fluid aspiration | Pleural fluid, ascitic fluid, cardiac fluid, cyst fluid |

**Table 15-3.** Therapeutic endoscopic ultrasound intervention.

| | |
|---|---|
| 1. EUS-guided injection | Celiac plexus neurolysis |
| | Botulinum injection in achalasia |
| | Upper GI bleeding |
| | Steroid injection in refractory GI-tract strictures |
| 2. EUS-guided drainage procedures | Pancreatic cysto-gastrostomy or duodenostomy |
| | Hepaticogastrostomy |
| | Percutaneous endoscopic gastrostomy |
| 3. EUS-guided resection | Mucosal and submucosal lesions |
| 4. EUS-guided tumor therapy | HIFU, microwave coagulation (MCT), cyto-implantation |

1. *EUS-directed intervention:* A procedure where the entire intervention, or part of it, is directly and simultaneously monitored by endoscopic ultrasound.
2. *EUS-assisted intervention:* A procedure that requires the aid of endosonography to be completed. EUS can be performed either immediately before or simultaneously with the interventional procedure. However, the EUS-assisted intervention is not directly monitored by ultrasound.

A *diagnostic EUS intervention* may comprise either fine-needle aspiration biopsy, histological needle biopsy, fluid aspiration for diagnostic purposes, or injection of contrast agents, also for diagnostic purposes (Table 15-2).

A *therapeutic EUS intervention* may comprise either EUS-guided injection for therapeutic purposes, EUS-guided drainage procedures, EUS-guided resection of various lesions, or EUS-guided tumor therapy (Table 15-3).

## Interventional EUS for Diagnosis
### EUS-Guided Fine-Needle Aspiration Biopsy

It is now possible to obtain cytological material by endosonography-guided fine-needle aspiration biopsy from most lesions identified during EUS (1). Both lesions within the gastrointestinal wall itself as well as lesions lying adjacent to the wall may be punctured through the esophagus, stomach, duodenum, or via the rectum. The overall sensitivity for malignant disease has been reported to be in the range of 80% to 85% with a positive predictive value of 100% and an accuracy for all diagnoses between 80% and 90%. However, the overall accuracy is in part dependent on the

site of the lesion biopsied as well as its particular pathological characteristics (2).

EUS-guided biopsy is addressed in Chapter 13 of this book. However, a brief discussion of future directions of this technique, based on results from a recently published multicenter study (2), is presented in the following section.

### GI Tract Lesions

EUS-guided biopsy of lesions within the gastrointestinal wall seems to have the lowest diagnostic values and the highest rate of inconclusive biopsies. In a recently published multicenter study with 457 patients having 554 lesions biopsied, a total of 115 lesions were located within the GI wall (2). Twelve of these lesions were submucosal tumors with five arising from the esophagus and seven from the stomach. The accuracy of EUS-guided FNA cytology of submucosal tumors was 50%, with half of the biopsy specimens being inadequate. Regarding smooth-muscle tumors, a single case of leiomyosarcoma was missed, although cytology demonstrated spindle cells in four of seven cases. EUS FNA was performed in 103 lesions arising in the gastrointestinal wall exclusive of stromal tumors (esophagus 32, stomach 52, duodenum 10, rectum 9) with a sensitivity, specificity, PPV, NPV and accuracy of 61%, 79%, 100%, 76%, 67%, respectively. The sensitivity of diagnosing gastric non-Hodgkin's lymphoma (89%, 8/9) was greater than gastric adenocarcinoma (40%, 10/25). The accuracy of EUS FNA for mucosal lesions in the esophagus, stomach, duodenum, and rectum was 69%, 62%, 60%, and 100%, respectively. It seems, therefore, that diagnosis of submucosal lesions may be better approached by EUS-directed histological needle biopsy. Future studies will undoubtedly answer this question.

## Lesions in Extraluminal Organs: Lungs, Mediastinum, Liver, Adrenal, Spleen, and Pancreas

The results of EUS-guided FNA biopsy of extraintestinal mass lesions have been described in a multicenter study that included 139 patients with 145 lesions of which 40 were benign and 105 were malignant. The site of the tumors included the liver (n = 12), pancreas (n = 124), abdomen (n = 7), and pelvis (n = 2). Within the subgroup of patients with liver, abdominal, or pelvic masses, 6 benign and 13 malignant lesions underwent EUS FNA with a sensitivity, specificity, and accuracy of 100%. The diagnostic values for pancreatic masses demonstrated a sensitivity of 86%, a specificity of 94%, a PPV of 100%, an NPV of 86%, and an accuracy of 88%. Other studies have demonstrated a nearly 100% rate of diagnostic success for EUS-guided FNA in patients with lung cancer located in the mediastinum (3). Whether EUS-directed histological needle biopsy might add anything to the diagnosis of pancreatic cancer seems questionable.

## Lymph Nodes

One of the major advances of EUS-guided biopsy is in examining lymph nodes that are suspicious for malignancy. In the multicenter study described previously, EUS FNA was performed in 171 patients with a total of 192 lymph nodes. Forty-six lymph nodes were found to be benign on follow-up and 146 were malignant. The diagnostic success of EUS-guided FNA of lymph nodes demonstrated a sensitivity, specificity, PPV, NPV, and accuracy of 92%, 93%, 100%, 86%, and 92%, respectively.

Benign disorders presenting in lymph nodes may be diagnosed by EUS FNA as well. A few authors have demonstrated that histoplasmosis and sarcoidosis can be identified by this technique (2,4). Recently, we diagnosed tuberculosis in a patient with enlarged retroperitoneal lymph nodes on a CT scan. The patient was referred for EUS FNA due to a suspicion of lymphoma. Therefore, it seems that the indications of EUS-directed biopsy of lymph nodes may expand to also include benign diseases where lymph nodes are involved.

## *EUS-Guided Histological Needle Biopsy*

### GI Tract Lesions, Extraluminal Organs, and Lymph Nodes

Until recently, EUS-guided histological needle biopsy has been difficult due to lack of suitable biopsy needles and EUS instruments with sufficiently large instrument channels. A few preliminary studies, including only a few patients have been published, reflecting the above-mentioned technical problems (5–7). Most of the patients included in these studies have had submucosal lesions biopsied. In a few cases, EUS-directed histological tissue sampling of extraluminal masses such as pancreatic tumors or lymph nodes has been attempted (5).

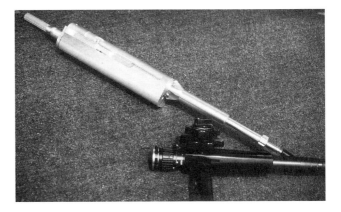

**Figure 15-2.** A prototype automated histological shutgun biopsy handle (Medi-Globe/GIP Medizin Technik) mounted on the biopsy channel inlet of a large channel echoendoscope (Pentax FG-38 UA).

Some of the technical limitations have been removed with the recent introduction of new EUS instruments with larger instrument channels, and new biopsy needle designs will soon be available (Figure 15-2). However, not all problems concerning EUS-guided tissue sampling may be solved with these developments. It is to be expected that larger needle diameters will increase the complication rate of EUS-guided biopsy, and the applications of EUS-guided histological biopsy may therefore be limited to fewer indications than expected. There is not much doubt that the diagnosis of mesenchymal tumors requires histological tissue sampling, but other indications for use of EUS-guided biopsy should be carefully established in the setting of well-controlled and clinically relevant trials.

## *EUS-Guided Injection for Diagnosis*

### CholangioPancreatography and Lymphography

It is relatively easy to define the pancreatic duct and the common bile duct with EUS. As a consequence, it is possible to inject contrast material into the common bile duct, the pancreatic duct, or even directly into lymph nodes outlined by EUS (8–12). The studies published to date are case studies involving only a few patients. As might be expected, this innovative technique has been used exclusively in patients in whom other more traditional methods such as ERCP or a standard percutaneous approach have failed. Wiersema was able to perform a successful EUS-directed ductography in 8 out of 11 patients in whom ERCP had been unsuccessful (11). The EUS-directed puncture of the CBD was performed either via the duodenal bulb or the second part of the duodenum, whereas the pancreatic duct was approached via the stomach. Further investigation is needed to define the risks and success rate of this new procedure.

A single author has reported on EUS-directed lymphography in a few patients in order to see whether

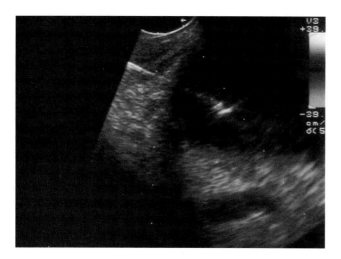

**Figure 15-3.** Endoscopic ultrasound image demonstrating guided aspiration of ascites. Echoes from the needle can be seen as the needle traverses the stomach wall. The needle tip is visualized in the echo-poor ascitic fluid. During aspiration, fluid flow at the needle tip can be seen by color Doppler imaging.

contrast enhanced lymphography may resolve the problems of false negative cancer diagnoses by EUS FNA of lymph nodes (12). No conclusion on this very preliminary study can be made, but the possibility of EUS-directed injection into even small lymph nodes underlines the potential of this technique.

### EUS-Guided Aspiration of Fluid

Aspiration and examination of pleural and ascitic fluid can reveal advanced disease in upper gastrointestinal tract cancer, but aspiration of cystic or cardiac fluid may also provide clinically important information in benign diseases. The anechoic ultrasonographic appearance of even small amounts of pleural, cardiac, and ascitic fluid is easily recognized on endoscopic ultrasonographic images. Extraluminal relationships allow the fluid to be distinguished from cystic lesions and by using color Doppler, blood vessels and lymphatic channels can be excluded. The EUS FNA aspiration technique of (thin) fluid is simple and often easier than obtaining adequate cytology during EUS FNAB (Figure 15-3). Preliminary data suggest that EUS-guided aspiration may reveal a diagnosis of malignant pleural and ascitic fluid and thereby change therapeutic strategy (13–17), but there are still some unanswered questions. EUS can detect very small amounts of fluid, which cannot be detected by CT (15) or percutaneous ultrasound, but is this fluid of clinical relevance? Second, but perhaps more important, the risk of seeding cancer cells during EUS-guided aspiration of fluid has not been evaluated. So far, there have been no reports of malignant seeding following EUS FNAB of lymph nodes, but some of these cases may

have been overlooked due to later resection of the area in question, or because the patients died of disseminated disease before the development of local problems following tumor seeding. If EUS-directed fluid aspiration through an endosonographically normal GI wall is planned, careful flushing of the needle and catheter during insertion and immediate suction may reduce the risk of malignant seeding (14), but patient selection for this technique must consider the potential risks of the procedure.

Nevertheless, in theory, there are no limitations to fluid aspiration in areas accessible to EUS FNA. For example, analysis of fluid from pancreatic cystic lesions obtained by EUS-guided aspiration has been helpful in the diagnosis of mucinous pancreatic neoplasms (17). Aspiration of gallbladder contents, diagnosis of abscesses, diagnosis and analysis of cardiac effusions, and characterization of malignant pleural effusion in primary lung cancer could also become routine uses of EUS-guided aspiration in the future, and the diagnostic and therapeutic benefits over existing methods is potentially dramatic.

## Interventional EUS for Therapy
### EUS-Guided Injection
#### Celiac Plexus Neurolysis
There is increasing evidence that celiac plexus neurolysis (CPN) in patients with carcinoma of pancreatic origin (19–21), and to a lesser extent, in patients with chronic pancreatitis, is of value (22). The superior staging and resectability assessment demonstrated by EUS in patients with pancreatic cancer, have already made EUS and EUS FNAB an important first-line imaging technique in these patients. As the majority of these patients will have nonresectable disease, and many of them also develop intractable pain, it is natural to consider performing an analgesic procedure such as EUS-directed CPN (EUS CPN), immediately after staging EUS is completed.

EUS CPN can be performed through a standard curved array echoendoscope (e.g., Pentax FG-32UA) with the same needle that is used for EUS FNAB. Following oropharyngeal anesthesia and intravenous sedation, as in a standard EUS staging procedure, the echoendoscope is advanced into the stomach. After the celiac axis has been identified (Figure 15-4) and positioned at the center of the ultrasound screen, the echoendoscope is advanced slightly and turned to the right until the celiac axis disappears, but the aorta is still visible. The needle is advanced into a position close to the aortic wall and a few ml of Bupivacaine is injected with careful endosonographic control, while at the same time monitoring the patient's level of pain. During injection of Bupivacaine a clear Doppler signal can be seen (Figure 15-5), and the area around

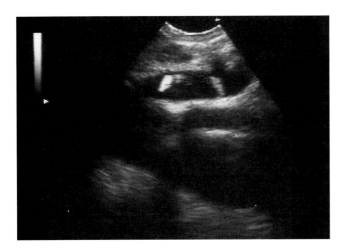

**Figure 15-4.** Endoscopic ultrasound image of the aorta visualized in the longitudinal plane. The coeliac axis is seen with color Doppler flow. The superior mesenteric artery is seen below the coeliac axis.

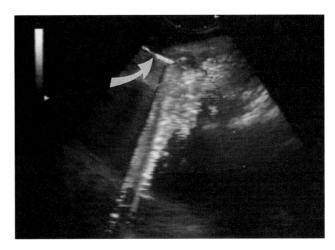

**Figure 15-5.** EUS-guided celiac plexus neurolysis. The transducer has been turned to the right. The needle echo can be seen traversing the stomach wall (*arrow*). The needle tip is positioned close to the aortic wall and a clear color Doppler signal is observed as the Bupivacaine is injected.

the needle tip becomes hyperechoic. After a few minutes, approximately 10 ml of absolute alcohol is injected at the same site. The procedure is then repeated on the left side of the aorta. Obviously, it is absolutely essential that the patient is exceptionally well sedated and remains calm and can lie motionless (patient may breathe normally) until the injections are completed.

Wiersema et al. performed EUS CPN in 30 patients with pain due to intra-abdominal malignancies. By injecting 3 ml of Bupivacaine followed by 10 ml of absolute alcohol on each side they were able to obtain a reduced pain score for a median follow-up of 10 weeks, and the procedures were performed on an outpatient basis (23,24). They also noted that patients with M1 disease had higher initial pain scores and a greater decline in pain scores after therapy patients with M0 disease.

A prospective study randomized 22 patients with chronic pancreatitis to either EUS CPN (n = 14) or CT-guided CPN (n = 8). Using 10 ml Bupivacaine followed by 3 ml triamcinolone on both sides, pre- and post-therapy pain scores were compared using the visual analogue scale (VAS). Forty-three percent of the patients in the EUS CPN group became pain free, with a mean post-procedure follow-up of 6 weeks. In comparison, only 25% of the patients in the CT-guided CPN group were pain free during a mean follow-up of 4 weeks. Also, although 15% in the EUS CPN group had persistent benefit after 12 weeks, none of the patients in the CT-guided group had persistent relief beyond 4 weeks (25). A subsequent cost comparison demonstrated EUS CPN to be less expensive than CT-guided CPN. Accumulated data on 90 patients treated in the same way showed similar results, and regression analysis suggested that patients who were younger than 45 years of age and those with a prior history of pancreatic surgery were unlikely to respond to EUS

CPN (26). These and other observations (27) indicate that pain related to chronic pancreatitis can be treated with EUS CPN, and as these patients represent a considerable therapeutic as well as economic burden to the health care system, the beneficial effects of the technique may be substantial. However, these patients also represent a very heterogeneous group with a variety of somatic complaints, other preexisting medical conditions, and several different psychiatric diagnoses. Under such circumstances, defining a group for study is difficult and proper patient selection for both control and treatment cohorts is mandatory.

Refining the technical aspects of EUS CPN (sequence of injections, substances, concentrations, needle type, and so forth) will require results from large, controlled studies, but EUS-directed application of some form of local anesthesia followed by injection of a potent cytotoxic agent makes common sense.

Only one complication (a peripancreatic abscess) has been attributed to EUS CPN (26). Furthermore, there have been no reports of damage to the wall of the aorta or the celiac trunk following injection of different substances. Minor episodes of hypotension during the injection procedure were reported by Wiersema et al. (23), but these cases responded well to saline infusion. The most prominent complication seen during immediate follow-up was transient diarrhea, probably due to neural release following injection of the celiac ganglion (23,25–27).

Practically speaking, a convincing argument can be made to support the use of EUS CPN rather than conventional percutaneous methods for chronic pain: the delivery/puncture route for EUS is short and the anatomical representation of the celiac area achievable with endosonography is unequalled by any other modality. (28,29). Some of the more severe potential complications (total or partial motor paralysis, paraplegia, pneumothorax, aortic dissection, and pseudoaneurysm) may be avoided by using the anterior approach (22,23). By mixing the injected substance with contrast during EUS CPN it has been demonstrated that the injected fluid remains in the anterior para-aortic region, thus avoiding the pleura, the spinal arteries, and the retro-crural space (23,27). Fluoroscopic guidance might provide an additional safety margin for the patient.

At this time, it is reasonable to conclude that EUS CPN, when performed by experienced endosonographers, is a safe and efficient procedure, but many additional studies are needed.

### Botulinum Injection in Achalasia

Achalasia is a motor disorder of the esophagus characterized by aperistalsis and an elevated lower esophageal sphincter (LES) pressure with incomplete relaxation after swallowing. In achalasia, a loss of ganglion cells within the myenteric plexus of the LES and destruction of the ganglion cells and postganglionic neurons that facilitate relaxation of the LES is seen. Accepted treatment for this disorder has been pharmacotherapy, balloon dilation of the LES, and surgical myotomy. Recently, injection of botulinum toxin into the LES during endoscopy has been reported as an effective and safe treatment, with a short-term symptomatic improvement of 90%, but apparently with lower sustained response at 6 months. It has been argued that treatment failure in some patients may be because a substantial portion of the dose of botulinum toxin is not delivered into the LES because the technique of delivery is "blind" (30). The LES can be accurately visualized by EUS as an echo-poor structure in the lower esophageal wall, and when using high-frequency transducers even the longitudinal and the circular anatomy of the muscle layer of the esophagus may be seen (31–36). Several authors have reported on the use of EUS in patients with achalasia, and preliminary data suggest that the LES may be thickened in these patients (30–36). A few studies have described the use of EUS-directed injection of botulinum toxin selectively into the LES in patients with achalasia (30,31,35). The authors suggest that needle placement with EUS guidance ensures that the entire toxin is injected into the LES rather than the surrounding esophageal area. However, because the exact mechanism by which botulinum toxin injection into the LES aids patients with achalasia is not known, the use of EUS in this situation should still be considered investigational.

### Injection Therapy in Upper GI Bleeding

The identification and treatment of upper gastrointestinal bleeding (UGIB) is usually performed by standard

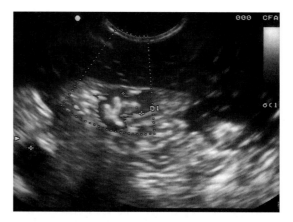

**Figure 15-6.** Power Doppler examination of a 1-cm submucosal hemangioma in the stomach wall in a patient with Osler's disease. The patient was successfully treated by EUS-guided injection with total eradication judged by loss of the Doppler signal.

endoscopy, but the task can prove troublesome in cases without distinct mucosal lesions or if endoscopic vision is reduced by massive bleeding. After having obtained hemostasis there is still a risk of rebleeding and it is often difficult to identify which patients are at the greatest risk of a new bleeding episode. Although the treatment and outcome may be different for UGIB caused by an ulcer, gastroesophageal varices, Dieulafoy's lesion, or aortoduodenal fistulas, the problems associated with endoscopic diagnosis and therapy are similar. The search for improved sclerotherapy techniques and systemic agents to aid endoscopists has been intensive and, as a consequence, EUS-guided therapy has also been evaluated in patients presenting with UGIB.

We have used EUS-directed sclerotherapy in UGIB when standard endoscopic therapy has failed. The same EUS method was used for ulcer bleeding, variceal bleeding, and bleeding from a Dieulafoy's lesion (Figure 15-6). First, if active bleeding was present the balloon of the curved array echoendoscope was used to slightly compress the suspected bleeding site, if possible. While slowly releasing pressure with close examination of the color Doppler signal, we then examined the wall for small calibre vessels. If a positive signal was identified, 5 ml of Polidocanol was then injected in different areas, as close as possible to the vessel, until the Doppler signal disappeared. After a few minutes, the area was reexamined and retreated if a Doppler signal redeveloped. EUS follow-up after two days revealed a hyperechoic area at the injection site, but no visible vessels.

Successful hemostasis has been observed using this technique, and similar observations have been made with radial EUS-assisted injection therapy in Dieulafoy's disease (37). Both miniprobes and echoendoscopes seem capable of locating a Dieulafoy lesion, but EUS-directed therapy has been described only with the echoendoscope (37,38). Miniprobes have also been used for assisting a conventional sclerotherapeutic procedure in ulcer patients: Kohler and Riemann were able to demonstrate superficial blood vessels in the ulcer base in 62% of 106 cases of acute ulcer bleeding. If these patients had sclerotherapy until the Doppler signal disappeared, a rebleeding rate of only 8% was observed (39,40). Another German group reported similar results in a smaller study (41), and also demonstrated the use of this technique in bleeding colorectal angiodysplasias (42).

There are no data available comparing directed with assisted sclerotherapy or comparing miniprobes with standard echoendoscopes. A possible explanation for the limited focus on EUS in acute ulcer bleeding may be the lack of available EUS equipment and expertise on short notice at the time when these patients need emergency endoscopy.

There has been considerable interest in the evaluation of varices by EUS, but whether EUS offers any genuine added benefit is unclear (43). Catalano and his group made some very interesting observations when comparing EUS-assisted sclerotherapy with band ligation in esophageal varices; in a small study of 14 patients, EUS-assisted sclerotherapy required significantly fewer sessions to achieve variceal obliteration, decreased the rate of rebleeding and mortality from recurrent variceal bleeding (44). Logistical problems with EUS-directed therapy in acute variceal bleeding are similar to those of acute ulcer bleeding and represent a significant handicap to application of EUS in this area.

## Steroid Injection in Refractory GI Tract Strictures

Endoscopic ultrasound miniprobe-assisted steroid injection in patients with refractory esophageal strictures has been reported recently in a preliminary study (45). In three patients not responding to dilation and subsequent blind injection of triamcinolone acetonide (40 mg/ml), a 12.5-MHz radial scanning miniprobe (Microvasive, Boston Scientific Corp.) was passed through a standard endoscope in order to examine the most optimal site of steroid injection. The thickness of the esophageal wall was measured during the ultrasonic examination along the entire length of the stricture and the distance from the incisors to the most thickened area was recorded. After dilation of the stricture, 0.5 ml aliquots of steroid solution were injected in each of four quadrants at the thickest site of the stricture as judged by endosonography. All three patients had symptomatic improvement but no long-term results are yet available. It should be noted that there are no controlled studies to date demonstrating that steroid injection is of any benefit in patients with benign esophageal strictures.

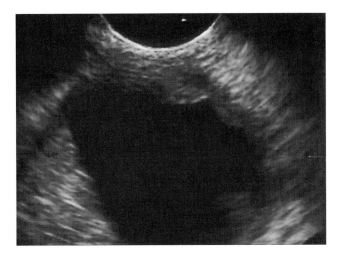

**Figure 15-7.** EUS image of a 3-cm anechoic pseudocyst in the tail of the pancreas. The scan is from the body of the stomach wall.

## EUS-Guided Drainage Procedures

### Pancreatic Cystogastrostomy or Duodenostomy

Endoscopically placed cystogastrostomy is a well-described alternative to surgical treatment of pancreatic pseudocysts. However, even in selected patients with an endoscopically visible bulge in the gastric or duodenal wall caused by the cyst, the technique has some limitations due to potential puncture of vessels interposed between the cyst and the gastric wall. EUS allows exact assessment of the cyst anatomy, including its location, possible feeding duct, and content, as well as the shortest path between the gastric or duodenal wall and the cyst (Figure 15-7). Thus, the most optimal puncture site can be selected and puncture of interposed vessels avoided (46–57). The initial endosonographic evaluation can be done using either a radial or curved array echoendoscope. A through-the-scope ultrasound catheter has also been used for pseudocyst localization in a patient without endoluminal bulging of the cyst (53). The current opinion is, however, that a curved array echoendoscope is preferable because of the possibility of direct real-time endosonographic guidance of the procedure, and because of its Doppler facilities, which may limit complications by preventing hemorrhage (48–49).

Three slightly different ways of endosonographically guided cystogastrostomy have been described. In one method the optimal site for cyst puncture is found by EUS-guided forceps marking of the mucosa (54). Subsequent stent placement is then performed "semiblindly" using the standard endoscopic approach. This technique must be considered to be EUS-assisted. In the second method, the pancreatic pseudocyst is punctured under direct endosonographic guidance (EUS-directed

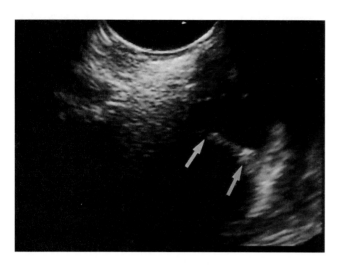

**Figure 15-8.** EUS-directed cystogastrostomy. The cystogastrostomy was created by means of a burning wire tip and the endoprosthesis was released entirely guided by endosonography. (*Arrows* = burning wire with the endoprosthesis.)

puncture) using a diathermy needle housed in a plastic catheter (47,49). Once inside the pseudocyst, the diathermy needle inside the catheter is replaced with a guide wire. The echoendoscope is then withdrawn and a large channel duodenoscope is inserted to perform an over-the-wire insertion of the endoprosthesis. A major drawback of both techniques is the need to exchange the ultrasound endoscope with a standard endoscope to allow introduction of an endoprosthesis of sufficient caliber.

In a case report, Wiersema described a completely EUS-directed cyst-duodenostomy procedure with a curved array ultrasound endoscope (52). A standard echoendoscope (Pentax 36 FG-UX) with a 2.4-mm instrument channel was used for placement of a 6 Fr endoprosthesis introduced over a guide wire after dilatation of the cyst duodenostomy site created by needle-knife puncture. We have recently tested a new EUS endoscope with a large instrument channel of 3.2 mm in diameter (Pentax FG 38 UX) (Figure 15-1). This channel allows the introduction of an 8.5 Fr endoprosthesis, which we feel is the minimal acceptable stent size for drainage of a pancreatic pseudocyst (58). With this instrument we were able to perform EUS-directed insertion of a stent with full ultrasonic monitoring of the procedure and without exchange of endoscopes (Figure 15-8). Thus, EUS-assisted or directed cystogastrostomy or duodenostomy is a possible alternative to conventional drainage procedures, and preliminary experience suggests that the technique is both safe and effective.

**HepaticoGastrostomy**
EUS-directed hepaticogastrostomy to palliate obstructive jaundice has been described in pigs on an experi-

mental basis (59). The common bile duct was ligated laparoscopically in five pigs. When the animals became jaundiced, a Pentax FG-32 UA linear array endoscope and a 22-gauge GIP/Medi-Globe needle was used to perform EUS-guided hepaticogastrostomy. In all cases, cholangiogram was obtained with the needle and a guide wire was passed into the biliary system under fluoroscopic control. A dilating catheter was then introduced and the needle tract was dilated over the guide wire, and a 5 Fr polyethylene, double pigtail biliary stent was deployed between the peripheral intrahepatic left biliary system and the stomach. The procedure was successfully completed in three animals, but in two animals technical problems were encountered. In two of these three cases, bilirubin normalized within 48 hours. The study concludes that biliary decompression can be obtained by EUS-guided hepaticogastrostomy, without causing significant intraperitoneal bleeding or bile leaks. Whether this procedure could be applied to humans is not known.

**Percutaneous Endoscopic Gastrostomy**
Endoscopic ultrasound-assisted placement of a percutaneous endoscopic gastrostomy tube (PEG) in an obese patient has been described in a single case study (60). In this patient, transillumination of the abdominal wall by a standard endoscope could not be achieved. A radial scanning ultrasound endoscope (Olympus, GF-UM20) was used to image the anterior abdominal wall from the stomach. The anatomy of the stomach wall layers and the echogenic abdominal wall adipose tissue were clearly seen. The optimal position for placement of the PEG tube was confirmed by both the visual and endoscopic ultrasound appearance of the proposed tract. The ultrasound image of a finger depressing the abdominal wall from outside the patient was demonstrated. No intervening bowel loops or liver parenchyma were seen, and this site was used for endoscopic PEG placement. Whether this technique may avoid the feared complication of perforation of interposed intestines is an open question.

## EUS-Guided Resection

Endoscopic resection (ER) of elevated mucosal and submucosal lesions in the upper gastrointestinal tract has become an attractive alternative to open surgery. Immediate recovery from an inexpensive and complete endoscopic procedure is highly cost effective compared to surgery and has obvious patient acceptance. However, problems with perforation and bleeding, and in cancer patients the crucial question of radicality, have reduced the initial enthusiasm. Following the introduction of dedicated echoendoscopes and EUS miniprobes, ER gained favor. At least theoretically, EUS might outline the lesions in question, and thereby aid the clinical de-

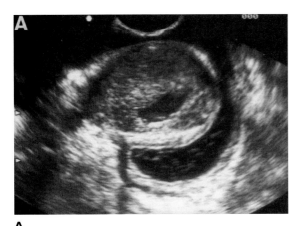

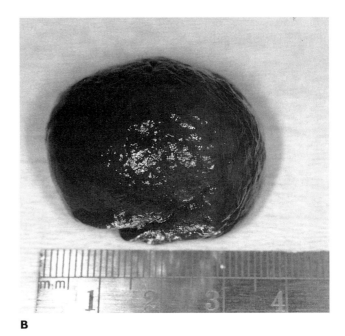

**Figure 15-9.** Leiomyoma in the stomach wall treated by EUS-assisted endoscopic resection. (A) EUS image of a 3.5-cm leiomyoma in the stomach wall. The transducer is placed in water in the stomach. (B) Photograph of the leiomyoma after endoscopic resection with normal gastric mucosa overlying the lesion.

cision as to whether ER is possible or not based on size, intramural location, and the location of interposed small caliber vessels. EUS can monitor the ER procedure by guiding the submucosal injection prior to resection (or decide that this is not necessary), and monitor the resection itself and the immediate follow-up after resection.

The ER technique can be performed with the use of EUS in several ways:

1. Initial endosonographic assessment with either a miniprobe or a standard echoendoscope is performed to determine whether ER can be successfully achieved.
2. A solution to elevate the lesion (saline, glycerine, epinephrine, etc.) is injected immediately after EUS evaluation (61–66), or via the echoendoscope under EUS direction using an EUS FNAB needle.
3. Following adequate elevation of the lesion, which may be monitored with EUS, the lesion is removed with an electro-cautery snare (65,67–69), or ligated using a band ligating device (61,64) prior to resection. The latter has been used in order to reduce the risk of bleeding, and in order to obtain EUS evidence that the mucosal layer was cleanly separated from the muscular layer prior to resection. A combination of injection and band ligation prior to ER has also been described (61,62)
4. Finally, EUS can monitor the area of resection as part of endoscopic follow-up (65).

EUS-assisted ER has been used for both benign and malignant lesions of the upper GI tract. Although the clinical impact of EUS-assisted ER in benign lesions

may be controversial (62), the procedure seems safe and applicable for many different lesions, including gastric adenoma (64), leiomyoma (61,62,70), gastrinoma (61,62), hemangioma (63) and lymphangioma (69). In these reports, lesions up to 15 mm in diameter have been removed by EUS-guided ER; however, the average reported specimen size was about 10 mm (61–70). If band ligation was used as part of the ER procedure, the diameter of the ligating device determined the maximal size of a lesion that could be removed. Our own experience with EUS-assisted endoscopic removal of submucosal tumors has allowed us to resect three leiomyomas and one leiomyosarcoma ranging from 3 to 4 cm in size without any complications (Figure 15-9). Tactile assessment of the tumor during initial EUS study as well as its relation to the proper muscle layer of the stomach wall is an added benefit of this technique.

Observations regarding EUS-assisted ER of malignant lesions have focused on early gastric cancer. Treating a malignant disease with local therapy is controversial, because inadequate treatment may reduce what would have been the high likelihood of cure with a surgical approach. Clearly, careful patient selection is absolutely essential. Based on a retrospective study, pretherapy EUS has a sensitivity and a specificity of 93% and 86%, respectively, for appropriate patient selection (67). Unfortunately, EUS failed to detect lymph node metastases in two patients (3%), but both patients had submucosal tumor infiltration on EUS and were not considered candidates for ER. The specificity regarding lymph node staging was 93% in the same study. Whether EUS FNAB has a role in the staging of early gastric cancer is unknown. Staging of these lesions can be performed with miniprobes as well as standard echoendoscopes (64–67). The results obtained in early gastric cancer following EUS-guided ER varies; whereas EUS seems able to select patients for ER, the presence of ulcerative changes makes the differentiation between mucosal and submucosal infiltration difficult (67). In addition, lack of radicality in horizontal direction of the specimen has been observed (64). Saline injection under direct endosonographic guidance has not been evaluated, but might add to the accuracy and safety of ER.

### EUS-Guided Tumor Therapy

The superior diagnostic and staging results reported by using EUS in patients with upper gastrointestinal tract cancer (UGIM) is largely due to the close proximity of the transducer to the tumor itself and the surrounding structures in the retroperitoneum and mediastinum. EUS has reduced the need for futile exploratory laparotomies (71) but has also focused attention on the large group of UGIM patients who have disseminated or unresectable disease at the time of EUS examination. Unfortunately, the therapeutic (palliative) options in these patients have not advanced significantly in the last decade. The search for more effective treatment strategies, including new techniques for directed tumor destruction, have intensified, and following the introduction of EUS FNAB, EUS-directed tumor therapy seems to be, at least in theory, a new option for more intensive and accurate targeted therapy. EUS-directed tumor therapy can be applied to the primary tumor (e.g., liver, pancreas, stomach), to malignant lymph nodes, or to metastases within the liver parenchyma. Because EUS-directed therapy is still experimental, the comments that follow do not refer to any specific anatomical areas, but offer a general appraisal of the technical possibilities and limitations that currently exist for this approach.

Local tumor destruction can be induced in several ways (Table 15-4), but most of them have definite technical limitations with regard to their current use in EUS-directed therapy.

Recently Chang et al. published their preliminary data from a phase I clinical trial using EUS-directed immunotherapy. The study demonstrated that local cytoimplantation was possible using EUS, but their conclusions regarding clinical utility require confirmation (72). The technique of simple injection of a toxic solution with the EUS FNAB needle has no immediate technical problems, but the pattern of distribution (diffusion) of the applied solution within the tumor is unknown. Percutaneous ultrasound-guided injection of absolute alcohol into hepatic carcinomas less than 50 mm in diameter has demonstrated increased patient survival when compared with surgery (73), but EUS-guided alcohol therapy for malignant disease has not

**Table 15-4.** Different methods for local tumor destruction.

Chemotherapy
Radiotherapy
Alcohol injection
Laser
Cryotherapy
Electrocautery
Microwave Coagulation Therapy (MCT)
High Intensity Focused Ultrasound tissue ablation (HIFU)

yet been tested. For large liver lesions, EUS would probably be inferior to the percutaneous route. Ultrasound-guided radiotherapy by implantation of radioactive seeds has been used for treatment of prostate cancer, but if this technique were adapted for EUS-directed tumor therapy, it would require the development of a shielded delivery system—a difficult goal given the size of the available working echoendoscope channels. Tio and colleagues have reported on one patient with anal carcinoma who was successfully treated with EUS-guided interstitial 192Ir implant (74).

Hyperthermic tumor therapy is possible using Neodymium YAG laser coagulation, electrocautery, or microwaves (see following paragraph), and cryoprobes with circulating nitrogen can create an ovoid freezing zone around the tip of the probe (75). All three methods have been used for local tumor destruction, but special devices for EUS-directed therapy are not available. An EUS-guided radiofrequency ablation technique has been recently tested in a porcine model (76). The authors were able to show that EUS could deliver predictable foci of coagulation within the pancreas, but no data on the risk of pancreatitis was provided.

Microwave coagulation therapy (MCT) is effective in the treatment of (small) liver tumors either with percutaneous ultrasound guidance or during laparoscopic ultrasonography (LUS) (77–79). The LUS-guided procedure has been performed under local anesthesia using a 1.6-mm thick microwave electrode (78). The MCT produced a clear echogenic area with an acoustic shadow, which could be seen easily during LUS. If the electrode (antenna) could be made long enough for the echoendoscope and still have sufficient rigidity to work like the EUS FNAB needle, it would be possible to perform EUS-directed MCT (80), and this could also be of clinical interest for ablation of nonhepatic tumors or malignant adenopathy.

High-intensity focused ultrasound (HIFU) represents a noninvasive method for inducing focal tissue destruction, but until recently the HIFU transducers were too large to be relevant for use with flexible endoscopes. Small HIFU transducers have been used in rabbits (81); the smallest probe had a width of only 11 mm, and could be mounted on a standard duodenoscope. The HIFU transducer consisted of two concentric elements, in which the central element was used like an A-mode scanner to control tissue depth after each "shot." By applying 66 pulses of 7.5W each for 4.5 seconds at five-second intervals, it was possible to obtain necrosis within the liver when the probe was used through the stomach wall (81). A major drawback to the use of HIFU in the upper GI tract is constant motion caused by gut peristalsis and respiration, which limits the ability to induce larger necrotic volumes with a mobile transducer. However, the use of an endoluminal HIFU system that uses longer ultrasound pulses and relies on local thermal diffusion and spontaneous tissue motion may be able to safely generate larger areas of tumor necrosis during a single treatment session. The combination of a highly accurate diagnostic imaging instrument with a noninvasive therapeutic tool is promising, and at present is perhaps the most interesting area of future development of EUS-directed tumor therapy.

## Conclusion

Many of the techniques described in this chapter are at an experimental stage. Larger trials are mandatory to provide evidence of their potential superiority when compared to other (conventional) diagnostic and treatment modalities. Some of the techniques reported here will undoubtedly disappear due to the introduction of better conventional imaging techniques or superior treatment modalities, but rapid progress is being made to overcome some of the remaining technical limitations of EUS. A larger working channel is essential for the future development of interventional EUS, because it will enable the use of larger and more sophisticated treatment and drug delivery systems. The present 3.2-mm working channel of a so-called large channel echoendoscope (Pentax FG-38 UX) allows the placement of an 8.5 Fr. endoprosthesis, but much work lies ahead, especially regarding further development of accessories for specific interventional EUS procedures. For example, EUS may replace ERCP as a less invasive diagnostic tool in several clinical settings, and by employing a larger working channel, routine tasks such as stenting of bile ducts and stone extraction currently limited to ERCP may become the domain of EUS.

Other innovative applications, including three-dimensional imaging using endosonographic instruments, are also on the horizon.

Future research in interventional EUS should probably meet a few basic, but important criteria:

- Terminology and definitions should be stringent in order not to confuse EUS-*directed* with EUS-*assisted* procedures.
- Prospective assessment of clinical outcomes and cost-effectiveness analyses are needed. The general lack of true EUS outcome studies has already been

noted (82), and cost-effectiveness evaluation is especially important for EUS, because it presents a radically different alternative to conventional therapy such as surgery. Reimbursement by third-party payors depends in large part on proving that, at the very least, EUS does not increase costs of medical care for certain diagnostic categories.
- Studies comparing EUS-directed/assisted procedures with established endoscopic therapeutic modalities (e.g., sclerotherapy for bleeding esophageal varices) must include sufficient patients and be statistically valid. Many therapeutic procedures can be performed during standard endoscopy and the addition of EUS may not necessarily improve outcome.
- Close follow-up and evaluation of patients undergoing interventional EUS in order to establish possible complications and potential contraindications is mandatory.

Interventional EUS is not a task for beginners in endosonography. As was true for interventional ERCP, formal or informal training standards are needed to define competence in interventional EUS and the technique itself must be used more widely to reduce the complication rate to as close to zero as possible. Defining the number of diagnostic and staging EUS studies completed independently by a fellow that meets the consensus for competency may be a first step in that process.

EUS and EUS FNAB have become important tools in modern gastroenterology and hepatology, but they are still in their infancy. In the years ahead, interventional EUS techniques will undoubtedly become a commonplace technique, combining the benefits of endoscopy and ultrasound and advancing a synergistic step forward in patient care.

### References

1. Vilmann P. Endoscopic ultrasonography with curved array transducer in diagnosis of cancer in and adjacent to the upper gastrointestinal tract—scanning and guided fine needle aspiration biopsy. Munksgaard 1998. Diss. 1–232.
2. Wiersema MJ, Vilmann P, Giovannini M, et al. Endosonography-guided fine needle aspiration biopsy: diagnostic accuracy and complication assessment. Gastroenterology 1997;112:1087–1095.
3. Pedersen BH, Vilmann P, Folke K, Jacobsen GK, et al. Endoscopic ultrasonography and real-time guided fine needle aspiration biopsy of solid lesions of the mediastinum suspected of malignancy. Chest 1996;110:539–544.
4. Wiersema MJ, Chak A, Wiersema LM. Mediastinal histoplasmosis: evaluation with endosonography and endoscopic fine needle aspiration biopsy. Gastrointest Endosc 1994;40:78–81.
5. Binmoeller KF, Thul R, Rathod V, et al. Endoscopic ultrasound-guided, 18-gauge, fine needle aspiration biopsy of the pancreas using a 2.8 mm channel convex

array echoendoscope. Gastrointest Endosc 1998;47:121–127.

6. Binmoeller KF, Jabusch HC, Seifert H, Soehendra N. Endosonography-guided fine needle biopsy of indurated pancreatic lesions using an automated biopsy device. Endoscopy 1997;29:384–388.

7. Harada N, Kouzu T, Arima M, Isono K. Endoscopic ultrasound-guided histologic needle biopsy. Endoscopy 1996;28:S47. Abstract.

8. Koito K, Nagakawa T, Murashima Y, et al. Endoscopic ultrasonographic-guided punctured pancreatic ductography: an initial and successful trial. Abdom Imag 1995;20:222–224.

9. Harada N, Kouzu T, Arima M, et al. Endoscopic ultrasound-guided pancreatography: a case report. Endoscopy 1995;27:612–615.

10. Gress F, Ikenberry S, Sherman S, Lehman G. Endoscopic ultrasound-directed pancreatography. Gastrointest Endosc 1996;44:736–739.

11. Wiersema MJ, Sandusky D, Carr R, et al. Endosonography-guided cholangiopancreatography. Gastrointest Endosc 1996;43:102–106.

12. Kojima S, Goto H, Hirooka Y, et al. Contrast echolymphography using EUS-guided puncture. 11th International Symposium on Endoscopic Ultrasonography, Kyoto, Japan 1998:P55. Abstract.

13. Chang KJ, Nguyen P, Erickson RA, et al. The clinical utility of endoscopic ultrasound (EUS) guided fine needle aspiration (FNA)—the UCI experience. Gastrointest Endosc 1996;43:S56. Abstract.

14. Chang KJ, Albers CG, Nguyen P. Endoscopic ultrasound-guided fine needle aspiration of pleural and ascitic fluid. Am J Gastroenterol 1995;90:148–150.

15. Nguyen P, Rezvani F, Chang KJ. Endoscopic ultrasound (EUS) and EUS-guided thoracocentesis of pleural fluid. DDW 1997:3380.

16. Canto M, Gislason G. Is extraluminal fluid (EFLUID) at endoscopic ultrasonography (EUS) an accurate marker of peritoneal carcinomatosis (PC)?: a prospective study. Gastrointest Endosc 1998;47:AB142. Abstract.

17. Nguyen P, Le J, Chang KJ. A large series of patients with ascites on endoscopic ultrasound (EUS). Gastrointest Endosc 1998;47:AB151. Abstract.

18. Mallery S, Quirk D, Lewandrowski K, et al. EUS-guided FNA with cyst fluid analysis in pancreatic cystic lesions. Gastrointest Endosc 1998;47:AB149. Abstract.

19. Polati E, Finco G, Gottin L, et al. Prospective randomized double-blind trial of neurolytic coeliac plexus block in patients with pancreatic cancer. Br J Surg 1998;85:199–201.

20. Lillemoe KD, Cameron JL, Kaufman HS, et al. Chemical splanchniectomy in patients with unresectable pancreatic cancer. A prospective randomized trial. Ann Surg 1993;217:447–457.

21. Eisenberg E, Carr DB, Chalmers TC. Neurolytic celiac plexus block for treatment of cancer pain: a meta-analysis. Anseth Analg 1995;80:290–295.

22. Fugere F, Lewis G. Coeliac plexus block for chronic pain syndromes. Can J Anaesth 1993;40:954–963.

23. Wiersema MJ, Wiersema LM. Endosonography-guided plexus neurolysis. Gastrointest Endosc 1996;44:656–662.

24. Harada N, Wiersema MJ, Wiersema LM. Endosonography-guided celiac plexus neurolysis. Gastrointest Endosc Clin N Am 1997;7:237–245.

25. Gress F, Ikenberry S, Gottlieb K, et al. A randomized prospective trial of endoscopic ultrasound guided celiac plexus block (CB) for the control of pain due to chronic pancreatitis (CP). Gastrointest Endosc 1996;43:432A. Abstract.

26. Gress F, Ciaccia D, Sherman S, Lehman G. Multicenter evaluation of endoscopic ultrasound (EUS)-guided celiac plexus neurolysis (CPN) for treating abdominal pain associated with chronic pancreatitis (CP). DDW 1998:4061.

27. Faigel DO, Veloso KM, Long WB, Kochman ML. Endosonography-guided celiac plexus injection for abdominal pain due to chronic pancreatitis. Am J Gastroenterol 1996;91:1675.

28. Wiersema MJ, Chak A, Kopecky KK, Wiersema LM. Duplex Doppler endosonography in the diagnosis of splenic vein, portal vein, and portosystemic shunt thrombosis. Gastrointest Endosc 1995;42:1926.

29. Mortensen MB, Hovendal CP. Video-documented endosonographic identification of the coeliac trunk area in the preoperative assessment of resectability in gastroesophageal cancer. Endoscopy 1994;26:440–441. Abstract.

30. Hoffman BJ, Knapple WL, Bhutani MS, et al. Treatment of achalasia by injection of botulinum toxin under endoscopic ultrasound guidance. Gastrointest Endosc 1997;45:77–79.

31. Schiano TD, Fisher RS, Parkman HP, et al. Use of high-resolution endoscopic ultrasonography to assess esophageal wall damage after pneumatic dilation and botulinum toxin injection to treat achalasia. Gastrointest Endosc 1996;44:151–157.

32. Van Dam J, Falk GW, Sivak MV, et al. Endosonographic evaluation of the patient with achalasia: appearance of the esophagus using the echoendoscope. Endoscopy 1995;27:185–190.

33. Miller LS, Liu J-B, Barbarevech CA, et al. High-resolution endoluminal sonography in achalasia. Gastrointest Endosc 1995;42:545–549.

34. Van Dam J. Endoscopic ultrasonography in achalasia. Endoscopy 1994;26:792–793.

35. Birk JW, Khan AM, Gress F. The use of endoscopic ultrasound to evaluate response to intrasphincteric botulinum toxin in the treatment of achalasia. Gastrointest Endosc 1998;47:AB141. Abstract.

36. Kim JO, Hong SJ, Moon JH, et al. High-resolution endoscopic ultrasonography with miniature probe in achalasia. Gastrointest Endosc 1998;47:AB148. Abstract.

37. Fockens P, Meenan J, van Dullemen HM, et al. Dieulafoy's disease: endosonographic detection and endosonography-guided treatment. Gastrointest Endosc 1996;44:437–442.

38. Nesje LB, Skarstein A, Matre K, et al. Dieulafoy's vascular malformation: role of endoscopic ultrasonography

in therapeutic decision-making. Scand J Gastroenterol 1998;33:104–108.

39. Kohler B, Rieman JF. The endoscopic Doppler: its value in evaluating gastroduodenal ulcers after hemorrhage and as an instrument of control of endoscopic injection therapy. Scand J Gastroenterol 1991;26:471–476.

40. Kohler B, Riemann JF. Endoscopic injection therapy of Forrest II and III gastroduodenal ulcers guided by endoscopic Doppler ultrasound. Endoscopy 1993;25:219–223.

41. Jaspersen D, Körner T, Wzatek J, et al. Endoscopic Doppler sonography in gastroduodenal ulcer bleeding. Clin Investig 1992;70:705.

42. Jaspersen D, Korner T, Schorr W, Hammar CH. Diagnosis and treatment control of bleeding colorectal angiodysplasias by endoscopic Doppler sonography: a preliminary study. Gastrointest Endosc 1994;40:40–44.

43. Caletti G, Fusaroli P, Bocus P. Endoscopic ultrasonography. Endoscopy 1998;30:198–221.

44. Catalano MF, Lahoti S, Alcocer E, et al. Obliteration of esophageal varices using EUS guided sclerotherapy with color Doppler: comparison with esophageal band ligation. DDW 1998:3472.

45. Bhutani MS, Usman N, Shenoy V, et al. Endoscopic ultrasound miniprobe-guided steroid injection for treatment of refractory esophageal strictures. Endoscopy 1997;29:757–759.

46. Savides TJ, Gress F, Sherman S, et al. Ultrasound catheter probe-assisted endoscopic cystgastrostomy. Gastrointest Endosc 1995;41:145–148.

47. Binmoeller KF, Soehendra N. Endoscopic ultrasonography in the diagnosis and treatment of pancreatic pseudocysts. Gastrointest Endosc Clin N Am 1995;5:805–816.

48. Gerolami R, Giovannini M, Laugier R. Endoscopic drainage of pancreatic pseudocysts guided by endosonography. Endoscopy 1997;292:106–108.

49. Grimm H, Binmoeller KF, Soehendra N. Endosonography-guided drainage of a pancreatic pseudocyst. Gastrointest Endosc 1992;38:170–171.

50. Etzkorn KP, DeGuzman LJ, Holderman WH, et al. Endoscopic drainage of pancreatic pseudocysts: patient selection and evaluation of outcome by endoscopic ultrasonography. Endoscopy 1995;27:329–333.

51. Chan AT, Heller SJ, Van Dam J, et al. Endoscopic cystgastrotomy: role of endoscopic ultrasonography. Am J Gastroenterol 1996;91:1622–1625.

52. Wiersema MJ. Endosonography-guided cystoduodenostomy with a therapeutic ultrasound endoscope. Gastrointest Endosc 1996;44:614–617.

53. Savides TJ, Gress F, Sherman S, et al. Ultrasound catheter probe-assisted endoscopic cystgastrostomy. Gastrointest Endosc 1995;41:145–148.

54. Fockens P, Johnson TG, van Dullemen HM, et al. Endosonographic imaging of pancreatic pseudocysts before endoscopic transmural drainage. Gastrointest Endosc 1997;46:412–416.

55. Catalano MF, Lahoti S, Geenen JE, Hogan WJ. Evaluation of pancreatic pseudocyst by EUS: can it determine the endoscopic modality treatment of choice? DDW 1997:1067.

56. Giovannini M, Perrier H, Seitz JF. Cystogastrostomy entirely performed under endosonography guidance for pancreatic pseudocyst. DDW 1997:631.

57. Norton ID, Clain JE, DiMagno EP, et al. Endoscopic management of pancreatic pseudocyst by EUS localization of puncture site and balloon dilatation of fistulae. DDW 1998:2253.

58. Grace PA, Williamson RCN. Modern management of pancreatic pseudocysts. Br J Surg 1993;80:573–581.

59. Sahai AV, Hoffman BJ, Hawes RH. EUS-guided hepaticogastrostomy for palliation of obstructive jaundice: preliminary results in a pig model. 11th International Symposium on Endoscopic Ultrasonography, Kyoto, Japan 1998: P54. Abstract.

60. Panzer S, Harris M, Berg W, Ravich W, Kalloo A. Endoscopic ultrasound in the placement of a percutaneous endoscopic gastrostomy tube in the non-transilluminated abdominal wall. Gastrointest Endosc 1995;42:88–90.

61. Chang KJ, Yoshinaka R, Nguyen P. Endoscopic ultrasound-assisted band ligation: a new technique for resection of submucosal tumors. Gastrointest Endosc 1996;44:720–722.

62. Nguyen P, Bastas D, Chang KJ. Endoscopic ultrasound-assisted endoscopic mucosal resection of deep gastric lesions. DDW 1997:1664.

63. Yoshikane H, Suzuki T, Yoshioka N, et al. Hemangioma of the esophagus: endosonographic imaging and endoscopic resection. Endoscopy 1995;27:267–269.

64. Akahoshi K, Chijiwa Y, Tanaka M, et al. Endosonography probe-guided endoscopic mucosal resection of gastric neoplasms. Gastrointest Endosc 1995;42:248–252.

65. Takemoto T, Yanai H, Tada M, et al. Application of ultrasonic probes prior to endoscopic resection of early gastric cancer. Endoscopy 1992;24(Suppl.1):329–333.

66. Mooto Y, Okai T, Songur Y, et al. Endoscopic therapy for early gastric cancer: utility of endosonography and evaluation of prognosis. J Clin Gastroenterol 1995;21:17–23.

67. Akahoshi K, Chijiwa Y, Hamada S, et al. Endoscopic ultrasonography: a promising method for assessing the prospects of endoscopic mucosal resection in early gastric cancer. Endoscopy 1997;29:614–619.

68. Nishimori I, Morita M, Sano S, et al. Endosonography-guided endoscopic resection of duodenal carcinoid tumor. Endoscopy 1997;29:214–217.

69. Hizawa K, Aoyagi K, Kurahara K, et al. Gastrointestinal lymphangioma: endosonographic demonstration and endoscopic removal. Gastrointest Endosc 1996;43:620–624.

70. Songur Y, Okai T, Fujii T, et al. Endoscopic ultrasonography as a guide to strip biopsy removal of esophageal submucosal tumors. J Clin Gastroenterol 1995;20:77–79.

71. Mortensen MB, Scheel-Hincke JD, Madsen MR, et al. Combined endoscopic ultrasonography and laparoscopic ultrasonography in the pretherapeutic

assessment of resectability in patients with upper gastrointestinal malignancies. Scand J Gastroenterol 1996;31:1115–1119.

72. Chang KJ, Nguyen PT, Thomson JA, et al. Phase I clinical trial of local immunotherapy (cytoimplant) delivered by endoscopic ultrasound (EUS)-guided fine needle injection (FNI) in patients with advanced pancreatic carcinoma. Gastrointest Endosc 1998;47: AB144. Abstract.

73. Livraghi T, Lazzaroni S, Pellicano S, et al. Percutaneous ethanol injection of hepatic tumours: single-session therapy with general anesthesia. AJA 1993: 161:1065–1069.

74. Tio L, Reddy A, Kuettel M. Trans-anal ultrasound guided interstitial implant for treating anal carcinoma. DDW 1998:2281.

75. Holm HH, Skjoldbye B. Interventional ultrasound. Ultrasound Med Biol 1996;22:773–789.

76. Mallery S, Goldberg SN, Brugge WR. EUS-guided radiofrequency ablation in the pancreas: preliminary results in a porcine model. DDW 1998:2315.

77. Sato M, Watanabe Y, Nakata T, et al. Sequential percutaneous microwave coagulation therapy for liver tumor. Am J Surg 1998;175:322–324.

78. Ido K, Isoda N, Kawamoto C, et al. Laparoscopic microwave coagulation therapy for solitary hepatocellular carcinoma performed under laparoscopic ultrasonography. Gastrointest Endosc 1997;45:415–420.

79. Sekiyama K, Ebisawa M, Fujita R. Laparoscopic treatment under ultrasonography for small hepatocellular carcinoma. 11th International Symposium on Endoscopic Ultrasonography, Kyoto, Japan 1998:95. Abstract.

80. Ponchon T, Napoleon B. EUS guided treatment with microwaves and HIFU. 11th International Symposium on Endoscopic Ultrasonography, Kyoto, Japan 1998:93–94. Abstract.

81. Prat F, Chapelon J-Y, Arefiev A, et al. High-intensity focused ultrasound transducers suitable for endoscopy: feasibility studies in rabbits. Gastrointest Endosc 1997;46:348–351.

82. Rösch T. Endoscopic ultrasonography. Br J Surg 1997;84:1329–1331.

# 16

# Training in Endoscopic Ultrasound

## Klaus Gottlieb and Frank G. Gress

Endoscopic ultrasound (EUS) is a relatively new technology that has gained considerable recognition for its ability to accurately stage gastrointestinal (GI) malignancies. Previous reports have shown the accuracy of EUS to be superior to other diagnostic imaging modalities such as computed tomography (CT), magnetic resonance imaging (MRI), and angiography (1–41). EUS appears to be evolving into an important diagnostic tool for evaluating certain kinds of GI disorders.

Unfortunately, as with any new technology, there is initially a lack of experienced physicians qualified to perform the new technique or procedure. Currently, the number of operational EUS systems exceeds the number of qualified individuals available to utilize these instruments. Due to this lack of skilled endosonographers, EUS is mainly limited to tertiary and academic medical centers. Furthermore, there are very few academic institutions in the United States offering training in EUS. In fact, some experienced endosonographers worry that this unique and valuable imaging technology may fall into decline due to a lack of endosonographers.

Until recently, most gastroenterologists interested in competently performing EUS have had to be self-taught. The majority of experienced endosonographers in the United States believe that the key to proficiency in EUS training is pattern recognition through repetitive examinations, which can only be acquired at a center performing a large volume of cases. Self-taught endosonographers therefore have to be very highly motivated and also have considerable free time apart from their existing workload.

Several years ago, some academic medical centers in the United States initiated formal EUS training fellowships. They hoped that their graduates would promote EUS by returning to their practices and providing EUS services to their patient base, as well as teaching others this new and important technique. Currently, only a few U.S. centers offer formal EUS training; we have listed some of these centers in Table 16-1.

Because formal teaching is severely lacking for this new technology, a few have questioned whether the observed variability in EUS interpretation reflects the type of training or experience obtained. Studies of this hypothesis are few. Several recent reports on inter- and intraobserver variation and reproducibility of endoscopic ultrasonography suggest that three major factors can influence the EUS interpretation. These are operator subjectivity and experience and machine-dependent factors which produce artifacts that can interfere with image interpretation (42–43). This data suggests that experience in performing EUS procedures is important for obtaining competency for accurately and consistently evaluating gastrointestinal diseases.

EUS is primarily used to diagnose and stage GI malignancies, and in the future may play a central role in clinical oncology. Consistency in evaluating the extent of malignant disease is critical in this setting. A recent study investigating interobserver agreement for EUS staging of esophageal and gastric cancer reported interobserver agreement to be generally good, especially for T1 and T4 tumors. Overall agreement for T2 lesions was poor. Unfortunately, the authors did not look at specific factors that might affect agreement, such as the type of EUS training, number of EUS procedures performed, and overall length of experience with EUS (44). In a study on submucosal masses, we evaluated each endosonographer by overall training experience (formal fellowship versus self-teaching), total EUS procedures performed, total esophageal EUS cases performed, and the number of years of EUS experience for each endosonographer. Our results showed that the ability to correctly and consistently identify submucosal lesions correlated best with years of experience (43).

**Table 16-1.** List of academic centers providing supervised training in EUS or formal training programs in EUS:

1. Brigham & Women's Hospital, Boston, MA
2. Cleveland Clinic, Cleveland, OH
3. Columbia Presbyterian Hospital, New York, NY
4. Georgetown University, Washington, D.C.
5. Indiana University Medical Center, Indianapolis, IN
6. Massachusetts General Hospital, Boston, MA
7. MUSC, Charleston, SC
8. University of California at Irvine, Irvine, CA
9. University Hospitals of Cleveland, OH
10. University of Pennsylvania, Philadelphia, PA
11. University of Washington, Seattle, WA
12. Winthrop University Hospital, State University of New York at Stony Brook, Long Island, NY

Several studies have recently enlightened us on the learning curve and training parameters for obtaining competency in general endoscopic procedures (45–50). Cass et al. reported on the necessary skills and experience required for obtaining competence in performing upper endoscopy and colonoscopy (45). Marshall et al. also provided us with similar important information for colonoscopy (46). More recently, some data on the experience and procedural volume necessary to perform endoscopic retrograde cholangiopancreatography (ERCP), an advanced endoscopic procedure, has been reported (51). At this time, such data is unavailable for EUS.

Because there is limited data available on the parameters necessary for obtaining competency in EUS, this chapter provides information from available sources, including previously published data for other endoscopic procedures, learning theory, the learning experiences from other fields of medicine, and personal experience. We hope this material can provide the needed framework for those with a particular interest in learning EUS.

## Learning Endoscopic Ultrasound

### Motivation

Physicians are experts in self-directed learning. Fox and coworkers have tried to conceptualize possible motivational complexes into ten broad fields (52):

Curiosity
Personal well-being
Financial well-being
Stage of career
Competence
Clinical environment
Relationships with medical institutions
Relating to others in the profession
Regulation
Family and community

This is a useful list to contemplate before learning EUS because it can be applied to any career. Curiosity is defined as a need to pursue, expand, or develop an often preexisting interest. Applied to EUS this could mean, as an example, that an "interest" in imaging, in general, may be evidenced by regularly reviewing CT scans of one's patients with the radiologist, because it is "interesting." Financial aspects are important in EUS, unfortunately more on the debit than the credit side, at least during the training or learning phase. In addition, the purchase price for both linear array and radial scanning equipment can be exorbitant and out of reach for most hospitals, let alone solo or group practices. Furthermore, reimbursement is evolving and currently is hardly commensurate with the effort provided by endosonographers.

For most physicians who have started to learn EUS or are considering it, enhanced clinical competence is the major motivational factor; however, competitive forces in the clinical environment need to be assessed closely. For example, how would you feel after having spent considerable time, effort, and money to learn EUS on your own or in a formal fellowship (that even may have been self-funded) only to find out that a new associate has been hired by the university program or a competing group, just out of fellowship, and announced with big fanfare in the local press as an EUS "expert"?

This leads to two other important areas: relationships with institutions and others in the profession. Is endoscopic ultrasound really useful for my community? It makes very little sense to try to establish EUS in an environment without the support of medical and surgical oncologists, interventional radiologists, and pancreaticobiliary endoscopists. How motivated are my colleagues, referral sources, and my primary hospital to support this endeavor? Here motivation and commitment are not a one-way street. In other words, if the physician learning EUS cannot communicate his long-term commitment to EUS, he will not be able to engender the support, trust, and feedback necessary to get started and develop his or her skills. Furthermore, the hospital administration must be supportive of the EUS program.

There must be a "genuine interest" in EUS that is the driving force behind those endoscopists interested in pursuing training in endosonography. In the past, these successful individuals have put 100% effort into learning this technology with many having endured long, lonely months away from family to pursue their training. More importantly, these same individuals have been the driving force behind the propagation of EUS to other centers and the research that has allowed EUS to become a recognized endoscopic technique.

## Dimensions for Learning EUS

A rapid and wide diffusion of EUS through the gastroenterology community will only become a reality if increased training options become available and self-trained individuals continue to supplement the fellowship-trained practitioners, until more of the latter become available. The value and competence of individuals without formal training in this transition period is evident from the earlier examples of ERCP, cardiac echography and laparoscopic cholecystectomy. Each of these examples has some similarities with endoscopic ultrasound, but differs from it in other important aspects. In contrast, the skill of maneuvering the echoendoscope into the desired position for accurate imaging is complicated by the experience that is also needed for interpretation of the resultant images. This cognitive component of the procedure is exceedingly difficult to learn. Only constant repetitive procedures can improve the pattern recognition necessary to differentiate normal from abnormal findings and ultimately perform and interpret EUS competently.

## Visual Perception and Reality

Sensory stimulation from an ultrasound image, consisting of gray-scale pixels, is translated into a description in the mind that is meaningful and not cluttered with useless information. We create an image based on what we "see." For example, the novice endosonographer cannot at first discriminate one simple shape from another. One must first create meaningful objects, such as the splenic vein, the pancreas, and the common bile duct from a flickering ultrasound image, which at first appears not unlike the radar image of a snowstorm (white noise). Gestalt theorists have worked out principles of visual organization of which the most general is referred to as *Prägnanz.* Implicit in the concept is that, given a complex visual stimulus, whenever possible, some figure or pattern is perceived. Thus, the novice endosonographer gradually learns to differentiate images of anatomical structures from ultrasound artifacts.

There are two major theories of perceptional learning. According to *enrichment theory,* perceptual learning consists of enriching sensory experience with specific associations and rules for its interpretation that is derived from past experience. The proponents of the *discovery theory* interpret perceptual learning as a process of discovering how to transform previously "overlooked potentials for sensory information" into effective information. Therefore, one discovers new aspects of the sensory stimulus and creates new "realities." Clearly, both theories are not mutually exclusive and both are valuable in conceptualizing what happens when one begins to learn EUS (53).

Perceptual styles differ among individuals. A person who resists contextual influences and perceives the world as highly differentiated is said to be "field independent." Field independent people are superior in locating a simple visual figure embedded in a complex pattern (i.e., hidden figure tests). Field independent individuals are able to counteract optical illusions more readily than field dependent persons. It would seem that this is a desirable trait in the acquisition of EUS skills. Field dependence appears to decline with increasing age as does the closely related susceptibility to optical illusions.

## Learning Curves

Most of the research associated with learning curves has been reported in the area of psychomotor skills acquisition. The dependent variable is a fairly simple and easy to observe parameter such as reaction time, number of errors, etc., whereas the independent variable is the number of trials. These curves can be described by second-order polynomials and show no stepwise plateaus of proficiency but obey the law of diminishing returns. In other words, the learning curve is initially steep (large and rapid gains) and flattens with time (small and slow gains).

It appears that results from these experiments are most appropriate for the acquisition of the specific task studied and may have limited relevance to perceptual visual learning, which is paramount for learning EUS. With this caveat, it may be useful to summarize some of the findings of this research: Practice alone does not make perfect, and relevant feedback is necessary. Feedback is most helpful when it is *simultaneous* with continuous, frequent, and specific skill acquisition tasks. The result of unreinforced practice is extinction of the correct response and a proliferation of errors (54). It would seem, therefore, that EUS training in a formal training program under the direction of a mentor would be the preferred method for learning EUS.

## Adult Learning Theory

Earlier theories of psychomotor learning yielded significant insights but are limited in scope. In addition, they have the advantage that they can be studied rigorously in the laboratory. This is not the case with more complex theories of human learning. One nonreductionist approach, Kolb's *experiential learning theory,* seems to be particularly useful for our purposes (55). Learning is a cycle that begins with experience, continues with reflection, and later leads to action. Kolb refined the concept into the stages of action: concrete experience, critical reflection, active experimentation, and abstraction (Figure 16-1), which continues in a spiral fashion. This model seems to describe the interaction between the EUS trainee, the echoendoscope, the

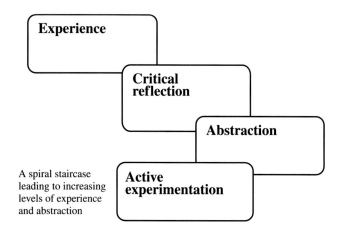

**Figure 16-1.** Kolb's Experiential Learning Model

EUS images obtained, and the preceptor/mentor in a meaningful way.

Learning as a process has been divided into stages, an intuitive conclusion reached by most physicians (56). Building upon prior experience, learning proceeds incrementally until eventually, a "comfort zone" is reached in which the operator is reasonably assured of his clinical and technical skills. A new learning task, e.g., EUS, creates tension and apprehension and disrupts the comfort zone. Learning a new task as complex as endoscopic ultrasound is stressful and can cause overall performance regression. This dip in the learning curve can be overcome if even the most skilled endoscopist accepts the fact that his ability to perform and interpret EUS images with confidence will be a long-term process requiring a large number of procedures despite preexisting proficiency in other advanced endoscopic techniques.

## *Published Data on Learning Experiences*

The ability to translate a 2-D ultrasound image into the three-dimensional reality required for image interpretation is a key requirement for successful EUS. This ability is similar to that required in surgery. Schuenemann and colleagues tested 120 general surgery residents with a neuropsychological battery and then rated them by attending surgeons, on surgical skills exhibited during the course of 1445 surgical procedures (57). Analysis of the neuropsychological battery resulted in three factors (complex visuo-spatial organization, stress tolerance, and psychomotor abilities) that were statistically unrelated to traditional measures such as the Medical College Admission Test and National Board scores. Multiple regression analyses indicated that academic predictors, taken alone, either did not correlate (National Board scores) or correlated negatively (Medical College Admission Test scores) with the surgery ratings. Conversely, neuropsychological

test scores showed significant positive correlation ($r = 0.68$) with the ratings. When both sets of predictor variables are combined, a multiple regression coefficient of 0.80 is found with the ratings, with more than two-thirds of the predictive power attributable to the neuropsychologic test scores.

The relationship between a specialized form of spatial ability known as "field articulation" and technical surgical skill was investigated by Gibbons et al. (58). This form of spatial ability is related to perceptual styles and field dependence. The latter can be defined as the ability to differentiate a simple figure from a complex configuration background. The relationship between hidden-figure test scores and average ratings of technical surgical skill made by 17 academic surgical faculty members in two independent institutions was highly significant.

Of course, the results of these studies are not directly applicable to the learning of endoscopic ultrasound; however, parallels can be drawn. Individuals hoping to learn EUS clearly have different visuo-spatial abilities, which are probably relevant to the speed with which they will be able to acquire the skills to perform EUS competently. There is very little data on the factors affecting one's ability to learn and perform the EUS procedure competently. Nevertheless, some interesting published data relating to the acquisition of general endoscopic skills do exist. Recently, Cass reported on findings from a prospective multicenter study evaluating competence parameters for upper endoscopy and colonoscopy (45). This study showed that certain criteria must be achieved before one can competently and independently perform these general procedures. Furthermore, they showed that a certain number of procedures for upper endoscopy and colonoscopy are necessary in order to achieve these milestones or competency criteria. Marshall et al. also showed similar findings, reporting a minimum number of colonoscopies were necessary to achieve overall competence (46). More recently, data from Duke University Medical Center reported on the minimum number of ERCP procedures necessary for a GI fellow to achieve competence in therapeutic ERCP, a technically advanced endoscopic procedure (51). Unfortunately, such important data is not yet available for EUS. However, EUS training studies are ongoing at this time and we look forward to these results. In the meantime, there are several reports exploring training issues pertaining to EUS.

Catalano and colleagues studied interobserver variation and reproducibility of EUS staging of esophageal cancer (42). As might be expected, they reported that experienced endosonographers were more accurate than inexperienced endosonographers at staging esophageal tumors. Fockens et al. reported that after completing 100 total EUS procedures for esophageal cancer staging, T-staging for esophageal tumors by EUS correlation with surgical staging increased from 58%

for the first 36 patients to 83% for the next 35. This significant study shows that a learning curve exists for EUS staging of esophageal cancer with a minimum of 100 EUS exams being required for this indication to achieve an acceptable level of accuracy (59).

Currently, there are no prospective, multicenter trials indicating the number of EUS procedures an individual must perform before he or she can be considered competent. Furthermore, endoscopy societies both in Europe and the United States have been unable to define a minimum number of procedures recommended for assessing competency. According to the European Society of Gastrointestinal Endoscopy "it is difficult to assess how many procedures are required in order to achieve sufficient skill and expertise, since this is dependent on many variables." This makes the task of hospital credentialing committees difficult, a subject we will bring up again later.

In a survey of endoscopic ultrasonographers reported by Boyce et al. the consensus was that approximately 150 procedures for staging luminal GI tumors are needed to acquire technical competence, defined as the ability to position the echoendoscope to obtain accurate imaging (60). They noted that more procedures are necessary for interpretative competence. It is not clear whether the acquisition of technical and interpretative competence is different for a third-year fellowship trainee compared to a seasoned endoscopist or an experienced biliary endoscopist. These are additional issues that deserve further study.

## Practical Aspects of Learning Endoscopic Ultrasound

Ideally, formal fellowship training in EUS will provide all aspects necessary for obtaining competence in this procedure. This section is dedicated to those interested in exploring EUS and those wishing to acquire these skills in a self-teaching program. However, these suggestions can be applied to anyone interested in learning EUS. The first step in learning endoscopic ultrasound is to immerse oneself in the subject. This includes utilizing all available educational materials. Trainees are urged to read a textbook on the subject from cover to cover. This first reading should be for overview purposes only. (A list of useful resources is given at the end of this section.) Second, it is imperative that the student conduct a thorough review of anatomy, both cross-sectional and traditional. There are excellent CT correlated anatomy texts available that provide a basic foundation for developing the conceptual thinking necessary for interpreting EUS. We recommend the text edited by Han and Kim (61), which provides superb CT anatomical imaging.

At this stage, the trainee should try to absorb as much as possible and observe actual endoscopic ultra-

sound procedures whenever possible. Observational practice means watching frequent and repetitive EUS procedures. If this is not practical, then a review of available videotapes is essential. Some videotapes are commercially available and many more are in the collections of accomplished endosonographers. In addition, observing transabdominal ultrasound procedures may be a useful way for some to become familiarized with gray-scale imaging and its peculiarities and pitfalls.

After an extended observation or self-study period, the student will naturally seek out hands-on experience. There can be little doubt that the best learning environment is found in a one-to-one preceptor-trainee relationship, ideally in a formal training program. However, other alternatives exist. The student can make personal arrangements with an EUS expert to observe procedures one day a week for a period of time. Eventually, the student will advance to a level where he or she can intelligently discuss or even anticipate the findings of the expert. At this stage, the student can proceed to performing EUS exams.

Additionally, two- or three-day hands-on courses are periodically sponsored by the American Society of Gastrointestinal Endoscopy (ASGE) and other GI societies and institutions. Although hands-on often involves animal models, it is a reasonable way to get started. The swine model for teaching endoscopic ultrasound is considered the model that best resembles the human anatomy of the GI tract, pancreas, and bile ducts (62).

We must mention, however, that taking a hands-on EUS course in no way certifies an endoscopist for privileges in endoscopic ultrasound. Credentialing can be granted only to those who can demonstrate acceptable competence in EUS. For example, one must be able to stage GI tumors using EUS at the same accuracy as that reported in the literature (see Tables 16-2 through 16-6). This can be done only over an extended period of time after adequate cases with surgical correlation have been achieved.

At the same time, the student will need to keep up-to-date with current developments in the field. *Gastrointestinal Endoscopy* and *Endoscopy* are two journals that publish many reports on EUS. In addition, several texts have been published on EUS, including the most recent text, *Gastrointestinal Endosonography* by Michael Sivak and Jacques Van Dam.

## Internet Resources for Learning Endoscopic Ultrasound

Internet Web sites have a short life and may not have been updated for a long time. Everybody who is familiar with the Net will know how to help themselves. Nevertheless, a few suggestions may be helpful. First of all, it is well worth periodically checking for

**Table 16-2.** Reported accuracy of EUS compared to histopathology in local staging of esophageal carcinoma.

| Reference | n | T stage | N stage |
|---|---|---|---|
| Murata (13)* | 173 | 88% | 88% |
| Tio (14) | 102 | 89% | 81% |
| Dittler (15) | 97 | 85% | 75% |
| Vilgrain (16) | 51 | 73% | 50% |
| Botet (17) | 50 | 92% | 88% |
| Grimm (18) | 49 | 89% | 90% |
| Rösch (19) | 44 | 82% | 70% |
| Ziegler (20)** | 37 | 89% | 69% |
| Sugimachi (21) | 33 | 90% | - |
| Rice (22) | 22 | 59% | 69% |
| Heintz (23)* | 22 | 77% | 86% |
| Schader (24) | 21 | 86% | 81% |
| Date (25)*** | 20 | 85% | - |
| Takemoto (26) | 18 | 72% | 79% |
| Total | 739 | 85% | 79% |

\* Only traversable tumors included
\*\* Linear scanning echoendoscope
\*\*\* Only adventitial and organ involvement (T3/4) was assessed

**Table 16-3.** Reported accuracy of EUS compared to histopathology in determining the T- and N-stages of patients with gastric carcinoma.

| Reference | n | T stage | N stage |
|---|---|---|---|
| Caletti (27) | 34 | 88% | 58% |
| Murata (28) | 146 | 79% | - |
| Grimm (29) | 118 | 80% | 88% |
| Akahoshi (30) | 74 | 81% | 50% |
| Tio (31) | 72 | 84% | 68% |
| Sanft (32) | 71 | 80% | 80% |
| Aibe (33) | 67 | 73% | 69% |
| Rösch (34) | 41 | 71% | 75% |
| Botet (35) | 50 | 92% | 78% |
| Yoshimi (36) | 40 | - | 73% |
| Saito (37) | 110 | 81% | - |
| Heintz (38) | 19 | 79% | 72% |
| Ohashi (39) | 174 | 67% | - |
| Yasuda (40) | 147 | 78% | - |
| Total | 1163 | 78% | 73% |

**Table 16-4.** Reported accuracy of EUS in the assessment of vascular invasion of the portal venous system by pancreatic carcinoma.

| Reference | n | Accuracy (%) |
|---|---|---|
| Yasuda (47) | 37 | 81 |
| Rösch (48) | 40 | 95 |
| Palazzo (49) | 38 | 87 |
| Sugiyama (50) | 5 | 100 |
| Amouyal (51) | 5 | 80 |
| Snady (52) | 30 | 97 |
| Gress ( ) | 81 | 93 |
| Total | 236 | 91 |

\* Only surgically confirmed cases are included.
Data express the correct prediction of the presence or absence of vascular involvement.

**Table 16-5.** Reported accuracy of EUS in the correct determination of depth of tumor invasion (T-stage) and lymph node metastases (N-stage) in ampullary carcinoma.

| Reference | n | T stage | N stage |
|---|---|---|---|
| Fujino (41) | 7 | 71% | - |
| Mukai (42) | 19 | 85% | 95% |
| Rosch (43) | 12 | 83% | 75% |
| Mitake (44) | 28 | 89% | 69% |
| Tio (45) | 24 | 88% | 54% |
| Barkun (46) | 4 | 75% | - |
| Total | 94 | 86% | 72% |

**Table 16-6.** Reported accuracy of EUS in the local staging of rectal carcinoma.

| Reference | n | T stage EUS | N stage EUS |
|---|---|---|---|
| Beynon (53) | 46 | - | - |
| Akasu (54) | 41 | 80% | 78% |
| Kramman (55) | 29 | 93% | - |
| Pappalardo (56) | 14 | 93% | 86% |
| Rotte (57) | 25 | 84% | - |
| Ruf (58) | 49 | 88% | - |
| Rifkin (59) | 81 | 67% | 80% |
| Waizer (60) | 48 | 77% | - |
| Goldman (61) | 32 | 81% | - |
| Beynon (62) | 44 | 91% | - |
| Strunk (63) | 10 | 70% | - |
| Total | 419 | 84% | 84% |

EUS-related resources by using general-purpose search engines, especially those that automatically perform simultaneous searches on several different search engines and combine the results (metasearches). The authors have found the following two search engines particularly fast and helpful: www.bytesearch.com and www.savvysearch.com. Relevant search terms are: endoscopic ultrasound, EUS, endosonography, and endoscopic ultrasonography.

The American Society for Gastrointestinal Endoscopy (ASGE) maintains a Web site (www.ASGE.org) with links to the American Endosonography Committee (AEC) home page. This may also in the future remain a good starting point for Web-related research. A promising Web site has also been created by members of the Munich EUS group for the European Society of Gastrointestinal Endoscopy (www.eus-online.org).

### Telemedicine

Another area that will certainly capture our attention is telemedicine. Telemedicine is currently in its infancy, but a variety of parties are expressing great interest in this area, and generous research funds seem to be available. The necessary infrastructure, basically the Internet, is already in place and regularly teleconferenced tumor board meetings are a reality in some areas of the country.

## Terminology

One of the characteristics of a new branch of learning is that it develops its own terminology. The use of a relatively standardized nomenclature in reporting endoscopic ultrasound findings is important for a variety of reasons. In contrast to transabdominal ultrasound or echocardiography, in which an ultrasound technician can obtain a series of standardized images that are later read by a radiologist or a cardiologist, obtaining and interpreting endoscopic ultrasound images is done simultaneously. The written report, dictated immediately after completion of the study, summarizing all relevant observations, is as important as, if not more important than, image documentation.

EUS is a very dynamic and operator-dependent procedure. Therefore, information obtained needs to be recorded in a way that is meaningful to other endosonographers, even if the referring physician is interested only in the overall impression. Accurate and comprehensive reporting is also an instrument of quality assurance and leads to an increasing refinement of what is seen. Furthermore, the use of standardized terms is a prerequisite for database creation and text-based searches and supports the ability to do research in EUS.

There is a direct relationship between the number of terms correctly understood and correctly used and the overall quality of the endoscopic ultrasound report and the quality of exams. We recommend using the recently prepared standard terminology for EUS. A "Minimal Standard Terminology in Endoscopic Ultrasonography, Version 1.0" has been developed by the International Working Group and was released in January 1998.

However, the use of standard terminology should not stifle the creativity of the endosonographer who chooses to use a more individualized text description of the findings, if appropriate. Personal or individualized descriptions should, however, be used together with and not instead of the accepted terminology.

## Hospital Privileges

Few hospitals have currently defined criteria for privileging physicians in endoscopic ultrasound. Presently, privileging depends mostly on a letter from a recognized expert stating that a certain level of competence has been achieved by the individual seeking privileges. This can be a thorny issue because the individual issuing such a letter puts his or her personal reputation at stake by doing so. Be that as it may, the lack of data and established criteria for assessing competency in EUS is a serious drawback.

**Table 16-7.** Privileging for Endoscopic Ultrasound (EUS).

**Level 1**

Diagnostic luminal EUS of esophageal, gastric, and rectal lesions
Requires: Privileges for diagnostic and therapeutic endoscopy of the upper and lower gastrointestinal tract and at least 100 EUS procedures for each indication performed under the supervision of an experienced endosonographer in the United States or Canada.

**Level 2**

Diagnostic EUS of pancreatic, biliary, and retroperitoneal lesions
Requires: Level 1 privileges and at least 100 EUS procedures with pancreatic, biliary, or retroperitoneal indications performed under the supervision of an experienced endosonographer in the United States or Canada.

**Level 3**

Interventional EUS, including, but not limited to, fine-needle aspiration, celiac plexus block, and pseudocyst puncture/cystgastrostomy
Requires: Level 1 and 2 privileges and the successful completion of a dedicated therapeutic endoscopic ultrasound training period under the supervision of an experienced endosonographer in the United States or Canada performing endoscopic ultrasound-guided fine-needle aspiration biopsies, celiac plexus blocks, EUS-guided pseudocyst cystgastrostomy, and so forth.

The ASGE Training Committee has developed preliminary guidelines for obtaining competence in EUS. For tumor staging, these guidelines use the important criteria of correlating a trainee's EUS staging ability to the gold standard measure of surgical pathology, or in the case of a lack of this standard, the staging of the trainee's mentor. Self-taught individuals would unfortunately be at a disadvantage, because they would have only the surgical pathology obtained from their own patients. A substantial number of cases would be required for each EUS indication (Tables 16-2 through 16-6) before an individual could be credentialled. Furthermore, EUS-guided fine-needle aspiration and other therapeutic EUS procedures such as celiac plexus block will require far more additional experience and training than diagnostic/tumor staging.

The ASGE guidelines for obtaining training and competency in endoscopic ultrasound is an important document that addresses some of the training issues we have mentioned. Credentialling criteria for endoscopic ultrasound have to be formulated in such a way that incompetent practitioners are excluded. At the same time, the hurdles must not be set too high to prevent reasonably trained individuals from getting started. One approach to this dilemma would consist of creating different levels of privileging, as outlined in

Table 16-7. This would permit some individuals who are mainly self-taught to gradually acquire competency in EUS in a succession of step-wise levels starting with basic staging.

### References

1. Tio TL, Cohen P, Coene PP, et al. Endosonography and computed tomography of esophageal carcinoma: preoperative classification compared to the new (1987) TNM system. Gastroenterology 1989;96:1478–1486.
2. Rösch T, Lorenz R, Zenker K, et al. Local staging and assessment of resectability in carcinoma of the esophagus, stomach and duodenum by endoscopic ultrasonography. Gastrointest Endosc 1992;38:460–467.
3. Murata Y, Suzuki S, Hashimoto H. Endoscopic ultrasonography of the upper gastrointestinal tract. Surg Endosc 1988;2;180–183.
4. Tio TL, Coene PPLO, den Hartog Jager FCA, Tytgat GNJ. Preoperative TNM classification of esophageal carcinoma by endosonography. Hepato-Gastroenterol 1990;37:376–381.
5. Dittler HJ, Bollschweiler E, Siewert JR. Was leistet die endosonograpie im präoperativen staging des ösophaguskarzinoms? Dtsch Med Wschr 1991;116:561–566.
6. Vilgrain V, Mompoint D, Palazzo L, et al. Staging of oesophageal carcinoma: comparison of results with endoscopic sonography and CT. AJR 1990;155:277–281.
7. Botet JF, Lightdale CJ, Zauber G, et al. Preoperative staging of esophageal cancer: comparison of endoscopic US and dynamic CT. Radiology 1991;181:419–425.
8. Grimm H, Maydeo A, Hamper K, et al. Results of endoscopic ultrasound and computed tomography in preoperative staging of esophageal cancer: a retrospective controlled study. Gastrointest Endosc 1991;37:279. Abstract.
9. Rösch T, Lorenz R, Zenker K, et al. Local staging and assessment of resectability in carcinoma of esophagus, stomach and duodenum by endoscopic ultrasonography. Gastrointest Endosc 1992;38:460–467.
10. Ziegler K, Sanft C, Zeitz M, et al. Evaluation of endosonography in TN staging of oesophageal cancer. Gut 1991;32:16–20.
11. Sugimachi K, Ohno S, Fujishima H, et al. Endoscopic ultrasonographic detection of carcinomatous invasion and of lymph nodes in the thoracic esophagus. Surgery 1990;107:366–371.
12. Rice TW, Boyce GA, Sivak MV Jr. Esophageal ultrasound and the preoperative staging of carcinoma of the esophagus. Surgery 1991;101:536–544.
13. Date H, Miyashita M, Sasajima K, et al. Assessment of adventitial involvement of esophageal carcinoma by endoscopic ultrasonography. Surg Endosc 1990;4:195–197.
14. Takemoto T, Itoh T, Fukumoto Y, et al. Endoscopic ultrasonography in preoperative staging of esophageal cancer. In Dancygier H, Classen M, eds. 5th International Symposium on Endoscopic Ultrasonography. Munich: Demeter Verlag, (Z Gastroenterol suppl) 1989:34–38.
15. Caletti GC, Brochhi E, Gibilaro M, et al. Sensitivity, specificity and predictive value of endoscopic ultrasonography in the diagnosis and assessment of gastric cancer. Gastrointest Endosc 1990;36:194–195. Abstract.
16. Murata Y, Suzuki S, Hashimoto H. Endoscopic ultrasonography of the upper gastrointestinal tract. Surg Endosc 1988;2:180–183.
17. Akahoshi K, Misawa T, Fujishima H, et al. Preoperative evaluation of gastric cancer by endoscopic ultrasound. Gut 1991;32:479–482.
18. Tio TL, Schouwink MH, Cikot RJLM, Tytgat GNJ. Preoperative TNM classification of gastric carcinoma by endosonography in comparison with the pathological TNM system: a prospective study of 72 cases. Hepatogastroenterol 1989;36:51–56.
19. Aibe T, Fujimara H, Noguchi T, et al. Endosonographic detection and staging of early gastric cancer. In Dancygier H, Classen M, eds. 5th International Symposium on Endoscopic Ultrasonography. Munich: Demeter Verlag, (Z Gastroenterol suppl) 1989: 71–78.
20. Botet JF, Lightdale CJ, Zauber AG, et al. Preoperative staging of gastric cancer: comparison of endoscopic US and dynamic CT. Radiology 1991;181:426–432.
21. Saito N, Takeshita K, Habu H, Endo M. The use of endoscopic ultrasound in determining the depth of cancer invasion in patients with gastric cancer. Surg Endosc 1991;5:14–19.
22. Ohashi S, Nakazawa S, Yoshino J. Endoscopic ultrasonography in the assessment of invasive gastric cancer. Scand J Gastroenterol 1989;24:1039–1048.
23. Yasuda K, Nakajima M, Cho E, et al. Benign versus malignant gastric ulcers: a role for endoscopic ultrasonography? In Dancygier H, Classen M, eds. 5th International Symposium on Endoscopic Ultrasonography. Munich: Demeter Verlag, (Z Gastroenterol suppl) 1989:50–56.
24. Rösch T, Braig C, Gain T, et al. Staging of pancreatic and ampullary carcinoma by endoscopic ultrasonography. Gastroenterology 1992;102:188–199.
25. Mitake M, Nakasawa S, Tsukamoto Y, et al. Endoscopic ultrasonography in the diagnosis of depth invasion and lymph node metastasis of carcinoma of the papilla of Vater. J Ultrasound Med 1990;9:645–650.
26. Tio TL, Tytgat GNJ, Cikot RJLM, et al. Ampullopancreatic carcinoma: preoperative TNM classification with endosonography. Radiology 1990;175:455–461.
27. Yasuda K, Mukai H, Fujimoto S, et al. The diagnosis of pancreatic cancer by endoscopic ultrasonography. Gastrointest Endosc 1988;34:1–8.
28. Rösch T, Braig C, Gain T, et al. Staging of pancreatic and ampullary carcinoma by endoscopic ultrasonography. Gastroenterology 1992;102:188–199.
29. Palazzo L, Roseau G, Gayet B, Vilgrain V, Belghiti J, Fekete F, Paolaggi JA. Endoscopic ultrasonography in the diagnosis and staging of pancreatic adenocarcinoma. Results of a prospective study with comparison to ultrasonography and CT scan. Endoscopy 1993 Feb;25(2):143–150.

30. Amouyal P, Amouyal G, Mompoint D, et al. Endosonography: promising method for diagnosis of extrahepatic cholestasis. Lancet II 1989:1195–1198.

31. Snady H, Cooperman A, Siegel JH. Assessment of vascular involvement by pancreatic disease: a comparison of endoscopic ultrasonography to computerized tomography and angiography. Gastrointest Endosc 1990;36:197. Abstract.

32. Grimm H, Maydeo A, Soehendra N. Endoluminal ultrasound for the diagnosis and staging of pancreatic cancer. Bailiere's Clin Gastroenterol 1990;4:869–887.

33. Snady H, Cooperman A, Siegel JK. Endoscopic ultrasonography compared with computed tomography and ERCP in patients with obstructive jaundice or small peripancreatic mass. Gastrointest Endosc 1992; 38:27–34.

34. Snady H, Bruckner H, Cooperman A, et al. Endoscopic ultrasonography criteria of vascular invasion by potentially resectable pancreatic tumors. Gastrointest Endosc 1994;39:69.

35. Akasu T, Sunouchi K, Sawada T, et al. Preoperative staging of rectal carcinoma: prospective comparison of transrectal ultrasonography and computed tomography. Gastroenterology 1990;98:268. Abstract.

36. Beynon J, McC Mortensen NJ, Foy DMA, et al. Preoperative assessment of local invasion in rectal cancer: digital examination, endoluminal sonography or computed tomography? Br J Surg 1986;73:1015–1017.

37. Kramann B, Hildebrandt U. Computed tomography versus endosonography in the staging of rectal carcinoma: a comparative study. Int J Colorect Dis 1986; 1:216–218.

38. Pappalardo G, Reggio D, Frattaroli FM, et al. The value of endoluminal ultrasonography and computed tomography in the staging of rectal cancer: a preliminary study. J Surg Oncol 1990;43:219–222.

39. Rotte KH, Kluhs L, Kleinau H, Kriedemann E. Computed tomography and endosonography in the preoperative staging of rectal carcinoma. Europ J Radiol 1989; 9:187–190.

40. Rifkin MD, Ehrlich SM, Marks G. Staging of rectal carcinoma: prospective comparison of endorectal US and CT. Radiology 1989;170:319–322.

41. Waizer A, Zitron S, Ben-Baruch D, et al. Comparative study for preoperative staging of rectal cancer. Dis Colon Rectum 1989;32:53–56.

42. Catalano MF, Sivak MV, Bedford RA, et al. Observer variation and reproducibility of endoscopic ultrasonography. Gastrointest Endosc 1995;41:115–120.

43. Gress F, Schmitt C, Savides T, et al. Interobserver agreement of endoscopic ultrasound (EUS) for evaluating submucosal masses. Gastrointest Endosc 1998; 47:421A.

44. Burtin P, Napoleon B, Palazzo L, et al. Interobserver agreement in endoscopic ultrasonography staging of esophageal and cardia cancer. Gastrointest Endosc 1996;43:20–24.

45. Cass OW, Freeman ML, Peine CJ, et al. Objective evaluation of endoscopy skills during training. Ann Int Med 1993;118:40–44.

46. Marshall JB. Technical proficiency of trainees performing colonoscopy: a learning curve. Gastrointest Endosc 1995;42:287–291.

47. Hawes R, Lehman GA, et al. Training resident physicians in fiberoptic flexible sigmoidoscopy: how many supervised examinations are required to achieve competence? Am J Med 1986;80:465–470.

48. Ransohoff DF, Lang CA. Sigmoidoscopic screening in the 1990's. JAMA 1993;269:1278–1281.

49. American Society for Gastrointestinal Endoscopy. Principles of training in gastrointestinal endoscopy. Manchester, MA, 1998.

50. Schoenfeld PS, Cash B, Kita J, et al. Effectiveness and patient satisfaction with screening flexible sigmoidoscopy performed by registered nurses. Gastrointest Endosc 1999;49:158–162.

51. Jowell PS, Baillie J, Branch S, et al. Quantitative assessment of procedural competence: a prospective study of training in endoscopic retrograde cholangiopancreatography. Ann Intern Med 1996;125:983–989.

52. Fox RD, Mazmania PE, Putnam RW. Changing and learning in the lives of physicians. New York: Praeger; 1989:6–27.

53. Sekuler R, Blake R. Perception. New York: McGraw Hill; 1994.

54. Kling JW, Riggs LA. Woodworth & Schlosberg's Experimental Psychology; 3rd ed. New York: Holt, Rinehart and Winston; 1971.

55. Kolb DA. Experiential learning: experience as the source of learning and development. Upper Saddle River, NJ: Prentice-Hall; 1983.

56. Bunker KA, Webb A. Learning how to learn from experience: impact of stress and coping (report no. 154). Greensboro, NC: Center for Creative Leadership; 1992.

57. Schuenemann AL, Pickleman J, Hesslein R, Freeark RJ. Neuropsychologic predictors of operative skill among general surgery residents. Surgery 1984;96: 288–295.

58. Gibbons RD, Baker RJ, Skinner DB. Field articulation testing: a predictor of technical skills in surgical residents. J Surg Res 1986;41:53–57.

59. Fockens P, Van den Brande, Van Dullemen H, et al. Endosonographic T-staging of esophageal carcinoma: a learning curve. Gastrointest Endosc 1996;44:58–62.

60. Boyce HW Jr. Training in EUS. 10th International Symposium on Endoscopic Ultrasonography, Cleveland, OH, 1995.

61. Han MC, Kim CW. Sectional human anatomy: transverse, sagittal, and coronal sections correlated with computed tomography and magnetic resonance imaging. Igaku-Shoin Medical Pub., 1995.

62. Bhutani M, Stills HF, Aveyard MA. Further development in the swine model for teaching diagnostic and interventional endoscopic ultrasound. Gastrointest Endosc 1998;47: AB44.

# Index